In A Page Pediatrics

In A Page Pediatrics

JONATHAN E. TEITELBAUM, MD
Editor-in-Chief
Assistant Professor of Pediatrics
Drexel University College of Medicine
Director, Pediatric Gastroenterology and Nutrition
The Children's Hospital at Monmouth Medical Center
Long Branch, New Jersey

SCOTT KAHAN, MD, MPH
Editor-in-Chief
Series Editor
Research Fellow, The Johns Hopkins University
School of Medicine
Department of Preventive Medicine and Public Health
Johns Hopkins Bloomberg School of Public Health
Baltimore, Maryland

KATHLEEN O. DEANTONIS, MD
Faculty, Department of Pediatrics
Mercy Hospital of Pittsburgh
Pittsburgh, Pennsylvania

Wolters Kluwer | Lippincott Williams & Wilkins
Health

Philadelphia • Baltimore • New York • London
Buenos Aires • Hong Kong • Sydney • Tokyo

Acquisitions Editor: Nancy Anastasi Duffy
Associate Managing Editor: Jessica Heise
Marketing Manager: Jennifer Kuklinski
Production Editor: Gina Aiello
Designer: Risa Clow
Compositor: Nesbitt Graphics, Inc.

Printed in the United States

Printed in the United States of America

Library of Congress Cataloging-in-Publication Data

In a page. Pediatrics / Scott Kahan, editor-in-chief; Jonathan E. Teitelbaum, Kathleen O. DeAntonis, [editors].—2nd ed.
   p. ; cm.
  Includes bibliographical references and index.
  ISBN-13: 978-0-7817-7045-3
  ISBN-10: 0-7817-7045-9
  1. Pediatrics—Handbooks, manuals, etc.   I. Kahan, Scott.   II. Teitelbaum, Jonathan E.
III. DeAntonis, Kathleen O.   IV. Title: Pediatrics.
  [DNLM: 1. Pediatrics—Handbooks. WS 39 I35 2008]
  RJ48.I5 2008
  618.92—dc22

                                                                        2007044969

To purchase additional copies of this book, call our customer service department at (800) 638–3030 or fax orders to (301) 223–2320. International customers should call (301) 223–2300.

Visit Lippincott Williams & Wilkins on the Internet: http://www.LWW.com. Lippincott Williams & Wilkins customer service representatives are available from 8:30 am to 6:00 pm, EST.

07 08 09 10
1 2 3 4 5 6 7 8 9 10

Preface

The idea for this series came from the difficulty that I experienced during medical school and residency in weeding through the massive amount of medical information that confronted me. The problem wasn't that the material was too complex; rather, it was the challenge of separating the forest from the trees. Indeed, I still often feel overwhelmed by all there is to know.

I wanted a resource that would streamline the abundance of medical knowledge into a manageable nucleus, or as a resident once described it to me, "a book that tells me exactly what I need to know so my attending won't think I'm an idiot!"

That became the goal of this series: to present medical diseases in a high-yield, understandable fashion that makes it easier for readers to concentrate on the "big picture," without being distracted by the mountain of surrounding detail.

Reviews from medical students, residents, fellows, and other health professionals have been excellent. I hope readers will find the *In A Page* series to be a valuable tool on rounds, for board review, and for independent study. As always, I welcome your questions, comments, and suggestions.

SCOTT KAHAN, MD
drkahan@gmail.com

Contributors

Karen Benedum, MD
Chair of Pediatrics
Mercy Hospital of Pittsburgh
Pittsburgh, Pennsylvania

Mary Carrasco, MD
International Health, Child Advocacy, and
Community Health
Mercy Hospital of Pittsburgh
Pittsburgh, Pennsylvania

Srinivas C. Chevuru, MD
Assistant Professor of Pediatrics
University of Kentucky School of Medicine
Kentucky Children's Hospital
University of Kentucky Medical Center
Lexington, Kentucky

Doug Cress, MD
Clinical Associate Professor
University of Pittsburgh Medical Center
Pittsburgh, Pennsylvania

Manisha Harpavat Dave, MD
Assistant Professor of Pediatrics
Department of Gastroenterology
Children's Hospital of Pittsburgh
Pittsburgh, Pennsylvania

Fatma Dedeoglu, MD
Instructor in Pediatrics
Harvard Medical School
Boston, MA
Attending Physician
Division of Immunology/Rheumatology
Children's Hospital Boston
Boston, Massachusetts

Anthony DiBartolomeo, MD (deceased)
Previous Associate Dean for Clinical Affairs
West Virginia University School of Medicine
Morgantown, West Virginia

Patricia Dubin, MD
Assistant Professor of Pediatrics
Children's Hospital of Pittsburgh
Pittsburgh, Pennsylvania

Tracy B. Fausnight, MD
Assistant Professor of Pediatrics
Division of Rheumatology, Allergy, and
Immunology
Penn State Children's Hospital
Hershey, Pennsylvania

Howard Ferimer, MD
Departments of Critical Care and Pediatrics
Mercy Hospital of Pittsburgh
Pittsburgh, Pennsylvania

Norman Ferrari, III, MD
Senior Associate Dean for Medical
Education
Professor of Pediatrics
West Virginia University School of
Medicine
Robert C. Byrd Health Sciences Center
Morgantown, West Virginia

Sarah Friebert, MD, FAAP
Director, A Palette of Care Program
Haslinger Division of Pediatric
Palliative Care
Associate Professor of Pediatrics
Pediatric Hematology/Oncology
Akron Children's Hospital
Akron, Ohio

Robin Gehris, MD
Clinical Associate Professor
University of Pittsburgh Medical Center
Pittsburgh, Pennsylvania

Amy Goldstein, MD
Clinical Assistant Professor
University of Pittsburgh School of Medicine
Division of Pediatric Neurology
Children's Hospital of Pittsburgh
Pittsburgh, Pennsylvania

Adda Grimberg, MD, FAAP
Assistant Professor of Pediatrics
University of Pennsylvania School
of Medicine
Division of Pediatric Endocrinology
The Children's Hospital of Philadelphia
Philadelphia, Pennsylvania

Robert Guthrie, MD
Professor of Pediatrics
Drexel University College of Medicine
Chief of Pediatrics
Allegheny General Hospital
Pittsburgh, Pennsylvania

Sara Hamel, MD
Behavioral/Developmental Pediatrician
Coordinator of Training
Associate Professor of Pediatrics
Department of Pediatrics
University of Pittsburgh School of Medicine
Child Development Unit
Children's Hospital of Pittsburgh
Pittsburgh, Pennsylvania

Marybeth Hummel, MD
Director of Medical Genetics
West Virginia Genetics Center
Department of Pediatrics
Robert C. Byrd Health Sciences Center
West Virginia University School of Medicine
Morgantown, West Virginia

Esther Jacobowitz Israel, MD
Assistant Professor, Pediatrics
Harvard Medical School
Associate Chief, Pediatric Gastroenterology
and Nutrition
MassGeneral Hospital for Children
Boston

Mambarath A. Jaleel, MD
Assistant Professor of Pediatrics
Division of Neonatal-Perinatal Medicine
University of Texas Southwestern Medical
Center at Dallas
Dallas, Texas

Margaret Jaynes, MD
Professor of Pediatrics
West Virginia University School of Medicine
Chief of Pediatric Neurology
West Virginia University Health
Science Center
Morgantown, West Virginia

Rachna Kapoor, MD
Attending Physician
Mercy Hospital of Pittsburgh
Pittsburgh, Pennsylvania

Nikolaos Kefalas, MD
Fellow, Pediatric Endocrinology
and Metabolism
HASBRO Children's Hospital,
Brown University
North Providence, Rhode Island

Anthony Lee, MD
Chief Resident, Internal Medicine
and Pediatrics
West Virginia University School of Medicine
Morgantown, West Virginia

Philana Ling Lin, MD, MSc
Assistant Professor of Pediatrics
Children's Hospital of Pittsburgh
Pittsburgh, Pennsylvania

Don Lujan, MD
Fellow, Orthopedic Surgery
University of Pittsburgh Medical Center
Pittsburgh, Pennsylvania

Sarah J. Marlin, MD
Resident, Department of Pediatrics
Baylor College of Medicine
Houston, Texas

Loreta Matheo, MD
Department of Adolescent Medicine
Children's Hospital of Pittsburgh
Pittsburgh, Pennsylvania

Kathryn Moffat, MD
Director, Cystic Fibrosis Center
Assistant Professor of Pediatrics
West Virginia University School of Medicine
Robert C. Byrd Health Sciences Center
Morgantown, West Virginia

Michele Monaco, MD
Professor of Pediatrics
Drexel University College of Medicine
Division of Pediatric Cardiology
Allegheny General Hospital
Pittsburgh, Pennsylvania
Geisinger Medical Center Pediatric
Subspecialties–Cardiology
Danville, Pennsylvania

Dawn Nolt, MD
Assistant Professor of Pediatrics
Pediatric Infectious Disease Specialist
Doernbecher Children's Hospital
Portland, Oregon

Sarah O'Brien, MD
Pediatric Academic Association
Columbus, Ohio

Paul Ogershok, MD
Associate Professor of Internal Medicine
and Pediatrics
West Virginia University School of Medicine
Morgantown, West Virginia

Jack Perkins, MD
Chief Resident, Combined Internal
Medicine and Emergency Medicine
University of Maryland
Baltimore, Maryland

Klara Posfay-Barbe, MD
Department of Pediatrics
Children's Hospital of Geneva
University Hospitals of Geneva
Geneva, Switzerland

Ellen Roh, MD
University of Pittsburgh Medical Center
Pittsburgh, Pennsylvania

Mustafa Sahin, MD, PhD
Attending Physician
Department of Neurology
Children's Hospital of Boston
Boston, Massachusetts

Mark Sangimino, MD
Professor, Orthopedic Surgery
Drexel University College of Medicine
Allegheny General Hospital Human
Motion Center
Pittsburgh, Pennsylvania

Luna Sharma, MD
West Virginia University Health
Sciences Center
West Virginia University School of Medicine
Morgantown, West Virginia

Dan Sheehan, MD, PhD
Associate Professor of Pediatrics
Children's Hospital of Buffalo
Buffalo, New York

Viyaji Sheshadri, MD
Pediatric Cardiologist
Attending Physician
Mercy Hospital of Pittsburgh
Pittsburgh, Pennsylvania

Shefali Vyas, MD
Associate Director of Pediatric Nephrology
and Transplantation
Saint Barnabas Medical Center
Livingston, New Jersey
Associate Professor of Pediatrics
Mount Sinai School of Medicine
New York, New York

Marty Weiss, MD
Chief of Pediatric Infectious Diseases
Professor of Pediatrics
Residency Program Director
West Virginia University School of Medicine
Robert C. Byrd Health Sciences Center
Morgantown, West Virginia

Garrett C. Zella, MD
Fellow, Pediatric Gastroenterology
and Nutrition
MassGeneral Hospital
Harvard Medical School
Boston, Massachusetts

Acknowledgments

We thank our friends and colleagues who shared their time and pearls of wisdom in helping make this book an outstanding resource.

We are also grateful to our parents and families for their support and understanding. In particular, Jonathan thanks his wife and best friend, Michelle, for her unconditional love, guidance, and encouragement, and his loving daughters, Gillian and Marissa, who make it hard to leave for work but a joy to return home. Kate thanks her wonderful husband Joe, a genuinely special person and a wonderful husband, and her beautiful children. And Scott extends his thanks to Meri for her love and support.

We are grateful to the staff of Lippincott Williams & Wilkins, especially Nancy Duffy, Liz Stalnaker, and Jessica Heisse.

Finally, this book is dedicated with love and respect to the memory of the late Dr. Anthony DiBartolomeo, a great teaching physician who educated with enthusiasm, healed with compassion, lived with joy, and died with dignity.

Contents

Section 3

Gastroenterology

Section 4

Nephrology/Urology

Section 5

Endocrinology

Section 6

Neurology

Infectious Disease

Section 8

Hematology/Oncology

Section 9

Dermatology

Section 10

Conditions of the Newborn

Section 11

Congenital/Genetic Diseases

Section 12

Metabolic Disorders

Contents

Section 13

Developmental Disorders

Section 14

Allergy/Immunology

Section 15

Orthopedics

AAP	American Academy of Pediatrics
ABCD	airway, breathing, circulation, dextrose
ABVD	doxorubicin, bleomycin, vinblastine, and dacarbazine
ACE	angiotensin-converting enzyme
Ach	acetylcholine
ACTH	adrenocorticotropic hormone
ADEM	acute disseminated encephalomyelitis
ADH	antidiuretic hormone (vasopressin)
ADHD	attention deficit hyperactivity disorder
ADPKD	autosomal dominant polycystic kidney disease
AIDS	acquired immunodeficiency syndrome
ALL	acute lymphocytic leukemia
ALPS	autoimmune lymphoproliferative syndrome
ALT	alanine aminotransferase
ALTE	apparent life-threatening event
AML	acute myelogenous leukemia
ANA	antinuclear antigen
ANC	absolute neutrophil count
ANCA	antineutrophil cytoplasmic antibody
AOM	acute otitis media
AP	anterior-posterior
APECED	autoimmune polyendocrinopathy–candidiasis–ectodermal dystrophy
APL	acute promyelocytic leukemia
AR	allergic rhinitis
AR	aortic regurgitation
ARB	angiotensin II receptor blockers
ARDS	adult respiratory distress syndrome
ARF	acute renal failure
ARPKD	autosomal recessive polycystic kidney disease
AS	aortic stenosis
ASCA	anti–*Saccharomyces cerevisiae* antibodies
ASD	atrial septal defect
ASO	antistreptolysin O

AST	aspartate aminotransferase
ATP	adenosine triphosphate
ATPase	adenosine triphosphatase
AVED	ataxia with vitamin E deficiency
AVPR	arginine vasopressin receptor
AZT	zidovudine
BH4	tetrahydrobiopterin
BP	blood pressure
BUN	blood urea nitrogen
BV	bacterial vaginosis
C	complement
CAD	coronary artery disease
CAH	congenital adrenal hyperplasia
cAMP	cyclic adenosine monophosphate
CAVH	continuous arteriovenous or venovenous hemofiltration
CBC	complete blood count
CDH	congenital diaphragmatic hernia
CF	cystic fibrosis
CFTR	cystic fibrosis transmembrane receptor
CGD	chronic granulomatous disease
CH_{50}	total serum hemolytic complement
CHARGE	coloboma of the eye, heart defects, atresia of the choanae, retardation of growth and/or development, genital and/or urinary abnormalities, and ear abnormalities and deafness
CHF	congestive heart failure
CKD	chronic kidney disease
Cl	chlorine
CMV	cytomegalovirus
CNS	central nervous system
CO_2	carbon dioxide
CPAP	continuous positive airway pressure
CPK	creatine phosphokinase
CPM	central pontine myelinolysis (CPM)
CPR	cardiopulmonary resuscitation
CRP	C-reactive protein
CRS	congenital rubella syndrome
CSF	cerebrospinal fluid
CT	computerized tomography
CVS	chorionic villous sampling
CVVH	continuous venovenous hemofiltration
CXR	chest X-ray

DDAVP	desmopressin
DHEA-S	dehydroepiandrosterone sulfate
DIC	disseminated intravascular coagulation
DIP	distal interphalangeal
DKA	diabetic ketoacidosis
DMSA	dimercaptosuccinic acid
DNA	deoxyribonucleic acid
Dx/HA	dextranomer/hyaluronic acid
EBV	Epstein-Barr virus
ECMO	extracorporeal membrane oxygenation
ED	emergency department
EDTA	ethylenediamine tetraacetic acid
EEG	electroencephalogram
EGD	esophagogastroduodenoscopy
EIA	enzyme immunoassay
EKG	electrocardiogram
ELISA	enzyme-linked immunosorbent assay
EMG	electromyelography
ER	emergency room
ERCP	endoscopic retrograde cholangiopancreatography
ESR	erythrocyte sedimentation rate
FDA	Food and Drug Administration
FENa	fractional excretion of sodium
FEV_1	forced expiratory volume in 1 second
FISH	fluorescent in situ hybridization
FSGS	focal segmental glomerulosclerosis
FSH	follicle-stimulating hormone
FTA-ABS	fluorescent treponemal antibody-absorption test
FTT	failure to thrive
FVC	forced vital capacity
G6PD	glucose-6-phosphate dehydrogenase deficiency
GAD	glutamic acid decarboxylase
GBM	glioblastoma multiforme
GBM	glomerular basement membrane
GBS	group B streptococcus
GCS	Glasgow coma scale
G-CSF	granulocyte colony-stimulating factor
GERD	gastroesophageal reflux disease
GFR	glomerular filtration rate
GGT	gamma glutamyl transpeptidase
GH	growth hormone

GHRH	growth hormone–releasing hormone
GI	gastrointestinal
GM-CSF	granulocyte-macrophage colony-stimulating factor
GnRH	gonadotropin-releasing hormone
GTPase	guanosine triphosphatase
H. pylori	*Helicobacter pylori*
H2	histamine-2
HA	headache
HAV	hepatitis A virus
Hb	hemoglobin
HbsAg	hepatitis B surface antigen
HBV	hepatitis B virus
hCG	human chorionic gonadotropin
HCV	hepatitis C virus
HEENT	head, eyes, ears, nose, throat
HEXA	hexosaminidase A
HGPRT	hypoxanthine-guanine phosphoribosyl transferase
HIAA	hydroxyindoleacetic acid
HIB	*Haemophilus influenzae* type B
HIV	human immunodeficiency virus
HLA	human leukocyte antigen
HMD	hyaline membrane disease
HPLC	high-performance liquid chromatography
HPV	human papillomavirus
HR	heart rate
HSV	herpes simplex virus
HTN	hypertension
HUS	hemolytic uremic syndrome
IANP	inappropriate atrial natriuretic peptide
IBD	inflammatory bowel disease
ICP	intracranial pressure
ICU	intensive care unit
ID	identification
IDM	infants of diabetic mothers
IFRT	involved-field radiation therapy
IgA	immunoglobulin A
IgE	immunoglobulin E
IGF	insulin-like growth factor
IGFBP	insulin-like growth factor binding protein
IgG	immunoglobulin G
IgM	immunoglobulin M

IL	interleukin
IM	intramuscular
INR	international normalized ratio
INSS	International Neuroblastoma Staging System
IPAA	ileo-pouch anal anastomosis
ITP	idiopathic thrombocytopenic purpura
IUFD	intrauterine fetal demise
IUGR	intrauterine growth retardation
IV	intravenous
IVC	inferior vena cava
IVH	intraventricular hemorrhage
IVIG	intravenous immunoglobulin
K/DOQI	Kidney Disease Outcomes Quality Initiative
KOH	potassium hydroxide
KUB	kidney, ureter, bladder
LA	left atrium
LD	learning disability
LDH	lactate dehydrogenase
LFT	liver function test
LGA	large for gestational age
LH	luteinizing hormone
LOH	loss of heterozygosity
LP	lumbar puncture
LV	left ventricle
MAS	meconium aspiration syndrome
MCH	mean corpuscular hemoglobin
MCV	mean corpuscular volume
MD	muscular dystrophy
MDR	multidrug resistance
MDS	myelodysplastic syndrome
MGN	membranous glomerulonephritis
MHA-TP	microhemagglutinin assay for *Treponema pallidum*
MI	myocardial infarction
MIBG	metaiodobenzylguanidine
MMR	measles, mumps, and rubella vaccine
MODY	maturity-onset diabetes of youth
MOPP	mechlorethamine, vincristine, procarbazine, and prednisone
MPGN	membranoproliferative glomerulonephritis
MR	mitral regurgitation
MRA	magnetic resonance angiogram
MRI	magnetic resonance imaging

MSAF	meconium staining of the amniotic fluid
MS-AFP	maternal serum alpha fetoprotein
MVP	mitral valve prolapse
NAC	N-acetylcholine
NAD	nicotinamide adenine dinucleotide
NADPH	nicotinamide adenine dinucleotide phosphate oxidase
NEC	necrotizing enterocolitis
NF	neurofibromatosis
NHBPEP	National High Blood Pressure Education Program Working Group
NHL	non-Hodgkin lymphoma
NOS	not otherwise specified
NPH	neutral protamine Hagedorn
NSAID	nonsteroidal anti-inflammatory drug
O_2	oxygen
OCPs	oral contraceptives
OTC	ornithine transcarbamylase
pANCA	perinuclear antineutrophil cytoplasmic antibodies
pCO_2	partial pressure of carbon dioxide
PCP	primary care physician
PCR	polymerase chain reaction
PDA	patent ductus arteriosus
PDD	pervasive developmental disorder
PEG	polyethylene glycol
PET	positron emission tomography
PFA	platelet function assay
PFO	patent foramen ovale
PFT	platelet function test
PID	pelvic inflammatory disease
PIP	proximal interphalangeal
PK	pyruvate kinase
PKU	phenylketonuria
PML-RAR	acute promyelocytic leukemia–retinoic acid receptor
PNET	peripheral neuroectodermal tumor
PNH	paroxysmal nocturnal hemoglobinuria
PO	by mouth
pO_2	partial pressure of oxygen
PPD	purified protein derivative
PPHN	persistent pulmonary hypertension of the newborn
PPS	peripheral pulmonic stenosis
PRN	as needed

PS	pulmonic stenosis
PT	protime
PT	prothrombin time
PTT	partial thromboplastin time
PTX	pneumothorax
PUBS	percutaneous umbilical blood sampling
PUVA	psoralen ultraviolet light A
PVR	pulmonary vascular resistance
RA	right atrium
RAST	radioallergosorbent test
RBC	red blood cells
RDS	respiratory distress syndrome
RDW	red cell distribution width
REM	rapid eye movement
RF	rheumatoid factor
RMSF	Rocky Mountain spotted fever
RNA	ribonucleic acid
RPGN	rapidly progressive glomerulonephritis
RPR	rapid plasma reagin
RS	Reed-Sternberg
RSV	respiratory syncytial virus
RUQ	right upper quadrant
RV	right ventricle
S_1	first heart sound
S_2	second heart sound
SBI	serious bacterial infection
SCID	severe combined immunodeficiency
SHOX	short stature homeobox
SIADH	syndrome of inappropriate antidiuretic hormone
SIDS	sudden infant death syndrome
SLE	systemic lupus erythematosus
STD	sexually transmitted disease
STING	subureteric transurethral injection
SVC	superior vena cava
SVT	supraventricular tachycardia
SW	Sturge-Weber disease
T_3	triiodothyronine
T_4	thyroxine
TA	tricuspid atresia
TAPVR	total anomalous pulmonary venous return
TB	tuberculosis

TcB	transcutaneous bilirubin
TEF	tracheoesophageal fistula
TGV	transposition of the great vessels
TIBC	total iron-binding capacity
TNF	tumor necrosis factor
TOF	tetralogy of Fallot
TORCH	toxoplasmosis, others, rubella, cytomegalovirus, and herpes simplex
TRH	thyrotropin-releasing hormone
TSB	total serum bilirubin
TSC	tuberous sclerosis complex
TSH	thyroid-stimulating hormone
TSS	toxic shock syndrome
TTF	thyroid transcription factor
TTN	transient tachypnea
TTP	thrombotic thrombocytopenic purpura
URI	upper respiratory infection
US	ultrasound
U.S.	United States
UTI	urinary tract infection
UVA	ultraviolet A light
UVB	ultraviolet B light
V/Q	ventilation/perfusion
VACTERL	vertebral, anorectal, cardiac, tracheoesophageal fistula, and renal and radial limb anomalies
VATS	video-assisted thoracic surgery
VCUG	voiding cystourethrogram
VDRL	venereal disease research laboratory
VHL	von Hippel-Lindau syndrome
VIP	vasoactive intestinal peptide
VIPoma	vasoactive intestinal peptide–producing tumor
VSD	ventricular septal defect
VT	ventricular tachycardia
vWD	von Willebrand disease
vWF	von Willebrand factor
VZIG	varicella zoster immunoglobulin
VZV	varicella zoster virus
WAGR	Wilms tumor, aniridia, genitourinary anomalies, mental retardation
WBC	white blood cell
WHO	World Health Organization
WPW	Wolff-Parkinson-White

Cardiology

Ventricular Septal Defect

INTRODUCTION

- Characterized by a defect in the interventricular septum
- The most common congenital cardiac defect; represents more than 20% of all congenital heart defects and 10% of congenital defects diagnosed in adults
- May be part of more complex congenital heart syndromes, including tetralogy of Fallot
- Most cases are surgically corrected or close spontaneously during childhood
- Most commonly diagnosed in infancy, either by physical examination or due to early onset of congestive heart failure
- This is a common cardiac defect in Down syndrome, either as the only cardiac defect or in association with other defects

ETIOLOGY, EPIDEMIOLOGY, & RISK FACTORS

- The ventricular septal defect (VSD) may occur in various areas along the septum
  - Defects in the membranous septum are most common (70–80% of cases)
  - Defects in the muscular septum (5–20%) may be multiple
  - Defects in the atrioventricular canal or inlet (<10%) are typically large and exist beneath the AV valves; often associated with Down syndrome
  - Defects in the outlet (also known as supracristal, infundibular, or subarterial) are usually associated with aortic regurgitation
- After birth, pulmonary vascular resistance decreases as fetal circulation transitions to postnatal circulation; in patients with a ventricular septal defect (VSD), left-to-right shunting across the VSD develops as pulmonary resistance decreases during the newborn period
- Left-to-right shunting develops across the VSD as pulmonary resistance decreases; pulmonary overcirculation associated with pulmonary hypertension may lead to the development of elevated pulmonary vascular resistance, which over time can become permanent (resulting in right-to-left shunting; this reversal of shunt direction is known as Eisenmenger syndrome)
- Often associated with other congenital heart defects, including atrial septal defect, patent ductus arteriosus, right aortic arch, bicuspid aortic valve, or pulmonic stenosis

PATIENT PRESENTATION

- Harsh holosystolic murmur
  - Heard best at the left lower sternal border
  - Radiates to the right lower sternal border
  - Intensity varies based on the size of the VSD and the pulmonary vascular resistance (smaller defects generally cause louder murmurs)
  - Very restrictive (small) defects, particularly if occurring in the muscular septum, are often audible in the newborn period
  - In large defects, the murmur may not be audible until pulmonary vascular resistance has decreased and shunting increases
- Small defects may be asymptomatic
- Large defects may result in dyspnea, poor feeding and growth, profuse perspiration, recurrent respiratory infections
- Exam may reveal a palpable precordial thrill

DIFFERENTIAL DX

- Right ventricular outflow tract obstruction (eg, tetralogy of Fallot, pulmonary stenosis)
- Left ventricular outflow tract obstruction (eg, aortic stenosis, subvalvular aortic stenosis)
- Mitral regurgitation
- Tricuspid regurgitation
- Primary pulmonary hypertension
- Vasculitis
- Left ventricular failure
- Chronic thromboembolic disease
- Functional murmur

DIAGNOSTIC EVALUATION

- EKG may reveal intraventricular conduction delay or right bundle branch block, right axis deviation, right atrial abnormalities, and right ventricular hypertrophy; however, in many cases, especially with small VSDs, the EKG is normal
- Echocardiography with Doppler is >90% sensitive and is usually diagnostic
  - Most sensitive for VSDs larger than 6 mm; less sensitive for muscular defects
  - Can calculate the degree of intracardiac shunting (pulmonary-to-systemic flow ratio, or QP:QS)
  - Also evaluates for other congenital abnormalities
- VSDs are classified as restrictive (QP:QS <1.5), moderately restrictive (QP:QS 1.5–2.5), or nonrestrictive (large defects)
  - Shunts with QP:QS <1.5 are hemodynamically insignificant
  - Shunts with QP:QS 1.5–2.0 are hemodynamically significant and can result in volume overload and arrhythmias
- Cardiac catheterization is useful if there is elevated pulmonary vascular resistance or associated defects (ie, left ventricular outflow tract obstruction) are suspected but not confirmed by echocardiography
- Chest X-ray may show cardiomegaly with increased pulmonary vascular markings
- Annual cardiac evaluation is indicated for adults with large uncorrected defects, late repairs, and Eisenmenger syndrome

TREATMENT & MANAGEMENT

- It is usually prudent to await spontaneous closure or reduction in size of the defect
  - Up to 50% of defects will spontaneously close during the first year of life
  - This is particularly true for small or asymptomatic VSDs and in patients with medically controlled CHF with good growth pattern and absence of increasing pulmonary vascular resistance
- Surgical closure is typically done before school age at 6–12 months if CHF or cardiomegaly is present; it may be performed earlier in infancy if CHF is not easily controlled or if there are concerns of pulmonary hypertension
  - May be performed earlier in infancy if CHF is not easily controlled
  - Surgical closure is indicated if QP:QS >1.5, pulmonary artery systolic pressure >50 mmHg, left ventricular and left atrial enlargement, or left ventricular dysfunction
  - Surgery may also be indicated in membranous or outlet VSDs with more than mild aortic regurgitation, or if more than two episodes of endocarditis have occurred
  - Small VSDs may be closed by a purse-string procedure; larger defects are closed with a patch
- CHF may be treated with digoxin, diuretics, and careful attention to nutrition
- Bacterial endocarditis prophylaxis should be used if the defect has not completely closed

PROGNOSIS & COMPLICATIONS

- 30–50% of cases will spontaneously close during the first year of life
  - Muscular defects are most likely to close spontaneously
  - Inlet and outlet defects rarely close spontaneously
  - Large and medium defects usually progress to heart failure if not corrected
- Large untreated lesions may result in CHF within 6–8 weeks
- The majority of cases do well after surgical closure
- Postoperative patients may have residual VSDs or may have arrhythmias after surgery
- Rarely, spontaneous closure can be complicated by the development of right ventricular outflow obstruction or aortic insufficiency; when these complications occur, surgical intervention may be necessary

Atrial Septal Defect

INTRODUCTION

- An abnormal communication between the atria due to a defect in the interatrial septum
- May result from an ostium primum defect, ostium secundum defect, or incomplete closure of the foramen ovale
- Accounts for 5–10% of cases of congenital heart disease
- The second most common congenital heart disease of adults, accounting for 30–40% of all congenital heart disease in adults

ETIOLOGY, EPIDEMIOLOGY, & RISK FACTORS

- Ostium secundum defect (most common, 75% of cases): Due to excessive resorption of the septum primum or inadequate development of the septum secundum
- Ostium primum defect: Due to incomplete fusion of the atrioventricular endocardial cushions
- May also result from incomplete closure of the foramen ovale
- The atrial septal defect (ASD) allows left-to-right shunting (acyanotic), resulting in volume overload of right atrium and right ventricle, increased pulmonary blood flow, and enlargement of the right atrium, right ventricle, and pulmonary artery; ultimately, pulmonary hypertension occurs
- Reversal of shunting may occur as pulmonary pressure exceeds systemic pressures, leading to a right-to-left shunt (known as Eisenmenger syndrome)
- Incidence is 6.4 out of 10,000 live births
- 2:1 female-to-male predominance

PATIENT PRESENTATION

- Systolic ejection murmur at the left lower sternal border
- Widely split and fixed S_2
- Occasionally, a loud S_1 and pulmonary ejection click may be heard
- Clinical findings vary with the size of the defect
  - Small defects may be asymptomatic
  - Large defects may result in dyspnea, poor feeding, poor growth, profuse perspiration, and recurrent respiratory infections
- Usually asymptomatic in childhood
- May present with exercise intolerance in older children

DIFFERENTIAL DX

- Ventricular septal defect
- Peripheral pulmonary stenosis
- Pulmonary stenosis
- Aortic stenosis
- Patent ductus arteriosus
- Coarctation of the aorta
- Mitral stenosis
- Mitral valve prolapse
- Tetralogy of Fallot
- Pulmonary embolism
- Primary pulmonary hypertension
- Functional murmur

DIAGNOSTIC EVALUATION

- EKG is the initial diagnostic test
  - Ostium secundum defects: Incomplete right bundle branch block and right axis deviation
  - Ostium primum defects: Right bundle branch block, left axis deviation, and 1st-degree atrioventricular block
- Chest X-ray may reveal pulmonary artery, right atrium, and right ventricular enlargement; left atrial enlargement may be present in ostium primum or long-standing ostium secundum defects
- Echocardiography with Doppler is used to confirm the diagnosis
- Cardiac catheterization may be indicated, particularly in adults with atrial septal defects
  - Right heart catheterization to determine the degree of shunting (pulmonary-to-systemic flow ratio, or QP:QS) and pulmonary hypertension
  - Left ventricular angiography may show a "gooseneck" deformity in the outflow tract (subaortic stenosis) in ostium primum defects
- MRI may be used to define the anatomic location and size of the defect and the surrounding anatomy (pulmonary venous drainage)

TREATMENT & MANAGEMENT

- Surgical closure of the defect is the definitive therapy
  - Surgical patch, suture-based closure, or catheter-based closure may be used
  - Ostium primum defect requires patch closure of the septal defect with mitral valve repair if a cleft mitral leaflet is present
  - Contraindications for repair of an ASD include severe pulmonary hypertension or reversal of intracardiac shunt (Eisenmenger syndrome) with resting oxygen saturation less than 90%
- Elective surgical repair is usually done during the preschool years or when diagnosed in older adults
  - Optimal repair should occur prior to age 25 with pulmonary artery systolic pressures less than 40 mmHg
- Endocarditis prophylaxis is not necessary

PROGNOSIS & COMPLICATIONS

- Spontaneous closure may occur during the first year of life
- Most patients are asymptomatic until adulthood
- Pulmonary hypertension, atrial arrhythmias, heart failure, and tricuspid and mitral regurgitation are potential late findings
- Prognosis is worsened with the development of pulmonary hypertension, right heart failure, atrial arrhythmias, or stroke
- Residual shunt occurs in 7–8% of surgical closures
- Catheter closure, when indicated, has 95% success rate with minimal residual shunting
- Operative mortality rates for uncomplicated secundum defects are approximately 1–3%

Patent Ductus Arteriosus

INTRODUCTION

- Oxygenation of fetal blood occurs in the placenta; the ductus arteriosus (connecting the pulmonary artery to the aorta) allows oxygenated blood from the placenta to bypass the nonfunctioning fetal lungs to enter the systemic circulation
- After birth, oxygenation of blood occurs in the lungs, so a conduit that allows blood to bypass the pulmonary circulation is no longer required
- If the ductus does not close as it should, blood flows from the aorta to the pulmonary artery as pulmonary vascular resistance decreases postnatally
- A resultant left-to-right shunt causes pulmonary vascular congestion and, ultimately, pulmonary vascular obstructive disease

ETIOLOGY, EPIDEMIOLOGY, & RISK FACTORS

- Flow through the ductus normally stops within 10–15 hours of birth; complete closure of the ductus generally occurs within 2–3 weeks of life
- Normally, closure is mediated by a reduction in E-type prostaglandins, as well as the acute rise in arterial oxygen that occurs immediately following birth
- Persistence of the ductus can occur as a result of relative hypoxemia secondary to birth at high altitude, pulmonary atresia, etc.
- The ductus may also maintain patency in certain congenital conditions in which it assists in supplying systemic circulation (eg, interrupted aortic arch, hypoplastic left heart syndrome)
- Accounts for 5–10% of all congenital heart disease
- Risk factors include female gender, maternal rubella infection, and prematurity
  - Particularly common in premature infants, but often resolves as term is approached
  - Occurs in 60% of infants born prior to 28 weeks gestation
- A hereditary form includes Char syndrome (patent ductus arteriosus [PDA], characteristic facial features, and an abnormal 5th digit)

PATIENT PRESENTATION

- Findings vary with the size of defect
  - Small defects may be inaudible, asymptomatic, and clinically inconsequential
  - Moderate to large defects generally result in variable signs and symptoms of CHF, including tachypnea, dyspnea, poor feeding and growth, profuse sweating with activities such as crying and feeding, and recurrent pneumonia
  - Large defects eventually result in CHF, which is characteristically unresponsive to ACE inhibitors and diuresis
- Continuous "machinery" murmur at the left upper sternal border (maximal at the midclavicular line) is the classic finding
- Premature infants may have a large patent ductus arteriosus without a murmur
- Active precordium and bounding pulses (wide pulse pressure)

DIFFERENTIAL DX

- Venous hum
- Coronary artery fistula
- Aortic stenosis with associated aortic insufficiency
- Systemic arteriovenous malformations
- Pulmonary artery atresia with collateral circulation
- Ventricular septal defect

DIAGNOSTIC EVALUATION

- Clinical examination
- EKG varies depending on age and the size of defect; it may show left ventricular hypertrophy, left atrial hypertrophy, and/or right ventricular hypertrophy
- Chest X-ray reveals cardiomegaly with increased pulmonary vascular markings and a prominent aortic knob; also may reveal left ventricular hypertrophy, left atrial enlargement, and large pulmonary arteries
- Echocardiography with Doppler is diagnostic
  - PDA is easily identified with color Doppler; reveals degree of retrograde flow in the pulmonary artery
  - The best images are generally obtained from a suprasternal notch view
  - Can also identify associated chamber enlargement (left ventricular hypertrophy and left atrial dilation)
- Cardiac catheterization with angiography, if necessary, is also diagnostic

TREATMENT & MANAGEMENT

- The PDA can be closed by several methods:
  - IV indomethacin: Used in early infancy of premature infants; less effective in term infants (IV ibuprofen can also be used, but is not available in the U.S.)
  - Surgical ligation, preferably done thoracoscopically: This is the treatment of choice in infants who fail indomethacin therapy (surgery is generally delayed for at least 7 weeks in patients with concurrent endocarditis)
  - Percutaneous closure using coil embolization
- Indomethacin given intravenously has been uniquely useful in the treatment of premature infants with patent ductus arteriosus complicating respiratory distress syndrome
- Persistence of the ductus arteriosus may be beneficial in certain congenital conditions in which the systemic circulation is compromised (eg, aortic interruption or coarctation, hypoplastic left ventricle); in these cases, infusion of prostaglandins may be indicated to preserve the defect

PROGNOSIS & COMPLICATIONS

- Spontaneous closure in term infants generally occurs in the first week of life; in premature infants, spontaneous closure may be delayed until postnatal corrected gestational age approaches term
  - It is rare for spontaneous closure to occur beyond the first year of life
- Moderate to large cases may be associated with CHF in term infants, while even smaller defects may contribute to pulmonary difficulties in premature infants with respiratory distress syndrome
- Small defects are generally asymptomatic, although they do pose an underlying risk for endocarditis
- Pulmonary hypertension may result in shunt reversal (Eisenmenger syndrome)

Tetralogy of Fallot

INTRODUCTION

- Consists of four congenital heart defects:
  - Ventricular septal defect
  - Overriding aorta (dextroposition of the aorta such that it is positioned toward the right side or middle of the heart, which receives blood flow from both ventricles)
  - Pulmonary outflow tract obstruction secondary to hypoplasia and stenosis
  - Right ventricular hypertrophy
- The most common cyanotic congenital heart defect after 1 year of age
- Accounts for 10% of all congenital heart disease

ETIOLOGY, EPIDEMIOLOGY, & RISK FACTORS

- Results in right-to-left shunt through the ventricular septal defect and cyanosis
- The degree of pulmonary outflow tract obstruction determines the onset and severity of symptoms and cyanosis
- Has been associated with a 22q11 chromosomal microdeletion also associated with thymic hypoplasia
- One of the 5 T's of cyanotic congenital heart disease
  - If an atrial septal defect is also present (10%), it is commonly called pentalogy of Fallot

PATIENT PRESENTATION

- Harsh systolic crescendo-decrescendo murmur along the left sternal border
  - Radiates to left upper sternal border
  - The intensity of the murmur depends on the degree of outflow obstruction (critical obstruction or atresia may exhibit little or no murmur)
- Most patients have substantial right-to-left shunting and resulting cyanosis, often at birth
- In other patients, CHF (dyspnea, poor feeding, poor growth, profuse perspiration, recurrent respiratory infections) occurs in infancy and cyanosis begins late in the first year of life
- Hypercyanotic ("Tet") spells consisting of intense cyanosis and hyperpnea result from decreased pulmonary blood flow, resulting in a greater right-to-left shunt to the aorta
  - Most commonly occurs from 2–9 months of age
  - Children often assume a squatting position

DIFFERENTIAL DX

- Cyanotic congenital heart defects with pulmonary outflow obstruction ("pink tetralogy of Fallot")
- Ebstein anomaly
- Eisenmenger syndrome
- Transposition of the great arteries
- Ventricular septal defect
- Subaortic stenosis
- Pulmonary valve stenosis
- Double outlet right ventricle with pulmonic stenosis

DIAGNOSTIC EVALUATION

- Clinical examination
- EKG reveals right axis deviation and right ventricular hypertrophy
- Chest X-ray may reveal a classic "boot-shaped" cardiac silhouette with a prominent right ventricle and concavity of the right ventricular outflow tract and main pulmonary artery; a right-sided aortic arch and large ascending aorta can also be seen
- Echocardiography with Doppler is diagnostic
- Cardiac MRI can also visualize the defects
- Cardiac catheterization is not needed for diagnosis but may be important in defining peripheral pulmonary artery size, coronary artery distribution, and the magnitude of the shunt

TREATMENT & MANAGEMENT

- In cases of severe obstruction, prostaglandin E_1 should be started in the neonatal period in order to maintain a patent ductus arteriosus
- Corrective surgery is most commonly performed before 1 year of age unless the pulmonary arteries are significantly hypoplastic
- If the pulmonary arteries are too hypoplastic to allow primary repair, then palliation is performed, usually by the placement of a modified Blalock-Taussig shunt, followed within 6–12 months by more definitive repair
- In patients who are not candidates for complete surgical repair, palliative surgeries can be performed, all of which are designed to increase pulmonary blood flow and thereby decrease cyanosis
  - Potts procedure: Anastomosis of descending aorta to the left pulmonary artery
  - Blalock-Taussig: Anastomosis of subclavian to the pulmonary artery
  - Waterston: Anastomosis of ascending aorta to right pulmonary artery
- Transventricular or transatrial repair of the ventricular septal defect can be performed
- Treat "Tet" spells with supplemental oxygen and morphine, and place the child in a knee-to-chest position
- Patients should be monitored regularly with echocardiography or MRI for evidence of heart failure and progression of pulmonary regurgitation

PROGNOSIS & COMPLICATIONS

- The majority of patients survive surgical intervention with good long-term cardiac function
- Patients with significant pulmonary artery hypoplasia will have poorer long-term right ventricular function and survival
- Pulmonary regurgitation is common following definitive repair and is generally well tolerated, although some patients (particularly those with significant tricuspid regurgitation) may require pulmonary valve replacement
- As with all cyanotic congenital heart defects, patients with unrepaired tetralogy of Fallot are at increased risk for bacterial endocarditis, cerebral abscess, and stroke

Transposition of the Great Vessels

INTRODUCTION

- A conotruncal abnormality that results in the right ventricle giving rise to the aorta and the left ventricle giving rise to the pulmonary artery
- Complete separation of systemic and pulmonary circulations occurs; the aorta circulates blood back to the left heart, and the pulmonary artery circulates blood back to the right heart
- The systemic circulation is desaturated (hypoxemic), while the pulmonary circulation recirculates saturated blood
- Even short-term survival after birth requires some mixing of pulmonary and systemic blood, usually via a patent foramen ovale and patent ductus arteriosus

ETIOLOGY, EPIDEMIOLOGY, & RISK FACTORS

- The most common cause of cyanosis in the immediate newborn period
- Accounts for 5% of all congenital cardiac defects
- Represents one of the 5 T's of cyanotic congenital heart disease
- Incidence of 4.8 in 10,000 live births
- 3:1 male-to-female predominance

PATIENT PRESENTATION

- Murmur is not a significant finding, unless associated with other defects (eg, VSD or pulmonic stenosis)
- A single, loud S_2 occurs because the anteriorly positioned aortic valve closure obscures the sound of pulmonary valve closure
- Cyanosis is the dominant finding immediately after birth, unless an associated VSD is present

DIFFERENTIAL DX

- Other cyanotic congenital heart defects without significant murmur (eg, pulmonary atresia)
- Persistent pulmonary hypertension of the newborn (PPHN)

DIAGNOSTIC EVALUATION

- Clinical examination
- EKG reveals right ventricular hypertrophy and right axis deviation
- Chest X-ray may show normal heart size or mild cardiomegaly and normal to mild increase in pulmonary vascularity
  - The classic cardiac silhouette appearance is termed an "egg on a string" (a narrowed mediastinum is visualized due to the anterior positioning of the aorta and posterior positioning of the pulmonary artery)
- Echocardiography with Doppler is diagnostic
- Cardiac catheterization is rarely needed for diagnosis; however, balloon septostomy can be used to allow for better atrial mixing to mitigate cyanosis, providing short-term palliation

TREATMENT & MANAGEMENT

- Prostaglandin E_1 is used to maintain patency of the ductus arteriosus and to decrease pulmonary vascular resistance, thereby increasing pulmonary blood flow; the resultant increase in pulmonary venous return augments mixing through the foramen ovale
- A restrictive patent foramen ovale and elevated pulmonary vascular resistance may benefit from balloon atrial septostomy, which opens the foramen ovale to increase mixing
- The arterial switch procedure is performed in the neonatal period or early infancy and is now the definitive procedure of choice

PROGNOSIS & COMPLICATIONS

- Despite intense cyanosis at birth, the success rate of early surgical repair is excellent
- Surgical mortality is low (2–5%) after the arterial switch operation, even in the presence of an associated VSD

Total Anomalous Pulmonary Venous Return

INTRODUCTION

- Abnormality of the formation of the pulmonary veins and their communication with the left atrium, resulting in abnormal return of pulmonary venous blood to the right atrium
- The pulmonary veins may feed directly into the right atrium or into vessels that connect to the right atrium, such as the superior (SVC) or inferior (IVC) vena cavae
- The abnormal communication of the pulmonary veins with the right atrium may occur above or below the diaphragm
- Pulmonary venous return to the right atrium may be obstructed (more common when communication is below the diaphragm) or unobstructed (more common when communication occurs with the SVC)

ETIOLOGY, EPIDEMIOLOGY, & RISK FACTORS

- A rare cardiac lesion accounting for less than 1% of all congenital heart disease
- One of the 5 T's of cyanotic congenital heart disease
- Classified according to the location of the anomalous return
  - Supracardiac (attaches to SVC)
  - Cardiac (attaches to the right atrium)
  - Infracardiac (attaches to the IVC), which is most severe
- The below the diaphragm type has 4:1 male-to-female predominance
- Atrial septal defect commonly occurs in association and allows mixed blood to flow from the right atrium to the left atrium; however, right ventricular hypertrophy and pulmonary edema result

PATIENT PRESENTATION

- Clinical findings vary depending on the specific type of anomalous pulmonary return, particularly the presence or absence of pulmonary venous obstruction
  - Nonobstructed type may present with murmur, mild cyanosis, and signs of CHF with right ventricular volume overload (eg, tachypnea, poor feeding, failure to thrive, hepatomegaly)
  - Obstructed type is dominated by cyanosis, poor cardiac output, and pulmonary edema, which develop early in the neonatal period

DIFFERENTIAL DX

- Other cyanotic congenital heart lesions resulting in pulmonary edema
- Severe left heart obstruction with pulmonary edema
- May be part of complex cardiac abnormalities (eg, asplenia with AV septal defect, pulmonary atresia)
- Neonatal pneumonia with sepsis
- Persistent pulmonary hypertension of the newborn
- Respiratory distress syndrome

DIAGNOSTIC EVALUATION

- Clinical examination
- EKG may reveal right ventricular hypertrophy
- Chest X-ray: When pulmonary veins are obstructed, heart size is not enlarged but lung fields often reveal a "whiteout" due to severe pulmonary edema; nonobstructed type may show the classic "snowman" appearance of the cardiac silhouette
- Echocardiography with Doppler is generally diagnostic
- Cardiac catheterization may be useful in delineating mixed or more complex forms of pulmonary venous abnormalities
- MRI or CT scan may also be useful in complex forms of disease but has no role in the critically ill neonate or infant

TREATMENT & MANAGEMENT

- Critically ill, symptomatic patients (generally those with obstruction) require urgent or surgical intervention
- Surgical repair depends upon the particular defect; the goal is to redirect the anomalous pulmonary vein to the left atrium
  - Preoperative stabilization requires mechanical ventilation with high inspiratory pressures/positive end-expiratory pressure, as well as volume and inotropic support
- Patients without obstruction benefit from digoxin and diuretic therapy in preparation for nonemergent surgical intervention
- This lesion is generally not benefited by the use of prostaglandin E_1; in fact, it may induce pulmonary edema due to increased pulmonary arterial flow

PROGNOSIS & COMPLICATIONS

- Variable prognosis depending on the presence of pulmonary venous obstruction, pulmonary hypertension, and degree of mixing
- Patients may be critically ill shortly after birth or develop symptoms in weeks to months
- If surgical repair is timely, outcomes are excellent
- Patients with delayed diagnosis or those who develop persistent pulmonary hypertension have a poorer prognosis

Truncus Arteriosus

INTRODUCTION

- A conotruncal abnormality resulting in the formation of a single arterial trunk that gives rise to both the systemic and pulmonary circulation
- Accounts for less than 1% of all congenital heart disease

ETIOLOGY, EPIDEMIOLOGY, & RISK FACTORS

- The defect results in massive pulmonary overcirculation as pulmonary vascular resistance decreases at birth
- Virtually always associated with a large ventricular septal defect
- May have associated truncal valve abnormalities, resulting in stenosis or regurgitation
- Incidence of 1 in 10,000 live births
- DiGeorge syndrome is present in 30% of cases
- One of the five T's of cyanotic congenital heart disease

PATIENT PRESENTATION

- Moderate systolic murmur heard best at the left sternal border
- Single loud S_2
- Bounding pulses early in infancy that become even more prominent as pulmonary vascular resistance decreases
- Diastolic murmur may be present if truncal valve regurgitation is present
- Cyanosis present after birth is usually mild
- Signs and symptoms of severe CHF (tachypnea, dyspnea, poor feeding, profuse perspiration at rest and with feeding) develop within the first few weeks of life as pulmonary vascular resistance decreases

DIFFERENTIAL DX

- Other cyanotic congenital heart defects with pulmonary overcirculation

DIAGNOSTIC EVALUATION

- Clinical examination reveals mild cyanosis, murmur, and bounding pulses
- EKG reveals left ventricular or biventricular hypertrophy with strain
- Chest X-ray reveals cardiomegaly, increased pulmonary vascularity, and pulmonary edema
- Echocardiography with Doppler is diagnostic

TREATMENT & MANAGEMENT

- Early surgical repair (usually in the first month of life) is necessary to control the congestive heart failure, avoid development of severe pulmonary vascular disease, and allow survival
- Treatment of CHF with digoxin and diuretics is generally ineffective

PROGNOSIS & COMPLICATIONS

- Early CHF is not usually responsive to medical management
- Pulmonary vascular disease occurs at an early age
- High mortality if surgical repair is not undertaken in the first few weeks of life
- Postoperative course depends on various aspects of anatomy, particularly the structure and function of the truncal valve

Hypoplastic Left Heart Syndrome

INTRODUCTION

- A group of anomalies that result in underdevelopment of the left side of the heart
- Left ventricle size ranges from borderline low volume to total atresia
- Associated with hypoplasia of the left atrium, mitral valve abnormalities, and aortic stenosis, coarctation, or atresia

ETIOLOGY, EPIDEMIOLOGY, & RISK FACTORS

- In these patients, systemic flow and postnatal survival depend on a patent ductus arteriosus (prior to surgery): Pulmonary venous return to the left atrium enters the right heart via a patent foramen ovale or atrial septal defect; blood then flows from the right ventricle to the pulmonary arteries and flows through the patent ductus arteriosus to the aorta (right-to-left shunting)
- Accounts for 1% of all congenital heart disease
- Among congenital heart diseases, this is the most common cause of death during the first month of life
- Coarctation of the aorta is generally a "hidden" feature of this complex

PATIENT PRESENTATION

- Murmur is usually absent (a nondescript systolic murmur may be present)
- Right ventricular parasternal lift
- Single, loud S_2
- Cyanosis may not be present at birth, but patients typically appear blue-gray after 48 hours of life
- As the ductus arteriosus begins to close, patients develop shock (poor pulses, clammy skin, lethargy, decreased urine output)
- Symptoms of CHF or shock develop in hours to days; it is rare for an untreated infant to live for more than a few days

DIFFERENTIAL DX

- Neonatal sepsis or pneumonia
- Persistent fetal circulation
- Other congenital heart defects, particularly left heart obstructions (eg, coarctation of the aorta)

DIAGNOSTIC EVALUATION

- Clinical examination: Signs of decreased systemic perfusion dominate the clinical picture
- EKG is not generally useful; will show the right ventricular dominance that is normal of newborns
- Chest X-ray reveals cardiomegaly (despite the small left ventricle) with increased pulmonary vascular markings and pulmonary edema (may be difficult to distinguish from diffuse neonatal pneumonia)
- Echocardiography with Doppler is diagnostic
- Fetal echocardiography is indicated if an obstetrical scan reveals an abnormal four-chamber view or a previous child was born with a congenital heart defect; it is useful in planning delivery and neonatal intervention

TREATMENT & MANAGEMENT

- Prostaglandin E_1 infusion is critical to maintain a patent ductus arteriosus; it should be initiated immediately after birth/diagnosis
- Medical treatment of shock and metabolic acidosis
- Cautious oxygen administration since it may precipitate further decrease in pulmonary vascular resistance, even in the face of prostaglandin E_1 infusion
- Surgical palliation occurs in stages:
  - Norwood procedure: Connects the pulmonary artery and the aorta to improve aortic outflow
  - Glenn shunt: Bidirectional cavopulmonary anastomosis to reduce the volume load on the right ventricle
  - Modified Fontan procedure: Surgical connection of the right atrium and pulmonary artery to improve blood flow in the lungs
- Heart transplantation, although limited by heart availability, may be done during the neonatal period or later in childhood, adolescence, or adulthood for patients with failing Fontan procedures

PROGNOSIS & COMPLICATIONS

- If not made prenatally, diagnosis is usually made in the first few hours to days of life or at autopsy after sudden neonatal death
- Untreated infants die in days to weeks as the ductus arteriosus closes or severe heart failure ensues
- 25–35% mortality is associated with the first stage of surgical repair
- Overall survival after Fontan procedure is about 50% at 4 years
- After cardiac transplantation, patients usually have normal cardiac function but face life-long medication side effects and the risk of rejection and infection
- Long-term results are improving as surgical techniques and postoperative care improve

Coarctation of the Aorta

INTRODUCTION

- Narrowing and constriction of the aorta near the ductus arteriosus, just after the left subclavian artery
  - The constricted area has been described as being above (preductal) or below (postductal) the entrance of the ductus arteriosus; however, it is now recognized that most cases are juxtaductal (across from the ductal opening in the aorta)
- There is increased blood flow proximal to the constriction (to the head and arms) and decreased blood flow beyond the constriction (to the lower extremities)

ETIOLOGY, EPIDEMIOLOGY, & RISK FACTORS

- Preductal coarctation is associated with other cardiac defects (eg, ventricular septal defect, patent ductus arteriosus, aortic stenosis)
- Postductal and juxtaductal coarctation are typically associated with a closed ductus arteriosus; thus, blood flow to the distal aorta is provided by collateral circulation
- Accounts for 8–10% of all congenital heart disease
- Incidence of 3.2 in 10,000 live births
- 2:1 male-to-female predominance
- 85% of affected patients also have a bicuspid aortic valve
- May be associated with Turner syndrome

PATIENT PRESENTATION

- Age and symptoms at presentation depend on location of constriction, size of the aortic lumen at and above the coarctation, and the extent of collateral circulation
- During the neonatal period, symptomatic neonates exhibit evidence of CHF or cardiogenic shock (eg, dyspnea, poor feeding, oliguria/anuria, acidosis, pulmonary edema) and typically have a gallop rhythm
  - Differential strength of pulses is less obvious until CHF/shock is treated
- Beyond neonatal period, there are delayed or weak femoral pulses, and blood pressure in the arms is greater than blood pressure in the legs
  - Murmur of bicuspid aortic valve at the right upper sternal border
  - CHF is less common
- In childhood and adolescence, hypertension is common

DIFFERENTIAL DX

- Sepsis/shock
- Other aortic arch anomalies
- Pulmonic stenosis
- Peripheral pulmonic stenosis
- Aortic stenosis
- Patent ductus arteriosus
- Essential hypertension
- Other causes of hypertension

DIAGNOSTIC EVALUATION

- Clinical examination
- Four-extremity blood pressures
  - Caution: Blood pressure in the left arm may not reveal as significant a difference from lower extremity pressure if the coarctation site extends to the base of the left subclavian artery; thus, the best method to recognize differential blood pressures is by measuring the pressures in the right arm and either lower extremity
- EKG may reveal right ventricular hypertrophy in neonates or left ventricular hypertrophy in older children and adolescents
- Chest X-ray is variable: Symptomatic infants may have cardiomegaly and pulmonary congestion; older, asymptomatic children may have "rib notching" due to enlarged subcostal collateral circulation
- Echocardiography with Doppler is diagnostic
- Cardiac catheterization further defines the anatomy of the coarctation and collateral circulation

TREATMENT & MANAGEMENT

- Surgery should be performed shortly after diagnosis in older infants, children, and adolescents, even if asymptomatic
  - Resection with end-to-end anastomosis
  - Graft is placed into the narrowed area to increase lumen size
  - Dilatation procedures have been used but may be complicated by aneurysm formation or restenosis
- Neonates manifesting CHF or cardiogenic shock should be treated medically prior to surgical repair: Correct hypoxemia and acidosis, control ventilation, infuse prostaglandin E_1 to maintain or "reopen" the ductus arteriosus for palliation until surgery can be performed, and provide inotropic support
- Balloon angioplasty may be performed, but it is better reserved for cases of restenosis that may occur many years after repair
- Lifelong bacterial endocarditis prophylaxis is beneficial

PROGNOSIS & COMPLICATIONS

- In mild cases, the diagnosis may be delayed until childhood or adolescence when hypertension with decreased femoral pulses is recognized
  - If not repaired or if repaired late, adults are at risk for complications of hypertension, endocarditis, and aortic rupture or dissection
  - Delay or failure to repair after the second decade of life is associated with premature development of cardiovascular disease
- In severe cases, CHF can be life threatening during early infancy
- There is a risk of restenosis at site of neonatal repair
- Patients require periodic follow-up for surveillance of blood pressure and aortic valve function

Aortic Stenosis

INTRODUCTION

- Narrowing in the area of the aortic valve, which may occur at (valvular), above (supravalvular), or below (subvalvular) the valve
  - Valvular stenosis has an abnormal valve shape, which may be bicuspid instead of tricuspid
  - Subvalvular stenosis generally consists of a fibrous ring below the valve
  - Supravalvular stenosis is a constriction or narrowing of the aorta directly above the valve

ETIOLOGY, EPIDEMIOLOGY, & RISK FACTORS

- Usually caused by a congenital malformation of the aortic valve that results in thickened, fused valve leaflets (bicuspid valve) with restricted systolic movement and left ventricular outflow tract obstruction
- Left ventricular outflow obstruction leads to left ventricular hypertrophy and, eventually, left ventricular failure, decreased cardiac output, and pulmonary congestion and edema
- Congenital left ventricular outflow tract obstruction may also be secondary to isolated or associated subvalvular or supravalvular aortic stenosis
- Congenital aortic stenosis represents 5% of all congenital heart disease
- Acquired aortic stenosis secondary to rheumatic heart disease is rare before adulthood
- 3:1 male-to-female predominance
- Bicuspid aortic value is common, occurring in 2% of population

PATIENT PRESENTATION

- Harsh systolic murmur located at the right upper sternal border
  - Radiates to the neck
  - May occur with a systolic ejection click or decreased first heart sound
  - The louder, harsher, and longer the murmur, the more severe the stenosis
- Symptoms vary with degree of stenosis
- Mild and moderate cases are generally asymptomatic, even during activity
- Severe cases may result in chest pain, fatigue, dizziness, or syncope during activity
- Critical aortic stenosis presents in early infancy with evidence of CHF or cardiogenic shock, including decreased cardiac output and pulmonary edema

DIFFERENTIAL DX

- Aortic valve stenosis
- Subvalvular aortic stenosis
- Supravalvular aortic stenosis
- Hypoplastic left ventricle
- Cardiomyopathy (hypertrophic or dilated)
- Coarctation of the aorta

DIAGNOSTIC EVALUATION

- Clinical examination
- EKG may reveal left ventricular hypertrophy
- Chest X-ray reveals normal heart size with prominent ascending aorta
- Echocardiography with Doppler is diagnostic and will define the severity of the defect
- Cardiac catheterization can further define anatomy and confirm severity of aortic gradient; may also allow for intervention with balloon aortic valvotomy in cases of severe stenosis

TREATMENT & MANAGEMENT

- Balloon valvotomy is used to treat valvular stenosis
  - Not useful in subvalvular or supravalvular disease
- Prosthetic valve replacement is not recommended in children due to the need for prolonged anticoagulation
- The Ross procedure may be used, in which a native pulmonary valve replaces the stenotic valve and a homograft is used in place of the pulmonary valve
- Neonatal patients with critical aortic stenosis require medical therapy prior to surgical intervention or balloon valvotomy
  - Medical therapy includes prostaglandin E_1, inotropic agents, ventilator support, correction of acidosis, and prophylaxis for bacterial endocarditis

PROGNOSIS & COMPLICATIONS

- Prognosis varies with severity of the lesion
- Some patients with severe disease die in the neonatal period; those who respond well to surgery may require reoperation later in life
- Mild to moderate cases should be followed for progression of stenosis; patients who require valve replacement in later decades generally have a very good prognosis
- Limitation of physical activity is recommended in some cases

Pulmonary Stenosis

INTRODUCTION

- Pulmonary stenosis is a narrowing of the pulmonary valve that separates the right ventricle and the pulmonary artery
- Results from thickened and fused pulmonary valve leaflets, which restrict systolic excursion of the valve
- Significantly increased resistance to outflow through the pulmonary valve results in decreased flow to the pulmonary artery circulation and right ventricular hypertrophy
- In severe cases of neonatal pulmonary stenosis, obstruction may result in significant cyanosis due to right-to-left shunting through a patent foramen ovale

ETIOLOGY, EPIDEMIOLOGY, & RISK FACTORS

- Accounts for 5–8% of all congenital heart disease
- Dysplasia of the pulmonary valve is commonly seen in Noonan syndrome

PATIENT PRESENTATION

- Symptoms vary depending on severity of stenosis
  - Mild cases are generally asymptomatic and recognized only by the characteristic murmur
  - Severe cases (critical aortic stenosis) are cyanotic due to decreased pulmonary perfusion and may demonstrate evidence of right heart failure (dyspnea, enlarged liver, edema)
- Systolic murmur with ejection click
  - Intensity varies with severity of stenosis; louder, longer murmurs indicate more severe pulmonary obstruction
  - Loudest at the left upper sternal border
  - Radiates to the left side of the back

DIFFERENTIAL DX

- Atrial septal defect
- Peripheral pulmonary stenosis
- Patent ductus arteriosus
- Coarctation of the aorta
- Subaortic stenosis
- Ventricular septal defect

DIAGNOSTIC EVALUATION

- Clinical examination is usually suggestive of the diagnosis
  - Caution: Cyanotic infants with critical pulmonary stenosis (particularly when right ventricular dysfunction or hypoplasia is present) will often not have a significant murmur
- EKG is normal or shows variable degrees of right ventricular hypertrophy
- Chest X-ray is often normal but depends on age and severity of the lesion; an enlarged cardiac silhouette, dilated pulmonary artery, and decreased pulmonary markings may be seen
- Echocardiography with Doppler is diagnostic
- Cardiac catheterization is now part of the therapeutic approach, leading to balloon valvotomy

TREATMENT & MANAGEMENT

- Patients with critical pulmonary stenosis should be started on prostaglandin E_1
- Balloon valvotomy is now the treatment of choice
  - Patients have a less competent valve after valvotomy; however, their cardiac function still improves overall
- Surgical intervention may still be needed, particularly in critical stenosis with a hypoplastic and/or dysplastic valve
- Bacterial endocarditis prophylaxis is indicated

PROGNOSIS & COMPLICATIONS

- Prognosis varies with severity of the lesion
- Critical stenosis may result in CHF in the first month of life
- Mild to moderate cases should be followed for progression of stenosis
- The majority of patients do well after dilatation or surgical repair
- Restenosis can still occur even after balloon dilatation or surgical repair

Mitral Valve Prolapse

INTRODUCTION

- Myxomatous changes leading to abnormality of the mitral valve, resulting in systolic billowing of one or both of the mitral leaflets into the left atrium
- May have associated regurgitation of the mitral valve

ETIOLOGY, EPIDEMIOLOGY, & RISK FACTORS

- Occurs in up to 5% of children
- More common in females
- Particularly common in patients with Marfan syndrome

PATIENT PRESENTATION

- Generally asymptomatic
- Some patients may complain of atypical chest pain or palpitations
- Rarely, syncope may occur
- Midsystolic click and mid-to-late systolic murmur

DIFFERENTIAL DX

- Mitral regurgitation secondary to other mitral valve abnormalities (eg, rheumatic fever, ostium primum atrial septal defect with cleft mitral valve)
- Small perimembranous ventricular septal defect
- Pulmonary or aortic ejection click
- Primary arrhythmia causing palpitations

DIAGNOSTIC EVALUATION

- Clinical examination
- EKG is usually normal, but there may be mild ST segment and T wave changes in the inferior and lateral leads, ectopy (atrial or ventricular), or occasionally tachyarrhythmias
- Chest X-ray is normal
- Echocardiography with Doppler is diagnostic

TREATMENT & MANAGEMENT

- No treatment is required in children
- Monitor for arrhythmias and cardiac function
- Patients with complicating arrhythmias may be treated with β-blockers or calcium channel blockers
- Bacterial endocarditis prophylaxis is indicated

PROGNOSIS & COMPLICATIONS

- May not be diagnosed until adolescence or adulthood
- Adult patients are more likely to be symptomatic with chest pain, palpitations, arrhythmias
- Sudden death has been reported but is rare

Rheumatic Heart Disease

INTRODUCTION

- Rheumatic fever (RF) is a nonsuppurative complication of untreated or partially treated group A β-hemolytic streptococcal pharyngitis that occurs due to an abnormal immune response to a component of the group A *Streptococcus*
- Generally considered a connective tissue disease, rheumatic fever is a multisystem disorder that occurs 1–5 weeks after streptococcal infection and usually affects heart, joints, and subcutaneous tissues
- May result in pathologic changes of various cardiac structures and valves: The mitral (75%) and aortic valves (20%) are most commonly affected, initially presenting as regurgitation, but then stenosis may develop after many years

ETIOLOGY, EPIDEMIOLOGY, & RISK FACTORS

- Most common in children age 5–15
- Clinical manifestations follow group A streptococcal infection of the tonsillopharynx
- Rheumatic strains involve certain structural characteristics of the M protein with resistance to phagocytes
- The acute phase of rheumatic fever is characterized by exudative and proliferative inflammatory reactions involving connective or collagen tissue
- The interstitial connective tissue becomes edematous and eosinophilic
- Susceptible hosts have a high incidence of class II HLA antigens
- The incidence and prevalence differ by country; remains a common cause of acute and chronic acquired cardiac disease in developing nations, with an incidence of about 100 per 100,000
- Uncommon in the U.S., with incidence of 2 per 100,000
  - The decreased incidence in the U.S. is due to improved nutrition, hygiene, and living conditions; a decrease in the prevalence of rheumatic strains of *Streptococcus*; and the widespread use of penicillin

PATIENT PRESENTATION

- Pharyngitis may precede symptoms by 1–5 weeks
- Fever
- Joint manifestations (75% of patients): Inflammation and pain, usually in larger joints
- Signs of heart failure (50% clinically, 90% by echo): Dyspnea, tachycardia, mitral regurgitation, aortic regurgitation, pericarditis, varying degree of atrioventricular block
- Erythema marginatum (10%): Serpiginous erythematous rash
- Subcutaneous nodules (2–10%): Hard, painless nodes under skin overlying joints
- Sydenham chorea (<5%): Rapid, purposeless movements that occur late and only while awake ("bag of worms" of tongue upon protrusion, squeezing/relaxing motion during handgrip, knee jerk)

DIFFERENTIAL DX

- Endocarditis
- Viral infection (rubella, hepatitis B)
- Septic arthritis (*Neisseria*)
- Acute rheumatoid arthritis
- Systemic lupus erythematosus
- Still disease
- Lyme disease
- Osteomyelitis
- Sickle cell disease

DIAGNOSTIC EVALUATION

- Diagnosis is made clinically based on a combination of clinical manifestations and specific laboratory tests known as the Duckett-Jones Criteria
- Diagnosis requires the presence of two major criteria or one major and two minor criteria, plus evidence of a preceding streptococcal infection
- Major criteria: Carditis, migratory polyarthritis, erythema marginatum, Sydenham chorea, subcutaneous nodules
  - Carditis: Pancarditis occurs in 50% of acute cases; valvulitis is the most common manifestation, and concomitant myocarditis may result in heart failure symptoms
  - Arthritis: Polyarthritis is the most common major manifestation of RF; it is almost always asymmetric, migratory, and involves the large joints
  - Chorea: Occurs in 20% of cases; results from inflammatory involvement of the CNS and may appear up to 3 months after the initial manifestation; characterized by purposeless and involuntary movements; usually resolves in 1–2 weeks
  - Erythema marginatum: Occurs in <5% of cases; an evanescent, erythematous, macular rash with pale centers and serpiginous margins
  - Subcutaneous nodules: Firm, painless, and freely movable; occur in 3% of patients
- Minor criteria: fever; arthralgias; elevated ESR, CRP, or WBC; first-degree heart block
- Echocardiography to assess valvular dysfunction and evidence of myocardial and pericardial involvement

TREATMENT & MANAGEMENT

- Treat group A streptococcal pharyngitis with either 10 days of an oral antibiotic (penicillin V) or a single IM dose of benzathine penicillin G
- Treat clinical manifestations as they arise
  - Salicylates can relieve the inflammation of the arthritis, and carditis and corticosteroids may be used to treat significant carditis; however, there is no evidence that either of these two therapies affects the course of the carditis
  - Symptomatic therapy and treatment of heart failure symptoms, if present, with diuretics, oxygen, and digitalis
- Long-term antibiotic prophylaxis to prevent recurrences of acute rheumatic fever should be used to avoid recurrent valve injuries that may lead to chronic valve damage
  - Prophylaxis should be continued for 5 years if there are no signs of carditis and 10 or more years if cardiac involvement is present
  - Life-long prophylactic antibiotics for all surgical procedures

PROGNOSIS & COMPLICATIONS

- Immediate mortality of acute rheumatic fever is 1–2%
- Prognosis is generally good; however, there is a significant risk of recurrence
- Untreated acute rheumatic fever lasts 3 months; if carditis occurs, may last up to 6 months
- Arthritis typically resolves in weeks
- Chorea typically resolves in weeks to months
- Carditis and/or valvulitis at initial diagnosis may vary from mild to severe, including congestive heart failure
- Long-term outcome is based on the severity of valvular heart disease
- Most patients who develop valvular dysfunction require intervention, including valvotomy, valve repair, or replacement

Bradyarrhythmias

INTRODUCTION

- Pathologic bradycardia is most often due to processes that result in hypoxemia, acidosis, hypotension, or increased vagal tone
- Symptoms result from a decrease in cardiac output (CO) due to the low heart rate (HR), despite the body's attempt to increase stoke volume (SV) (CO = HR × SV)
- Severe bradycardia or asystole, rather than ventricular fibrillation, is the more common terminal event provoking a need for neonatal/pediatric resuscitation

ETIOLOGY, EPIDEMIOLOGY, & RISK FACTORS

- Common etiologies include atrioventricular (AV) node dysfunction, hypoxia, and prematurity
- AV node dysfunction (second- or third-degree AV block) may be caused by congenital or acquired causes
  - Congenital causes include maternal autoimmune disease (eg, SLE), maternal collagen vascular disease, and congenital heart disease
  - Acquired causes include infections (eg, Lyme disease), endocrine disorders, drugs, and cardiac surgery
- Hypoxia may occur due to any form of respiratory compromise or any cardiac condition that impairs oxygenation

PATIENT PRESENTATION

- Symptoms of decreased cardiac output (eg, fatigue, syncope, dizziness, dyspnea, CHF)
- Patients with pathologic, severe sinus bradycardia also manifest symptoms of the underlying illness (eg, respiratory distress, hypoxia, acidosis)
- Congenital complete heart block may result in fetal distress (eg, hydrops fetalis, fetal loss) or CHF early in the neonatal period
  - Infants and children with congenital complete heart block in the absence of structural cardiac defects are often asymptomatic (particularly if the heart rate is >55 bpm)

DIFFERENTIAL DX

- Physiologic bradycardia (due to a healthy, low resting heart rate)
- Pathologic bradycardia (due to hypoxemia and other disorders)
- AV nodal dysfunction (first-, second-, or third-degree heart block)

DIAGNOSTIC EVALUATION

- Pathologic bradycardia can be diagnosed based on the clinical presentation
- EKG is diagnostic for AV nodal dysfunction
- Echocardiography with Doppler may be useful in the diagnosis of associated congenital or acquired cardiac/myocardial disease
- Specific laboratory tests or endomyocardial biopsy may be required to diagnose the etiology of acquired AV block

TREATMENT & MANAGEMENT

- Pathologic bradycardia may be corrected with cardiopulmonary resuscitation, epinephrine, and treatment of the underlying condition
- Symptomatic neonates with congenital complete heart block may require pacing after stabilization with infusion of chronotropic agents (eg, isoproterenol, epinephrine), correction of acidosis, and support of respiration
- Adolescents and young adults with congenital or acquired complete heart block may require pacing if symptomatic with exertional dyspnea, chronic fatigue, or syncope

PROGNOSIS & COMPLICATIONS

- Prognosis varies with the underlying etiology
- In critically ill or injured children, severe bradycardia or asystole may be fatal despite adequately performed resuscitative efforts because it usually develops as a result of prolonged hypoxia or acidosis
- Acquired complete heart block may require pharmacologic and/or temporary pacing until the underlying cause is effectively treated (eg, Lyme disease, endocarditis, myocardial contusion)
- Prognosis for congenital complete heart block in the absence of underlying complex congenital cardiac defects is generally good

Tachyarrhythmias

INTRODUCTION

- Tachyarrhythmias include supraventricular tachycardia, sinus tachycardia, and ventricular tachycardia (VT), atrial flutter, and atrial fibrillation among others
- Supraventricular tachycardia (SVT) can be defined as an abnormally rapid heart rhythm originating above the ventricles, often (but not always) with a narrow QRS complex
- Atrial flutter may be a stable rhythm or a bridge between sinus rhythm and atrial fibrillation
- Symptoms develop when the excessively elevated heart rate disrupts effective ventricular filling and coronary perfusion, resulting in poor contractility, decreased cardiac output, and myocardial ischemia

ETIOLOGY, EPIDEMIOLOGY, & RISK FACTORS

- The prevalence of SVT is estimated to be between one in 250–25,000 children
  - SVT may be caused by myocarditis, toxins or drugs, hypoxia, electrolyte imbalances, coronary anomalies, or MI
  - SVT is a reentrant rhythm involving two distinct pathways for conduction, with unidirectional block in one of the two pathways creating a circuit through which an electrical impulse can cycle repetitively in one direction (antegrade or retrograde), with consequent rapid, regular ventricular contractions
  - In infants, SVT is usually associated with structurally normal hearts
  - Wolff-Parkinson-White syndrome (WPW) is more common in older children and adolescents (10–15% of children with WPW have Ebstein anomaly)
- Sinus tachycardia may be caused by fever, pain, dehydration, and anxiety
- VT may be caused by myocarditis, toxins or drugs, hypoxia, coronary anomalies, or MI; however, it is much less common in children than adults
- Atrial fibrillation and atrial flutter are uncommon in infants and children, almost always occurring in association with structural heart disease
  - The incidence is greatest when underlying heart disease is associated with left atrial enlargement or left ventricular or biventricular failure

PATIENT PRESENTATION

- Sudden sensation of rapid heart rate
- SVT: If prolonged (>24 hours) or associated with congenital cardiac defects, patients will likely develop CHF (tachypnea, weakened pulses, hepatomegaly, poor feeding) or cardiogenic shock (pallor, hypotension, respiratory insufficiency)
  - CHF and shock are more common in infants
  - Syncope associated with WPW syndrome may signal atrial fibrillation with rapid atrioventricular (AV) conduction along the accessory pathway
- VT: Usually presents with signs and symptoms of underlying critical illness or trauma
  - May be the presenting sign of drug or toxin exposures or inflammatory disease (eg, myocarditis)
  - Hypotension may cause sudden collapse
  - V fib or torsades de pointes may occur

DIFFERENTIAL DX

SVT
- Sinus tachycardia of sudden onset
- Atrial flutter
- Chaotic atrial rhythm

VT
- SVT with aberrant conduction
- SVT due to antegrade conduction (WPW)

DIAGNOSTIC EVALUATION

- EKG is diagnostic
- It may be difficult to differentiate SVT from intense sinus tachycardia clinically, but EKG or monitor rhythm strips will usually make the diagnosis
  - Both are narrow-complex (QRS <0.08 sec) rhythms
  - SVT is typically greater than 180 bpm in older children and adults and greater than 220 bpm in infants and young children; rhythm strips show a rapid rate with little R-R (beat-to-beat) variability
  - In sinus rhythm, patients with WPW exhibit preexcitation with a characteristic delta wave, widening of the QRS, and short PR interval
  - Cardiopulmonary exercise testing may be helpful in children whose symptoms are triggered by exercise; SVT can be elicited at times of increased adrenergic tone resulting from exertion
  - Electrophysiologic studies are often performed as part of the diagnostic evaluation of clinically significant SVT in children; this is especially true if catheter ablation is planned to treat the arrhythmia, although in some cases, a diagnostic procedure only may be performed (ie, to evaluate the effect of drug therapy)
- VT is a wide-complex (QRS >0.08 sec) tachycardia with regular rhythm and rate of 120–400 bpm

TREATMENT & MANAGEMENT

- An infant or child who presents with a tachyarrhythmia should have an immediate hemodynamic assessment and a 15-lead EKG (12 standard leads plus leads V3R and V4R [right-sided leads analogous to V3 and V4 on the left] and V7 [at the left posterior axillary line at the V4 level])
- Acute cases of SVT can be treated with vagal maneuvers, rapid infusion of adenosine, or electrical cardioversion (if unstable)
  - Vagal maneuvers (if stable), include induced gag reflex, rectal exam, or covering the face and nose with a bag of ice
- Chronic SVT can be treated with antiarrhythmic medications (eg, digoxin, propranolol, procainamide) or radiofrequency ablation of the accessory pathway
- Acute VT is treated with electrical cardioversion
  - Antiarrhythmic agents (eg, lidocaine, procainamide, amiodarone) may be used in stable patients and in patients with recurrent VT following electrical cardioversion
- Chronic VT is treated with antiarrhythmic medications (eg, quinidine, procainamide, propranolol)
- Electrophysiologic studies can be used to map the aberrant pathway and then ablate that pathway to result in a cure

PROGNOSIS & COMPLICATIONS

- The majority of patients with SVT do well on medical therapy or after ablation
  - Recovery of myocardial function is usually rapid after return to normal heart rate
  - Those patients with SVT who present younger than 3 to 4 months of age have a lower incidence of reoccurrence
- VT may be fatal upon presentation
  - The specific clinical course varies with the underlying etiology

Pulmonology

Asthma

INTRODUCTION

- A disease of chronic airway inflammation, bronchial hyperreactivity, and reversible airway obstruction
- May be extrinsic (due to hypersensitivity to allergens) or intrinsic (nonimmune triggers)
- The National Institutes of Health/National Heart Lung and Blood Institute has a severity rating and treatment system called *Guidelines for Diagnosis and Management of Asthma*, which can be accessed at www.nhlbi.nih.gov
- The severity of asthma is characterized as mild intermittent, mild persistent, moderate persistent, severe persistent, and exercise induced

ETIOLOGY, EPIDEMIOLOGY, & RISK FACTORS

- Asthma affects 5–10% of the population; it is the most common chronic disease of childhood, accounting for the most hospital days, missed school days, and parental missed work days
- Half of cases have onset before age 10, but can develop at any age
- Gender differences are age related: Males are more commonly affected than females before puberty, but not afterward
- Asthma occurs due to a combination of genetic and environmental factors
  - There is often a personal or family history of asthma or atopic diseases (allergies, hay fever, eczema)
  - Tobacco exposure has been linked to the development of worse and more persistent asthma episodes
- Respiratory syncytial virus (RSV) bronchiolitis may directly cause increased risk of asthma; airway hyperreactivity after RSV infection may persist for months to years

PATIENT PRESENTATION

- Signs and symptoms are due to narrowing of the intrathoracic airways
- Cough
- Polyphonic expiratory wheeze
- Shortness of breath
- Sputum production (mucorrhea)
- Sleep disturbance and nocturnal awakenings
- Exercise limitation
- Expiratory prolongation
- Increased anterior-posterior chest diameter
- Hyperinflation on percussion or X-ray
- Retractions (subcostal) and accessory muscle use
- Tachycardia and tachypnea during episodes

DIFFERENTIAL DX

- If unresponsive to asthma therapy, consider:
  - Airway malacia (AM)
  - GERD
  - Vascular anomalies
  - Lymphadenopathy
  - Tumors
  - Intraluminal masses
  - Foreign body
  - Vocal cord dysfunction
- If frequent/recurrent infections, consider:
  - Cystic fibrosis
  - Immune deficiencies
  - Primary ciliary dyskinesia

DIAGNOSTIC EVALUATION

- History and clinical examination
- Reversible airway obstructions measured by spirometry:
  - Peak expiratory flow <80% predicted
  - FEV_1 or FEV_1/FVC <80% predicted
  - Forced expiratory flow between 25% and 75% of FVC ($FEF_{25-75\%}$) <80% predicted
  - Demonstration of reversible airway dysfunction after bronchodilator therapy
  - 15% increase in FEV1 after β-agonist therapy
  - Bronchoconstriction in response to a methacholine or cold air challenge
- Chest X-ray may reveal hyperinflation, flattened diaphragms, and atelectasis
- Arterial blood gas (ABG) may reveal respiratory alkalosis in mild exacerbations, hypoxemia, and metabolic acidosis in severe disease
- Sputum culture reveals increased eosinophils and possible secondary infection

TREATMENT & MANAGEMENT

Acute Exacerbations
- Inhaled short-acting β-agonists for bronchodilation
- Anticholinergics (eg, ipratropium bromide)
- Oral or IV corticosteroids
- Supplemental oxygen

Prophylaxis
- Oral leukotriene inhibitors
- Inhaled corticosteroids should be used for chronic therapy if the patient is using bronchodilators more than twice weekly
- Long-acting β-agonists in combination with inhaled steroids
- Inhaled mast cell stabilizers (eg, cromolyn, nedocromil)
- Anti-IgE therapy
- Avoid aggravating factors (eg, tobacco exposure, causes of allergic rhinitis, otitis media, sinus infections, GERD)
- Appropriate vaccinations, including yearly influenza vaccine
- Allergy shots are controversial

PROGNOSIS & COMPLICATIONS

- Follows an episodic course with acute exacerbations separated by symptom-free periods
- Severity and response to treatment is followed by measuring pulmonary function
- Prognosis ranges from minimal symptoms to significant morbidity and mortality
- Prognostic factors: Severity of asthma, adherence to therapy, level of control, comorbidities (eg, allergies, sinus disease, recurrent/chronic otitis media, obesity, GERD)
- The likelihood of "growing out of asthma" may depend on genetics, etiology (eg, "RSV-induced" asthma), Severity, compliance, and exposure to triggers
- Status asthmaticus is a prolonged, severe attack that does not respond to initial therapy; it may lead to respiratory failure and death
- Mortality has been increasing, perhaps due to overreliance on bronchodilator drugs

Bronchiolitis

INTRODUCTION

- Inflammation and edema of the airways that may occur with or without bronchoconstriction
- The inflammation and edema of the airways result in wheezing and often crackles
- The most important identifiable cause is respiratory viruses (RSV)
- Typically affects infants

ETIOLOGY, EPIDEMIOLOGY, & RISK FACTORS

- The most important clinical etiology is RSV
  - RSV invades nasopharyngeal epithelial cells and spreads to the lower respiratory tract by cell-to-cell transfer; sloughing of dead bronchial cells and increased mucus production lead to plugging of airways, atelectasis, and hyperinflation
  - Significant association with respiratory failure, resulting in intensive care admission or death
  - May result in bronchial reactivity that can last for years after resolution of the infection
- Other identifiable viral pathogens include parainfluenza virus, influenza virus, adenovirus, and rhinovirus
- Bacterial etiologies include *Chlamydia pneumoniae* and *Mycoplasma pneumoniae*
- Occurs primarily during the winter months
- Peak incidence of hospitalization is in ages 1–4 months
- Infants at increased risk for severe disease include those with congenital heart disease, chronic neonatal lung disease, history of prematurity, and immunodeficiencies

PATIENT PRESENTATION

- Profuse rhinorrhea
- Cough
- Coryza
- Fever
- Tachypnea
- Nasal flaring and retractions
- Hyperinflation on percussion
- Crackles
- Wheezing and prolonged expirations
- Hemoglobin desaturation is common on pulse oximetry
- Severe disease (10–20% of cases) may result in grunting, apnea, cyanosis, and respiratory failure

DIFFERENTIAL DX

- Asthma
- Bacterial or viral pneumonia
- Foreign body
- Cystic fibrosis
- Interstitial pneumonitis

DIAGNOSTIC EVALUATION

- History and physical examination are often diagnostic
- Laboratory testing includes nasopharyngeal swab sample for RSV and other viruses, immunofluorescent antibody testing, ELISA testing, and cultures
- Chest X-ray may reveal patchy hyperinflation, atelectasis, consolidation, and peribronchial cuffing

TREATMENT & MANAGEMENT

- Administer supplemental oxygen to achieve oxygen saturations above 90% to minimize the work of breathing
- Administer intravenous fluids if tachypnea compromises oral feeding
- Nebulized albuterol may achieve bronchodilation; however, it is not effective in all patients and should only be used if a clinical response is observed
- Nebulized racemic epinephrine may decrease airway edema and may be superior to albuterol
- Corticosteroids and nebulized ipratropium have not been shown to be effective
- Patients with severe recurrent apnea or respiratory failure require assisted ventilation
  - Apnea and respiratory failure are much more likely in patients with risk factors (eg, young age, history of prematurity, heart or lung disease)

PROGNOSIS & COMPLICATIONS

- Prognosis is generally excellent, but there is an overall mortality rate of 1–4%
- Apnea tends to resolve within a few days; home monitoring after hospitalization is not needed
- Some studies suggest that up to 75% of infants will experience recurrent cough and wheezing

Cystic Fibrosis

INTRODUCTION

- A genetic disorder of the exocrine glands caused by a defect in the cystic fibrosis transmembrane receptor (CFTR) protein
- This defective protein causes abnormal sodium and chloride ion transport in the exocrine glands, resulting in thickened secretions in the sweat glands, respiratory tract, and pancreas
- May be discovered through routine newborn screening or during evaluation of chronic respiratory infections, malabsorption, or failure to thrive

ETIOLOGY, EPIDEMIOLOGY, & RISK FACTORS

- Thickened secretions in the lungs causes thick, poorly cleared mucus, resulting chronic bacterial colonization, recurrent respiratory infections, and chronic inflammation
- The chronic inflammation impairs lung function and eventually leads to respiratory failure
- Thickened secretions in the pancreas result in retention of pancreatic enzymes, steatorrhea, inflammation, and chronic pancreatitis with an eventual destruction of the pancreas
- A genetic disorder with autosomal recessive transmission
  - More than 1200 mutations exist, each with differing phenotypes
  - The most common mutation (two-thirds of all cases) is the ΔF508 deletion
- Far more common in whites (1 in 3000 individuals) than in blacks (1 in 15,000 individuals) or Asians (1 in 30,000 individuals)
- It is the most common severe recessive genetic disease among whites in the U.S.

PATIENT PRESENTATION

- Pulmonary presentations include chronic cough, wheezing, shortness of breath, hemoptysis, nasal polyps, and recurrent bouts of sinusitis, pneumonia, and pneumothorax
  - Pulmonary exacerbations may result in fever, increased cough and sputum production, weight loss, and diminished pulmonary function
- Gastrointestinal presentations include meconium ileus, malabsorption of fats and proteins, obstruction and/or intussusception, failure to thrive, GERD, and rectal prolapse
- Endocrine and reproductive tract presentations include diabetes mellitus, growth failure and delayed puberty due to malabsorption, obstructive azoospermia, and reduced fertility in women
- Hepatobiliary presentations include cholelithiasis, hepatosplenomegaly, elevations of liver transaminases, and biliary cirrhosis
- Clubbing

DIFFERENTIAL DX

- Asthma
- Ciliary dyskinesia
- Pneumonia
- Immunodeficiency
- Other causes of failure to thrive (eg, congenital heart disease, hyperthyroidism, chronic infection)
- Gastrointestinal disease (eg, chronic diarrhea, food allergy, gastroenteritis, pancreatic insufficiency, liver disease)

DIAGNOSTIC EVALUATION

- History and physical examination are often suggestive of the diagnosis
- Prenatal testing may include chorionic villous sampling at 10 weeks gestation or amniocentesis at 15–18 weeks gestation
- Newborn screening via immunoreactive trypsinogen in a dry blood heel-stick sample is done in some states (there are many false-positives)
- Sweat testing may be diagnostic and can be performed in infants as young as a few days old
- DNA analysis may be useful if the diagnosis is in doubt and for prognostic value
- Supportive evidence may come from sinus films, chest X-ray, pulmonary function testing, and stool analysis
  - Sinus films may reveal pansinusitis
  - Chest X-ray may reveal right upper lobe involvement, atelectasis, hyperinflation, increased AP diameter, bronchial dilatation, cysts, linear shadows ("tram lines"), and infiltrates
  - Pulmonary function testing shows an obstructive pattern (decreased FEV_1, increased lung volumes)
  - Stool analysis reveals increased fecal fat due to fat malabsorption

TREATMENT & MANAGEMENT

- Early aggressive treatment can significantly improve outcomes
- Yearly influenza vaccination in all patients
- Regular mobilization and clearance of secretions via chest physiotherapy, nebulized α-dornase (DNase) and/or bronchodilators, nebulized hypertonic saline, mechanical vibrating vest, positive airway pressure mask, and/or flutter valve
- Intermittent administration of inhaled tobramycin improves lung function and decreases exacerbations in patients colonized with *Pseudomonas*.
- Azithromycin orally three times weekly decreases airway inflammation in patients with *Pseudomonas*
- Prolonged courses of antibiotics (oral or IV), including antipseudomonal therapy, and more intensive airway clearance may be necessary during exacerbations
- Pancreatic enzyme replacement
- Gastric acid suppression (H2-receptor blockers or proton-pump inhibitors)
- Fat-soluble vitamin supplements
- Ursodeoxycholic acid for treatment of biliary disease
- Bilateral lung transplantation is an option for patients with end-stage lung disease

PROGNOSIS & COMPLICATIONS

- Follows a chronic course with acute exacerbations
- Median survival is now approaching 40 years
- Respiratory failure is the leading cause of death
- 2–5% die due to complications of liver disease
- Increased survival in those who receive early, aggressive care at specialized centers
- The most common infectious agents in children are *Staphylococcus aureus*, *Haemophilus influenzae*, and *Pseudomonas aeruginosa*
- An accelerated decline in lung function and poor prognosis are associated with poor physical fitness, poor nutritional status, lack of health insurance, female gender, and respiratory tract colonization or infection with *Pseudomonas* or *Burkholderia cepacia*

Pneumonia

INTRODUCTION

- A lower respiratory tract infection involving the alveolar spaces and airways (bronchopneumonia) that results in inflammation, alveolar exudates, and consolidation
- Presentation, pathogens, and prognosis vary depending on age
- The specific etiology is often not determined

ETIOLOGY, EPIDEMIOLOGY, & RISK FACTORS

- Neonatal pneumonia is often bacterial (eg, group B *Streptococcus, Escherichia coli, Klebsiella, Staphylococcus aureus, Pseudomonas aeruginosa, Haemophilus influenzae, Serratia marcescens*)
- Infant pneumonia may be viral or bacterial (eg, *S. pneumoniae, H. influenzae, Chlamydia*)
- Pneumonia in school-age children and adolescents may be viral or bacterial (eg, *S. pneumoniae, S. aureus, H. influenzae*, group A strep, *Bordetella pertussis, Mycoplasma pneumoniae*)
- Immunocompromised patients are at risk for fungal pneumonia
- Risk factors include narrowed airways, chronic airway inflammation, functional or anatomic abnormalities predisposing to aspiration, immunodeficiency syndromes, sickle cell disease, and airway hardware (eg, tracheostomy, endotracheal tube)
- Pathogens may lead to diagnosis of underlying problems (eg, *Pneumocystis carinii* and AIDS, *P. aeruginosa* and cystic fibrosis)

PATIENT PRESENTATION

- "Typical" pneumonia is characterized by acute or subacute onset of fever, dyspnea, and productive cough
- Signs of respiratory distress (tachypnea, nasal flaring, grunting, retractions, accessory muscle use, dyspnea)
- Cyanosis
- Pleuritic chest pain
- Abdominal pain
- Apnea
- Lethargy and ill appearance
- Auscultation findings include crackles, tachypnea, decreased breath sounds, tubular breath sounds, fremitus, bronchophony, wheezing, and dullness on percussion

DIFFERENTIAL DX

- Upper respiratory infection
- Malignancy
- Foreign body
- Thoracic trauma
- Congenital anomalies (eg, sequestration)
- Asthma
- Bronchitis

DIAGNOSTIC EVALUATION

- History and physical examination
- Pulse oximetry reveals hemoglobin desaturation
- Laboratory testing includes complete blood count with differential, blood cultures (more commonly positive when the pathogen is *S. pneumoniae*), and sputum or tracheal culture and Gram stain
  - Good-quality sputum cultures are difficult to collect in young children
- Chest X-ray findings range from diffuse patchy infiltrates to lobar consolidation
  - May be bilateral or unilateral
  - May occur with pleural effusion or cavitation
  - The initial chest X-ray may not show infiltrates in a dehydrated patient; be sure to repeat the X-ray after IV hydration
- Consider testing for cystic fibrosis or HIV testing in young patients with repeated cases of pneumonia

TREATMENT & MANAGEMENT

- Supportive therapy, including rest and fluids
- Bacterial pneumonia is treated with empiric antibiotics based on age and other host factors; tailor antibiotic therapy to the specific organism once discovered
- Viral pneumonia may be treated with antiviral medications, especially in immunocompromised patients
- Fungal pneumonia is treated with broad-spectrum antifungal medications in high-risk patients (eg, neonates, transplant patients, AIDS patients, or intensive care patients)
- Consider supplemental oxygen, ventilation, and/or cardiovascular support in severely ill patients
- Check local hospital resources for antimicrobial resistance profiles and formulary medications

PROGNOSIS & COMPLICATIONS

- Morbidity and mortality depend on the organism and interaction with host factors
- Prognosis is excellent for uncomplicated community-acquired pneumonia
- In neonates and immunocompromised patients, untreated or incompletely treated pneumonia can be fatal

Chronic Cough

INTRODUCTION

- Chronic cough is defined as a cough lasting more than 3 weeks
- Cough can be stimulated by:
  - Irritant receptors in the larynx that act to prevent or minimize aspiration
  - Irritant receptors in the large airways that respond to irritation (eg, inhalation of dust, smoke, foreign bodies) or respiratory infections
  - Stretch receptors in lung parenchyma that respond to distention of lung
  - Or, cough can be voluntarily initiated, psychogenic, or tic-related
- Chronic cough is one of the most common reasons for pulmonology referrals

ETIOLOGY, EPIDEMIOLOGY, & RISK FACTORS

- Asthma, GERD, and postnasal drip due to allergies are the most common causes
- Other causes include: postviral irritability, chronic exposure to an inhaled irritant (such as tobacco smoke), sinusitis, and other types of postnasal drip
- Less common causes include: tuberculosis, pertussis, congestive heart failure, and cystic fibrosis
- Postnasal drip can be caused by: environmental allergies, acute or chronic sinus infections, foreign body in the nose, deviation of the nasal septum, cold weather or dry air, or pregnancy

PATIENT PRESENTATION

- Productive or nonproductive cough
- Symptoms related to specific causes:
  - Failure to thrive (cystic fibrosis, heart failure, chronic infection)
  - "Allergic shiners," transverse nasal crease, boggy nasal mucosa, postnasal drip (allergies)
  - Nasal polyps, sinus tenderness (cystic fibrosis, sinusitis)
  - Dyspepsia, belching (GERD)
  - Hyperinflation, wheezing (asthma, cystic fibrosis, foreign body)
  - Crackles (suppurative lung disease or infection, aspiration, heart failure)
  - Murmur, gallop (heart failure)
  - Clubbing (suppurative lung disease)

DIFFERENTIAL DX

- Viral upper respiratory infection
- Asthma, exercise-induced asthma
- Environmental allergy
- Aspiration (dysfunctional swallow, foreign body or secondary to GERD)
- Physical or chemical irritation (smoke, dust, volatile chemicals)
- Psychogenic or habit cough ("tic")
- Cystic fibrosis
- Congenital anomalies (tracheoesophageal fistula, vascular ring, tracheomalacia)
- Suppurative lung disease (bronchiectasis, abscess)

DIAGNOSTIC EVALUATION

- History and physical examination
- Laboratory testing includes CBC (reveals lymphocytosis in cases of pertussis)
- PCR or serology for *B. pertussis, Mycoplasma,* or *Chlamydia*
  - Quantitative immunoglobulins $+/-$ IgG subclasses, antibodies to immunizations (immunodeficiency)
- Chest X-ray may reveal infection, cystic fibrosis, vascular ring, or foreign body
- Airway fluoroscopy may reveal tracheomalacia or vascular ring
- Sinus films if suspect sinusitis
- Barium esophagram may be indicated if suspect vascular ring or tracheoesophageal fistula
- Esophageal pH and impedance monitoring to diagnose GERD
- Other studies may include:
  - Swallowing evaluation and/or salivagram (aspiration)
  - Sweat test (cystic fibrosis)
  - Nasal or carinal biopsy for cilia (ciliary dyskinesia)
  - PPD (tuberculosis)
  - Bronchoscopy and bronchoalveolar lavage (tracheobronchomalacia, laryngomalacia, foreign body)
  - Pulmonary function testing (asthma, cystic fibrosis)
  - Allergy skin testing

TREATMENT & MANAGEMENT

- Nonspecific agents (do not take the place of specific therapies) include antitussives, expectorants, mucolytics
- Treat the underlying cause
  - Postnasal drip: Antihistamine (eg, diphenhydramine) and decongestants (eg, pseudoephedrine)
  - Sinusitis: Appropriate antibiotics, decongestants, nasal steroids, and/or surgery for chronic or intractable cases
  - Cough-variant asthma: Remove allergens; use bronchodilators, inhaled steroids, leukotriene antagonists, and mast cell stabilizers as needed
  - GERD: Lifestyle measures, histamine receptor blockers, proton pump inhibitors
  - Postviral: Antihistamine plus decongestant; add β-agonist and inhaled/systemic steroids as needed

PROGNOSIS & COMPLICATIONS

- Most cases (eg, environmental allergies, GERD, asthma) have resolution of symptoms with appropriate workup and treatment
- Asthma, while usually manageable, is the most common chronic disease of childhood and accounts for substantial amount of health care dollars and missed time from work and school
- Pertussis has been an increasing public health concern due to a growing reservoir of teenagers with fading immunity

Whooping Cough (Pertussis)

INTRODUCTION

- A potentially severe lower respiratory infection caused by *Bordetella pertussis*, a Gram-negative bacteria
- Characterized by an acute respiratory illness with paroxysmal cough; paroxysms are followed by a stridorous inspiration, the "whoop"
- Pertussis is a growing public health concern despite efforts to improve vaccination rates in infants and provide booster shots (Tdap) to adolescents

ETIOLOGY, EPIDEMIOLOGY, & RISK FACTORS

- A whooping cough–like syndrome may also be caused by *Bordetella parapertussis*, *Bordetella bronchiseptica*, *Mycoplasma pneumoniae*, *Chlamydia trachomatis*, *Chlamydia pneumoniae*, or adenovirus
- Infants younger than 6 months of age but not old enough to receive the three doses of pertussis vaccine are at the highest risk
- Many adults are unimmunized, and teenagers and young adults may have fading immunity; this reservoir of infection results in greater morbidity among the adult/adolescent population, as well as a greater threat to unimmunized or partially immunized infants
- Infants usually catch the disease from an unimmunized caregiver or a household member with fading immunity
- More than 90% of nonimmune household contacts of affected patients will develop the disease
- Transmission from person to person occurs via respiratory tract secretions
- Communicability may persist for 3 weeks or more after onset of cough

PATIENT PRESENTATION

- Three stages of pertussis infection:
  - Catarrhal stage (1–2 weeks): Mild upper respiratory tract symptoms (low fever, cough, coryza)
  - Paroxysmal stage (2–6 weeks): Severe paroxysms of cough, often with a characteristic inspiratory stridor ("whoop"), and occasionally followed by vomiting
  - Convalescent phase (2–4 weeks): Symptoms gradually lessen; the cough may persist for several months
- In infants younger than 6 months, the "whoop" is often absent; inability to feed, tachypnea, apnea, and cyanosis are common
- Adolescents and adults tend to present with an upper respiratory infection–type syndrome with persistent cough but without a "whoop"
- Post-tussive emesis can occur in any age group

DIFFERENTIAL DX

- Habit cough (cough tic)
- Asthma
- Tracheomalacia
- Bronchomalacia
- Large airway compression
- Bronchitis
- Foreign body aspiration
- Gastroesophageal reflux

DIAGNOSTIC EVALUATION

- The gold standard for diagnosis is culture of *B. pertussis* from nasopharyngeal secretions
- Leukocytosis and lymphocytosis are consistent with pertussis infections
- PCR of nasopharyngeal secretions
- Serologies (antibodies to *B. pertussis*)
  - Confirmation of pertussis infection is most reliably indicated by a 4-fold rise in IgG or IgA or a 4-fold rise or fall in IgM antibodies in paired specimens
  - Immunization induces serologically detectable IgG and IgM, but not IgA
  - IgM titers typically rise after immunization but then rapidly fall; IgM titers do not reliably increase after infection in immunized children
  - IgG titers are long lasting

TREATMENT & MANAGEMENT

- Standard antibiotic for treatment and prophylaxis is erythromycin for 14 days or clarithromycin for 7 days
- Infants less than 6 months of age and other patients with potentially severe disease often require hospitalization for supportive care of apnea, cyanosis, coughing paroxysms, vomiting, and dehydration
- Hospitalized patients should be isolated for 5 days after initiation of antibiotic therapy
- There is no clear benefit of corticosteroids or albuterol
- All household and other close contacts (eg, childcare) should receive prophylaxis with erythromycin
- Close contacts younger than 7 years should receive pertussis immunization according to the recommended schedule

PROGNOSIS & COMPLICATIONS

- Antibiotic treatment limits transmissibility; however, treatment will not shorten the duration of illness if given beyond the catarrhal phase (ie, must be given before "whoop" appears)
- Children may return to daycare 5 days after initiation of antibiotic therapy
- The duration of classic pertussis is 6–10 weeks; however, more than half of primary cases last less than 6 weeks
- Typically, there are no permanent pulmonary sequelae
- Severe complications include pneumonia, seizures, encephalopathy, and death

Foreign Body Aspiration

INTRODUCTION

- Foreign body aspiration is an important cause of illness and death in children, especially under the age of 6
- It is one of the leading causes of accidental death or injury in the home in any age group and the leading cause of unintentional injury and death for children less than 1 year of age
- It should be suspected when a child has acute onset of coughing, choking, gasping, or wheezing; however, it may present more subtly, such as ongoing increased work of breathing or a cough

ETIOLOGY, EPIDEMIOLOGY, & RISK FACTORS

- Peak incidence is between 1 and 3 years of age
- Twice as common in boys as girls
- Most aspirations occur when a child with food or a small toy in his/her mouth is startled, falls, or bumps his/her head
- Older children may place objects into the mouths of younger siblings or give infants inappropriate toys or food
- Neurologically impaired children with dysfunctional swallowing are prone to aspiration
- Obstruction may be partial or complete
- Peanuts and other nuts are most common; also vegetables, hard candy, hot dogs, grapes, metal objects, balloons, plastic objects, and bones
- Dependent lung lobes (commonly the right lower lobe) are most often affected, but location depends on the patient's position when aspiration occurs

PATIENT PRESENTATION

- Abrupt onset of coughing or wheezing in a previously healthy child is the hallmark symptom
  - Unilateral wheezing occurs due to obstruction and inflammation of the affected side
  - Bilateral wheezing may occur due to peanut-induced inflammation following peanut aspiration
- Triad of cough, wheeze, and decreased breath sounds is present in 40% of cases
- Chronic cough may also be a presentation
- Exam findings may include:
  - Mechanical "ball-valve" sound on auscultation
  - Hyperinflation upon percussion of the affected side
  - Decreased aeration of affected side
- Hemoptysis, recurrent or persistent pneumonia, or lung abscess can also occur

DIFFERENTIAL DX

- Asthma
- Bronchiolitis
- Pneumonia
- Croup
- Tracheobronchial tumor
- Endobronchial infection with mycobacteria
- Tracheomalacia or bronchomalacia
- Psychogenic cough

DIAGNOSTIC EVALUATION

- History and physical examination
- Obtain a lateral neck film if laryngeal, tracheal, or esophageal foreign body is suspected
- Chest X-ray may reveal radiopaque objects; however, most aspirated foreign bodies are not radiopaque
- Inspiratory and expiratory chest X-rays will show less emptying in the affected lung lobe(s)
  - Partial obstruction: Infiltrate or hyperinflation beyond the obstruction; may result in ball-valve obstruction, such that the mediastinum and heart shifts *away from* the affected side
  - Total obstruction: Atelectasis occurs beyond the obstruction; the mediastinum shifts *toward* the affected side
- In children younger than 2–3 years of age who cannot exhale on command, right and left lateral decubitus films and fluoroscopy of inspiration and expiration are indicated
- Rigid bronchoscopy may be therapeutic as well as diagnostic if the obstruction can be removed during the procedure

TREATMENT & MANAGEMENT

- Initiate immediate first aid for the choking child who cannot breathe, cough, or talk
  - Age <1 year: Back blows followed by chest thrusts
  - Age >1 year: Abdominal thrust or Heimlich maneuver
  - Blind finger sweep is contraindicated in infants because the foreign body may become more deeply lodged, resulting in complete obstruction
- Attention to airway, breathing, and circulation
- Supplemental oxygen as needed
- Rigid bronchoscopy and removal of foreign body with McGill forceps
- Send specimens that cannot be clearly identified for microbiology (including mycobacteria) and pathology
- Thoracotomy is rarely needed

PROGNOSIS & COMPLICATIONS

- Foreign bodies can be removed by rigid bronchoscopy in more than 95% of cases
- Potential airway complications include acute airway obstruction due to edema, pneumo-mediastinum, pneumothorax, laryngeal edema or laceration, bronchial stenosis, bronchiectasis, and tracheoesophageal fistula

Pneumothorax

INTRODUCTION

- Pneumothorax (PTX) is caused by the introduction of air into the pleural space causing partial or complete lung collapse
- Results in pain, V/Q mismatch, and hypoxemia
- May be caused by trauma, by barotrauma, or may be spontaneous
- A tension pneumothorax (1–3% of cases) may occur as a complication of an existing pneumothorax; it occurs when air enters the pleural space during each breath but the air is unable to be released during expiration; it results in significant increase in intrapleural pressure that impedes venous return to heart, resulting in cardiovascular collapse

ETIOLOGY, EPIDEMIOLOGY, & RISK FACTORS

- Traumatic pneumothorax occurs due to penetrating or nonpenetrating chest trauma, including iatrogenic causes (eg, central line placement, CPR) and barotrauma
- Spontaneous pneumothorax usually occurs at rest
  - First-degree pneumothorax (70% of cases) is due to rupture of apical pleural blebs in patients with no underlying lung disease
  - Second-degree pneumothorax occurs in patients with existing lung disease (especially asthma, cystic fibrosis, infections, tumors), foreign body, congenital lung malformations, and Marfan syndrome
  - Risk factors include a history of smoking, positive family history of spontaneous pneumothorax, and tall, thin body habitus
  - Spontaneous neonatal pneumothoraces occur in 1–2% of newborns

PATIENT PRESENTATION

- Acute onset of focal pleuritic chest pain, which may radiate to the ipsilateral shoulder
- Dry cough
- Dyspnea
- Tachypnea
- Tachycardia
- Decreased or absent breath sounds on the affected side
- Hyperresonance and decreased tactile fremitus
- Tension pneumothorax may present with hypotension, absent breath sounds, distended neck veins, tracheal deviation to opposite side, diaphoresis, cyanosis, or cardiovascular collapse

DIFFERENTIAL DX

- Costochondritis
- Pulmonary embolus/infarction
- Rib fracture
- Pneumonia
- Chest trauma
- Viral pleuritis
- Myocardial ischemia
- Asthma
- Psychogenic pain
- Lobar emphysema
- Aortic dissection

DIAGNOSTIC EVALUATION

- History and clinical examination
  - The diagnosis is suggested by a patient with a predisposing condition or a precipitating event and the associated symptoms
  - Tension pneumothorax is a clinical diagnosis marked by a patient in acute severe respiratory distress with tracheal deviation, decreased or absent breath sounds, hypoxia, and hypotension
- Upright posterior-anterior and lateral chest X-rays will reveal the presence of a thin radiolucent pleural line, absence of vascular lung markings peripheral to the radiolucent line, and tracheal deviation to opposite side of pneumothorax
  - Expiratory or lateral decubitus films usually accentuate pneumothoraces and help detect smaller collections of gas
- Spiral CT scan of the chest may be used in recurrent cases or if chest X-ray is inconclusive
- Arterial blood gas (ABG) reveals hypoxemia due to V/Q mismatch
- EKG may reveal tachycardia, nonspecific ST changes, and T wave inversion

TREATMENT & MANAGEMENT

- Supplemental oxygen at 100%
- For smaller pneumothoraces, supplemental oxygen and observation with follow-up chest X-ray may be sufficient
  - Small-bore catheter aspiration may be necessary
  - Chest tube insertion may be necessary if catheter aspiration fails
- Symptomatic patients with large pneumothorax should be treated with a chest tube attached to an underwater seal device; chest tube suction (-20 cm H_2O) should be maintained until no air exits
  - Do not remove chest tubes for at least 24 hours
- Tension pneumothorax requires *immediate* needle decompression and chest tube; do not wait for radiologic verification
- Consider spiral CT scan once the lung is reexpanded in order to evaluate for apical blebs
- Treat underlying causes and associated conditions (eg, asthma, infection)

PROGNOSIS & COMPLICATIONS

- 100% oxygen increases the rate of air reabsorption; nearly 2% of intrapleural air is normally reabsorbed daily, but supplemental oxygen therapy increases reabsorption 4-fold
- Recurrence rate for spontaneous pneumothorax is 40–50%
- Consider recurrence prevention therapy (pleurodesis, video-assisted thoracic surgery [VATS], or thoracotomy) after the first or second pneumothorax

Gastroenterology

Infantile GERD

INTRODUCTION

- Gastroesophageal reflux is the involuntary passage of gastric contents into the esophagus
- This is a physiologic event occurring in all individuals through the day and is asymptomatic
- Gastroesophageal reflux disease (GERD) occurs when a patient develops symptoms or complications related to the reflux
- The lower esophageal sphincter, the diaphragmatic pinchcock, and the angle of His represent the first line of defense against acid reflux; the second line of defense is esophageal clearance, including gravity and peristalsis; the third line of defense is esophageal mucosal resistance

ETIOLOGY, EPIDEMIOLOGY, & RISK FACTORS

- The majority of cases in infants occur due to increased episodes of transient relaxations of the lower esophageal sphincter
- Other causes include reduced lower esophageal sphincter pressure, large hiatal hernias, protein allergy, and/or delayed gastric emptying
- GERD can begin during the first few weeks of life and peaks at 4–6 months
  - Daily regurgitation is present in 50% of infants less than 3 months, more than 66% at 4 months, and only 5% at 1 year
- In infants with GERD, less than 20% of pH probe-detected reflux events produce emesis
  - Emesis is more common in infants with reflux versus adults due to the short length of the esophagus and its smaller capacity (10 mL) in the newborn
  - 40% of healthy infants regurgitate more than once a day without pathologic sequelae
- Premature infants are more likely to have pathologic GERD versus full-term infants
- Genetics may play a role because two gene loci on chromosomes 9 and 13 have been identified in cases of severe, familial GERD
- Reflux-associated obstructive apnea, although somewhat controversial, is due to a combination of aspiration events or vagally mediated laryngospasm

PATIENT PRESENTATION

- Regurgitation is the classic symptom
- Vomiting
- Excessive crying or irritability, presumably due to esophageal acid exposure and injury
  - May result in difficulty sleeping
- Weight loss or poor weight gain, often secondary to inadequate caloric intake due to behavioral refusal to feed resulting from pain associated with acid reflux during meals
- Recurrent respiratory disease (eg, apnea, cough, stridor, wheezing)
- Bradycardia secondary to obstructive apnea
- Sandifer syndrome: Lateral head tilt and back arching secondary to esophageal irritation
- Hematemesis (very rare among infants)

DIFFERENTIAL DX

- Metabolic disease (eg, amino acidurias, urea cycle defects)
- Structural obstruction (eg, malrotation, pyloric stenosis, duodenal web or stenosis, tracheoesophageal fistula)
- Drugs/toxins (eg, ipecac, acetaminophen overdose)
- Seizures (if apnea is present)
- Increased intracranial pressure (eg, Chiari malformation, hydrocephalus, brain tumor)
- Food antigen allergy
- Viral gastritis
- Colic (when irritable)

DIAGNOSTIC EVALUATION

- History and physical examination are often diagnostic
  - The clinician must separate physiologic reflux from reflux that results in pathologic disease
- Barium radiography (upper GI series) is useful to define the gastrointestinal anatomy; has sensitivity of 30–85%, specificity of 20–80%, positive predictive value of 80% (vs. pH probe)
- Scintigraphy to evaluate for delayed gastric emptying, aspiration, and reflux will detect both acid and nonacid reflux
- pH probe to document esophageal pH over 24 hours is considered the gold standard, but it is not a great test and is not always reproducible
  - Normal values in infants less than 11 months: Average of 73 reflux episodes, 9.7 reflux episodes lasting beyond 5 minutes, 11.7% of time the esophageal pH is less than 4
  - Only 50% of children with an abnormal reflux index will have esophagitis; 95% of infants with esophagitis will have abnormal pH probes
  - Esophageal impedance monitoring can detect acid and nonacid reflux but is still experimental and has limited normal data available
- Endoscopy with esophageal biopsy to assess for esophagitis and allergic (eosinophilic) esophagogastroduodenitis

TREATMENT & MANAGEMENT

- Conservative therapy is often effective
  - Avoid seated and supine positions after feeding (the prone position in the awake child is correlated with reduced amounts of reflux)
  - Thicken feeds with 1 tablespoon of rice cereal per ounce of formula, and use a cross-cut nipple, which will reduce the amount of vomiting (but not the amount of esophageal reflux) but may result in constipation (use oatmeal to reduce constipation) and may be associated with increased choking with feeds
- Consider a 1- to 2-week trial of protein hydrolysate formula if allergy is suspected
- Pharmacotherapy is warranted when conservative therapy has not resolved the symptoms:
  - Histamine-2 (H2) blockers to suppress acid production
  - Proton pump inhibitors are not FDA approved in this age group but have proven effective
  - Prokinetic agents (eg, metoclopramide, erythromycin) to improve motility; however, the risk of side effects may outweigh the potential benefits
  - Erythromycin may be useful (thought to work via stimulation of the motilin receptor)
- Resistant or recurrent episodes require further diagnostic evaluation
- Surgical intervention via Nissen fundoplication may be required
  - Nissen fundoplication may be associated with adverse side effects, including dumping syndrome and gas bloat syndrome

PROGNOSIS & COMPLICATIONS

- Complete resolution of regurgitation is expected in 55% of infants by 10 months, 60–80% by 18 months, and 98% by 24 months
- Excessive acid reflux can cause esophageal ulceration and possible stricture formation
- Barrett's esophagus has not been described in the infant age group
- Studies suggest that infants with GERD may be more likely to become older children and adults with GERD
- Some children develop tachyphylaxis to the effects of H2 blockers and erythromycin
- Side effects of H2 blockers include headache, irritability, and change in bowel habits

Esophageal Atresia

INTRODUCTION

- Esophageal atresia is defined as a congenital anomaly resulting in interrupted continuity of the esophageal lumen
- Type A: Esophageal atresia without fistula (8%)
- Type B: Atresia with fistula between the upper esophagus and trachea (2%)
- Type C: Atresia with fistula between lower esophagus and trachea (85%)
- Type D: Atresia with a fistula between the upper and lower portions of the esophagus and trachea (1%)
- Type E: H-type with an isolated fistula between the esophagus and trachea (4%)
- The disease was universally fatal prior to the advent of surgical repair in 1941

ETIOLOGY, EPIDEMIOLOGY, & RISK FACTORS

- The underlying embryologic defect is thought to be excessive ventral invagination of the ventral pharyngoesophageal fold; developmental disorders of circulation have also been proposed
- Genes of the HOXD group have been linked to these disorders
- Overall incidence is 1 in 3000–4000 live births
- Highest rate occurs among Caucasians
- There is a 0.5–2% risk of recurrence among siblings
- Prolonged maternal use of contraceptive pills and progesterone and estrogen exposure during pregnancy have been implicated as teratogens
- 50–70% of patients have associated gastrointestinal anomalies, including anorectal malformations, duodenal atresia, malrotation, jejunoileal atresia, intestinal duplication, and hiatal hernia
- Various syndromes are associated with esophageal atresia, including CHARGE syndrome (coloboma, heart anomaly, choanal atresia, retardation, and genital and ear anomalies), Fanconi syndrome, McKusick-Kaufman syndrome, trisomy 21, and VACTERL syndrome (vertebral, anorectal, cardiac, tracheoesophageal fistula, and renal and radial limb anomalies)

PATIENT PRESENTATION

- At birth, infants are mucusy and require frequent suctioning
- Fistulas typically open into the trachea at the carina, resulting in respiratory symptoms (eg, cough, cyanosis, increased work of breathing) due to aspiration
- Coughing, vomiting, and/or cyanosis with feeds
- Pneumonitis may develop if the diagnosis is delayed
- Progressive abdominal distention may occur due to a distal fistula to the gastrointestinal tract
- An H-type fistula may result in delayed presentation, coughing and choking with feeds, and recurrent pneumonia

DIFFERENTIAL DX

- Duodenal atresia
- Ileal or jejunal atresia
- Malrotation
- Cardiac anomalies
- Esophageal stenosis
- Esophageal web
- Gastroesophageal reflux
- Protein antigen allergy
- Laryngotracheoesophageal cleft
- Diaphragmatic hernia
- Swallowing disorder

DIAGNOSTIC EVALUATION

- Atresia should be suspected prenatally when there is polyhydramnios and a smaller than usual gastric bubble (positive predictive value of 55%)
  - May also see an anechoic structure in the fetal neck representing the upper pouch
- In types A, B, C, and D, a suction catheter will not pass beyond the upper esophagus
- In type E, a barium swallow study with barium given under pressure or bronchoscopy may identify the fistula; however, the introduction of barium into the proximal pouch is typically not warranted in other types because it may result in aspiration
- In type A, there will be no intestinal air on initial X-rays because the gastrointestinal tract is not in continuity with the environment
- Preoperative bronchoscopy is recommended by some authorities to identify the location of the fistula
- Preoperative echocardiography may be indicated to identify associated cardiac defects, including atrial septal defect (8%), ventricular septal defects (28%), tetralogy of Fallot (13%), and patent ductus arteriosus (13%); echocardiography will also identify the laterality of the aortic arch to aid in the surgical approach (right-sided aortic arch occurs in less than 2% of cases)

TREATMENT & MANAGEMENT

- Surgical repair is the recommended treatment; the surgery includes extrapleural thoracotomy with division of the fistula and end-to-end anastomosis of the patent esophagus
- If possible, avoid endotracheal intubation prior to surgery because it may result in excessive abdominal distention via the fistula and possible perforation
- Long gap atresia (>2.5 cm) may prevent primary re-anastomosis and may require colonic interposition or pulling the stomach proximally into the chest
- In type A atresia, a gastrostomy tube may be placed for feeding until the surgery is completed
- Repair using minimally invasive techniques have been described but are not yet widely available
- Be sure to investigate for and manage associated gastrointestinal and cardiac anomalies

PROGNOSIS & COMPLICATIONS

- Postoperative leaks may occur at the site of anastomosis in up to 20% of cases; they may respond to prolonged parenteral nutrition, ventilatory support, and antibiotics
- Anastomotic strictures may occur after the immediate postoperative period; they may require dilatation or re-anastomosis
- Gastroesophageal reflux is common (occurs in 25–40% of cases clinically, up to 70% of cases by pH probe) secondary to distal esophageal dysmotility and may result in strictures or pneumonia
- Tracheomalacia or other tracheal anomalies occur in 75% of cases
- 97% survival rate in patients without other anomalies or complications

Peptic Ulcer Disease

INTRODUCTION

- In the early 20th century, psychological stress and diet were thought to cause ulcers
- In the 1950s, gastric acid was thought to play a major role
- More recently, we now know that there is a strong association between *Helicobacter pylori* infection and peptic ulcer disease; adult studies suggest that 15–20% of infected individuals will develop an ulcer

ETIOLOGY, EPIDEMIOLOGY, & RISK FACTORS

- Gastritis and peptic ulcer disease may be primary (usually associated with *H. pylori*) or secondary (usually due to NSAIDs, aspirin, systemic disease, burns, or head injury)
  - *H. pylori* is most often acquired before 5 years of age; 60% of affected children have been infected by 10 years of age
  - It is unclear how *H. pylori* causes ulcers, but duodenal gastric metaplasia appears to be essential for ulcerogenesis; *H. pylori* colonizes the metaplastic epithelium, resulting in acute inflammation and ulcer
- The prevalence of peptic ulcers is very low in children younger than 10 years old
- There is no evidence to suggest that any dietary factors contribute
- There appears to be a genetic predisposition attributed to blood group O and HLA type B
- Emotional stress alone is unlikely to cause ulceration
- Cigarette smoking predisposes to ulcer formation and complications, likely secondary to inhibition of prostaglandin synthesis, inhibition of duodenal bicarbonate, and stimulation of gastric acid secretion
- There is little evidence that alcohol causes ulceration

PATIENT PRESENTATION

- *H. pylori* gastritis is usually asymptomatic; occasionally, epigastric pain, vomiting, nausea, anorexia, and iron deficiency anemia have been reported
- Symptoms usually occur only in patients with duodenal ulcer disease
- Dyspepsia
- Epigastric pain
- Vomiting
- Nocturnal awakening
- Pain is associated with meals in 50–75% of cases
- Hematemesis may occur

DIFFERENTIAL DX

- Gastritis (eg, allergic, NSAID-related, uremic gastropathy, chronic varioliform, bile gastropathy, Henoch-Schönlein purpura, corrosive gastropathy, radiation gastropathy)
- Crohn disease
- Pancreatitis
- Cholelithiasis
- Nonulcerative dyspepsia
- Ulcerative esophagitis
- Pill esophagitis
- Allergic esophagitis
- Gastric volvulus
- Chronic granulomatous disease
- Zollinger-Ellison syndrome

DIAGNOSTIC EVALUATION

- Upper GI endoscopy (esophagogastroduodenoscopy) is diagnostic
- Biopsy should be taken during endoscopy for histologic evidence of gastritis
- Urease testing of the antral mucosa is often positive (*H. pylori* produces high levels of urease)
- Upper GI X-rays are only moderately sensitive in detection of ulcers but can be used to exclude anatomic causes of vomiting
- *H. pylori* detection can be accomplished noninvasively via serologies, urea breath testing, or stool ELISA testing; however, testing may prove the existence of infection but not ulcer
  - Serology for IgG antibodies may detect *H. pylori*; however, IgG persists for at least 3 months (longer than 1 year in some cases) following successful antimicrobial therapy, so this is not a good test to monitor response to therapy
  - Urea breath test: The patient swallows radiolabeled urea; infected patients exhale high amounts of radiolabeled carbon dioxide
  - Stool ELISA testing
- Because acid blockade is very effective in treating many forms of dyspepsia, it is often cost effective to give a trial of a proton pump inhibitor prior to invasive procedures
- Ultrasound is useful in ruling out gallbladder disease as a cause of dyspepsia
- Serologic testing of amylase and lipase can rule out pancreatitis

TREATMENT & MANAGEMENT

- The goal of therapy is to hasten ulcer healing, relieve pain, and prevent complications
- Triple-therapy combination (eg, omeprazole-clarithromycin-amoxicillin for 7–14 days) is highly effective
  - There are increasing reports of drug-resistant forms of *H. pylori*
  - The addition of bismuth may improve efficacy
  - Probiotics have been shown to decrease the number of infecting gastric organisms
- Sucralfate may also be effective; it forms a paste at the ulcer surface and helps to protect the mucosa and promote healing
  - In children with renal failure, the aluminum component may not be adequately excreted
- Proton pump inhibitors block parietal cell H^+/K^+ ATPase enzymes and have been shown to be highly effective in reducing acid secretion
  - Administer 30–60 minutes prior to breakfast or dinner
  - H2 antagonists and antacids are not as effective as proton pump inhibitors
- Misoprostol may be used in chronic NSAID users to prevent secondary ulcers
- For secondary ulcers, remove the offending agent
- Diet plays little role in the prevention or treatment of ulcer
- Patients with a bleeding ulcer may benefit from endoscopic hemostasis with ablation of the bleeding vessel by cautery, epinephrine injection, or clipping

PROGNOSIS & COMPLICATIONS

- Complications include bleeding (hematemesis or melena), perforation, or partial gastric outlet obstruction
- Failure of treatment is usually due to poor compliance, inadequate drug delivery, and/or antimicrobial resistance
- Failure to eradicate *H. pylori* results in a high ulcer recurrence rate
- 3 months of proton pump inhibitor will heal 95% of ulcers

Gluten-Sensitive Enteropathy

INTRODUCTION

- Celiac disease, also called gluten-sensitive enteropathy, is a permanent intestinal intolerance to dietary wheat gliadin and related proteins
- The incidence appears highest in regions of the world where wheat represents a substantial part of the diet (eg, England, Ireland, Italy, United States)
- It is a relatively common disease in the United States, affecting 1 in 145 people
- Celiac disease has not been described among the Japanese, who lack the genetic predisposition and environmental exposure to wheat

ETIOLOGY, EPIDEMIOLOGY, & RISK FACTORS

- Celiac disease is a T-cell mediated, chronic inflammatory disorder with an autoimmune component
- The inflammatory reaction occurs in the epithelial layer and the lamina propria and results in small intestinal villous atrophy with mucosal lesions and lymphocytic and plasma cell infiltration
- The adaptive immune response is preceded by altered processing of the gliadin protein by intraluminal enzymes, changes in intestinal permeability, and activation of the innate immune system
- At least 95% of affected individuals are HLA-DQ2 and HLA-DQ8 positive
- Increased incidence in children with IgA deficiency, trisomy 21, insulin-dependent diabetes mellitus, Turner syndrome, and dermatitis herpetiformis
- Prevalence among first-degree relatives of probands is 8%
- 75% of monozygotic twins are concordant with the disease
- Concordance rate among HLA-identical siblings is 30%
- Prevalence is greater in women than in men

PATIENT PRESENTATION

- May be asymptomatic
- Presentation varies in part with age
- Children 2 years or younger may present with diarrhea, anorexia, protuberant abdomen, wasted extremities, failure to thrive, irritability, or vomiting
- Among older individuals, the presentation may include short stature, pubertal delay, microcytic iron deficiency anemia, osteoporosis, ataxia, or infertility
- Constipation and large stools occur in 10% of cases
- Dental enamel hypoplasia

DIFFERENTIAL DX

- Cystic fibrosis
- Milk protein enteropathy
- Giardiasis
- Pancreatic enzyme deficiency
- Immunodeficiency
- Abetalipoproteinemia
- Sucrase-isomaltase deficiency
- Lactose intolerance
- IBS; toddler diarrhea
- Whipple disease
- Bacterial overgrowth
- Eosinophilic gastroenteritis
- Crohn disease
- Intestinal lymphoma
- Neuroblastoma
- Carcinoid syndrome
- Anorexia nervosa
- Gastroesophageal reflux

DIAGNOSTIC EVALUATION

- Diagnosis is suggested by the constellation of diarrhea, failure to thrive, and irritability
- Screening antibody testing for anti-tissue transglutaminase IgA is recommended
  - This test is commercially available and has a sensitivity and specificity up to 95%
  - May get a false-negative result in patients with IgA deficiency
  - If total serum IgA is low, anti-tissue transglutaminase IgG may be a better test
  - Anti-endomysial IgA is equivalent or mildly superior to tissue transglutaminase, but because this is a bioassay, it is expensive and relies on operator interpretation
  - Anti-gliadin and anti-reticulin antibodies have poor sensitivity and specificity
- HLA testing (DQ2, DQ8) is positive in 95% of affected patients and 30% of Americans
- Small intestinal biopsy is diagnostic and is the gold standard for diagnosis
  - Reveals partial villous atrophy with crypt hyperplasia and increased intraepithelial lymphocytes
  - Disease is typically proximal in the duodenum and can be reached endoscopically
  - Multiple biopsies are recommended as the disease may be patchy
- The intestine may appear scalloped; thus, capsule endoscopy may be diagnostic
- Serologic testing for complications of celiac disease (eg, anemia) can be performed
- Some authorities recommend bone density testing because osteoporosis is common
- Repeat biopsies on a gluten-free diet to demonstrate resolution of disease may rarely be indicated to document true disease
- A trial of gluten-free diet without diagnostic biopsy is *not* recommended

TREATMENT & MANAGEMENT

- Once the diagnosis is made by biopsy, the patient should be placed on a lifelong gluten-free diet
  - Foods such as wheat, barley, and rye should be avoided
  - Oats do not contain gluten, although in many countries, they are farmed with wheat, and therefore, many eliminate them from the diet as well due to concerns of contamination
  - A trained dietician should help the patient initiate the diet
- Vitamin and mineral supplementation to replace deficiencies
- Patients in celiac crisis (severe malnutrition) require volume depletion and correction of electrolyte imbalances; steroids may be helpful as well
- Future therapy may include enzyme supplement therapy with bacterial endopeptidases to destroy antigenic epitopes
- Transgenic agriculture is working on producing gluten-free wheat
- Family members should be screened for celiac disease once a proband has been identified
- Some advocate universal screening programs for all infants at 3 years of age

PROGNOSIS & COMPLICATIONS

- Patients generally respond quickly to a change in diet
- Adolescent patients may find it difficult to comply with dietary restrictions
- Failure to avoid gluten may result in growth failure, delayed puberty, small bowel lymphoma, small bowel adenocarcinoma, diabetes, or thyroid disease
- Normalization of serologic testing and histology generally occur by 6 months on a gluten-free diet

Chronic Diarrhea

INTRODUCTION

- Chronic diarrhea is often defined as the passage of 4 or more watery stools per day for a period of 2 weeks or more
- However, this definition may be too rigid; diarrhea can alternatively be defined as:
  - A significant increase in numbers of stools per day above baseline, *or*
  - A significant change in the form of stool to a looser consistency, *or*
  - Passage of greater than 10 cc/kg in stool volume per day
- Often, stratifying patients by age is helpful in making a diagnosis; additionally, separating patients into categories of bloody diarrhea, diarrhea with weight loss or poor weight velocity, and those without blood or weight issues aids in the diagnosis

ETIOLOGY, EPIDEMIOLOGY, & RISK FACTORS

- The mechanisms of diarrhea include secretory, osmotic, and inflammatory processes and motility disturbances
  - Osmotic diarrhea occurs due to malabsorption of a nonabsorbable solute, typically a dietary sugar, such as lactose (congenital lactase deficiency is rare and typically seen only in Finland), fructose (the use of high-fructose corn syrup as a sweetener has dramatically increased the incidence of fructose intolerance), sorbitol (excessive gum chewing with gums containing sorbitol), sucrose, or trehalose (found in mushrooms)
  - Secretory diarrhea occurs due to abnormal secretion of water and electrolytes into the intestinal lumen, even if the patient is not being fed
  - Inflammatory diarrhea (eg, ulcerative colitis, Crohn disease) occurs due to release of various cytokines that "loosen" the tight junctions in the gastrointestinal tract, intestinal protein loss, and a secretory component
  - Motility disorders cause decreased intestinal transit time
- Formula intolerance or allergy is the most common cause of chronic diarrhea in infants
- Toddler's diarrhea (nonspecific diarrhea of infancy) is typically related to excessive ingestion of fructose in juices or limited fat intake to slow intestinal transit
- Chronic infectious diarrhea is the most common cause of prolonged diarrhea in all ages

PATIENT PRESENTATION

- Grossly bloody diarrhea suggests colitis or enteritis and is often associated with crampy abdominal pain, urgency, and frequency
- Diarrhea with weight loss often indicates enteritis and may be associated with malodorous stools and fat malabsorption
  - Affected patients may be edematous due to low serum protein/albumin
- Diarrhea without blood and normal weight
  - Watery stools may be indicative of an osmotic diarrhea, which may be due to a sugar intolerance
  - Pain relieved by defecation and symptoms aggravated by stress are often due to functional disorders, such as irritable bowel
- Presence of ill contacts with a similar diarrhea suggests infection
- The color of stool is not helpful, unless bloody

DIFFERENTIAL DX

- Infants
  - Formula protein allergy
  - Congenital chloridorrhea
  - Glucose-galactose malabsorption
  - Sucrase-isomaltase deficiency
- Toddler
  - Toddler's diarrhea
  - Protracted viral enteritis
  - Giardiasis
  - Celiac disease
  - Cystic fibrosis
  - Constipation with encopresis
  - Bacterial overgrowth
- Children/adolescents
  - Inflammatory bowel disease
  - Celiac disease; IBS
  - Lactose/fructose intolerance

DIAGNOSTIC EVALUATION

- Stool studies
  - *Salmonella*, *Shigella*, and *E. coli* typically do not cause diarrhea for months; parasitic infections and *Clostridium difficile* can be more prolonged
  - Taking three stool samples from separate days will identify only 75% of *Giardia* infections
  - 72-hour stool fat collection is difficult but can identify fat malabsorption when the percentage of excreted fat is calculated using fat intake (normal is 90% absorption or more)
  - Fecal elastase on a single stool sample can identify patients with pancreatic insufficiency
  - Stool for occult blood can identify patients with mucosal injury
  - Testing for α1-antitrypsin will identify patients with protein-losing enteropathy
- Screening for inflammatory bowel disease should be done in those patients with a suggestive family history
  - Testing includes complete blood count, albumin, ESR, and C-reactive protein
  - Testing for anti-*Saccharomyces cervisiae* antibodies (ASCA) and ANCA may be helpful
  - Stool for inflammatory products, such as lactoferrin and calprotectin, may be helpful
- Screen for celiac disease with anti-tissue transglutaminase IgA
- Hydrogen breath test for disaccharidase deficiency and bacterial overgrowth
- Consider testing for hyperthyroidism, if clinically indicated
- Test for neuroendocrine tumors in cases of secretory diarrhea using serum VIP (VIPoma), gastrin (Zollinger-Ellison syndrome), and urine 5-HIAA (carcinoid) levels
- Endoscopy will identify patients with gross or microscopic inflammation

TREATMENT & MANAGEMENT

- Treatment is based on the underlying etiology
- Adequate nutrition and hydration for those patients with dehydration or malnutrition
- Prescribe hypoallergenic formulas for infants with milk-protein allergy
  - 30% of children with cow's milk allergic colitis will be allergic to soy protein
  - 95% of patients will tolerate complete hydrolysate formulas (eg, Alimentum, Nutramigen)
  - Amino acid–based formulas (eg, Neocate, Elecare) are universally effective but expensive
- Lactose-free diet or lactase supplements for patients with lactose intolerance
- Sucraid for patients with sucrase-isomaltase deficiency
- Gluten-free diet for patients with celiac disease
- Pancreatic enzymes for patients with cystic fibrosis or other pancreatic insufficiency
- Limitation of juice intake for those with toddler's diarrhea; increasing dietary pectin or fat has also proven beneficial
- Anti-inflammatory medicines for inflammatory bowel disease
- Low-dose tricyclic antidepressants for patients with irritable bowel syndrome
- Nonabsorbable antibiotics (eg, rifaximin) may be useful in postinfectious disease
- Administer appropriate antibiotics for those with infectious causes
  - Metronidazole is first-line therapy for *C. difficile*
  - Probiotics may help prevent recurrences

PROGNOSIS & COMPLICATIONS

- Variable prognosis, depending on the underlying etiology
- Milk-protein allergy usually resolves by 1–3 years of age
- Celiac disease and lactose intolerance require lifelong dietary restriction
- Patients with cystic fibrosis require lifelong enzyme replacement and nutritional support

Vomiting

INTRODUCTION

- Vomiting is a complex reflex behavior to a variety of stimuli that can result from abnormalities in the gastrointestinal system, urinary tract, central nervous system, or metabolic pathways
- It is thought that the ability to vomit developed as a protective mechanism to rid the body of ingested toxins
- Clinically, vomiting is distinguished from regurgitation because the former does not have prodromal events or retching and the gastric contents are expelled effortlessly

ETIOLOGY, EPIDEMIOLOGY, & RISK FACTORS

- Vomiting occurs after stimulation of either the vomiting center in the medulla or the chemoreceptor trigger zone in the floor of the fourth ventricle
- The emetic reflex has three phases: A prodrome, retching, and vomiting
  - A prodromal period occurs during which a sensation of nausea and signs of autonomic nervous system stimulation are present; there is inhibition of spontaneous contractions and dilation of the proximal stomach, the esophageal skeletal muscle shortens pulling the proximal stomach into the chest cavity, and a large-amplitude contraction from the jejunum propagates to the stomach at 8–10 cm/sec
  - Retching is involuntary, often rhythmic spasms as one attempts to vomit
  - Vomiting or forceful expulsion of stomach contents into the oral cavity is produced by coordinated action of the respiratory, pharyngeal, and abdominal muscles resulting in rhythmic changes in abdominal and thoracic pressures
- Anticipatory vomiting and vomiting due to psychological stress occur via pathways through the cerebral cortex and limbic system to the vomiting center
  - Motion sickness–induced vomiting occurs when the vomiting center is stimulated through the vestibular system from the labyrinth of the inner ear
- Bilious vomiting is caused by obstruction distal to the ligament of Treitz

PATIENT PRESENTATION

- Signs of autonomic nervous system stimulation (eg, cutaneous vasoconstriction, sweating, pupil dilation, increased salivation, tachycardia)
- Note the quality of the vomitus
  - Blood signifies inflammation to the mucosal surface of the GI tract (eg, peptic ulcer disease, erosive esophagitis, variceal bleeding)
  - Bilious vomiting is consistent with a mechanical obstruction of the GI tract
  - Vomiting of undigested, nonacidic food may represent an obstruction of the esophagus (eg, achalasia, stricture, Schatzki ring)
  - Vomiting of mucus or "egg whites" has been described in cases of allergic esophagitis
- The presence of colicky abdominal pain may suggest obstruction of a hollow lumen
- Early morning vomiting upon rising can be seen in patients with increased intracranial pressure

DIFFERENTIAL DX

Nonbilious Vomiting
- Acute gastroenteritis
- Toxins
- Gastroesophageal reflux
- Cholecystitis
- Pancreatitis
- Elevated intracranial pressure
- Cyclic vomiting/migraines
- Obstructive uropathy
- Adrenal insufficiency
- Food sensitivities
- Inborn errors of metabolism
- Labyrinthitis
- Behavioral disorders
- Pyloric stenosis

Bilious Vomiting
- Intestinal atresia, stenosis, malrotation/volvulus, duplication

DIAGNOSTIC EVALUATION

- Detailed history and physical examination
  - Assess the degree of dehydration based on alteration of vital signs (tachycardia, ortho-static hypotension), loss of weight, moisture of mucus membranes, and urine output
  - Note the color of the emesis: Bloody vomiting signifies mucosal inflammation and may require hemodynamic stabilization and subsequent esophagogastroduodenoscopy (EGD) to control bleeding; bilious vomiting requires an initial obstructive series and subsequent contrast studies (upper GI series or CT scan) to define anatomic obstructions
  - A decrease in bowel movements suggests intestinal obstruction; diarrhea suggests an acute infectious etiology
  - Abdominal exam may localize a point of tenderness representing underlying inflammation
  - Bowel sounds may be heard in rushes and tinkles in cases of intestinal obstruction; bowel sounds are absent in cases of intestinal ileus
  - Perform neurologic exam
- Further diagnostic tests (eg, head CT scan or MRI, abdominal ultrasound, contrast studies) may be necessary depending on history and physical exam findings

TREATMENT & MANAGEMENT

- Correct electrolytes and dehydration
- Subsequent treatment is largely based on the suspected etiology
- Medications that act on the chemoreceptor trigger zone may be helpful (eg, phenothiazines, haloperidol); recent evidence suggests these may allow for home treatment of acute gastroenteritis
- Prokinetic agents (eg, metoclopramide, erythromycin) may be used when there is gastric stasis; however, their efficacy is questionable, and tachyphylaxis may occur
  - Erythromycin acts as a prokinetic through stimulation of the motilin receptor
- Antihistamines and anticholinergics may be used for vestibular disturbances and motion sickness
- Emesis due to chemotherapy agents often responds to serotonin antagonists (eg, ondansetron)
- Migraine syndromes/cyclic vomiting may be treated with common analgesics, antidepres-sants, propranolol, cyproheptadine, or sumatriptan
- Intestinal obstruction ultimately requires surgical intervention but may acutely benefit from nasogastric decompression

PROGNOSIS & COMPLICATIONS

- Variable prognosis depending on the etiology
- Major sources of morbidity and mortality are inadequate hydration and hypovolemic shock and inadequate hemostasis due to significant GI blood loss
- Electrolyte disturbances result from varying losses of gastric hydrochloric acid, pancreatic bicarbonate, and sodium chloride
- Preoperative restoration of electrolyte balance reduces perioperative morbidity

Constipation

- Constipation is defined as either less than normal frequency of defecation, excessively hard stool consistency, or difficulty in stooling resulting in painful defecation or bleeding
- Stooling frequency varies widely and changes from infancy to adulthood
- The average number of stools during infancy is 4 per day; at 2 years, it is 2 per day; and during adulthood, it is slightly more than 1 per day (ranging from 3 per day to 3 per week)
- Constipation may be a symptom of a systemic illness but is most commonly an isolated, functional disorder
- Accounts for 25% of referrals to pediatric gastroenterologists and 5% of all visits to pediatric clinics

ETIOLOGY, EPIDEMIOLOGY, & RISK FACTORS

- Functional constipation is defined as a delay or difficulty in defecation present for at least 2 weeks and sufficient to cause significant distress to the patient but without evidence of structural, endocrine, or metabolic disease; the underlying cause is unclear; affected children may have a higher threshold for sensing rectal distension and thus an infrequent urge to defecate
- Functional fecal retention (the withholding of stool by a child to avoid repeating a traumatic stooling experience) is the most common cause of childhood constipation; it may result in loss of rectal muscle tone and may not resolve until complete evacuation of the lower colon is achieved, which allows muscle tone to be restored and continence to be established
- Encopresis (fecal soiling or incontinence) occurs as a result of loose stool leakage or overflow from a rectum that has been distended by retained stool; it typically presents between 3 and 7 years of age
- Obesity may be a risk factor for functional constipation and encopresis

PATIENT PRESENTATION

- Abdominal pain, typically in the lower quadrants or periumbilical
- Hard, pebble-like (scybalous) stools
- Large stools causing toilet blockage
- Encopresis
- Stool-withholding behavior (eg, scissoring legs, squatting, extended legs, standing on tiptoes)
- Mild rectal bleeding secondary to anal fissures
  - Blood is typically bright red and located on the toilet paper, painted across the stool, or dripping into the toilet water
- Anorexia associated with abdominal discomfort or feeding refusal
- Mild abdominal distension
- Delayed first meconium passage (approximately 95% of normal full-term infants pass meconium within 24 hours of life)

DIFFERENTIAL DX

- Functional: Functional fecal retention, constipation-predominant irritable bowel syndrome
- Neurologic: Hirschsprung disease (colonic aganglionosis), spinal cord dysraphism, intestinal neuronal dysplasia, botulism
- Structural: Meconium ileus, anal ring stenosis
- Endocrine/metabolic: Hypothyroidism, hypocalcemia, cystic fibrosis, malnutrition, celiac disease, congenital pseudo-obstruction
- Toxins/drugs: Diuretic use, chronic laxative abuse, iron or lead poisoning, narcotic use

DIAGNOSTIC EVALUATION

- Detailed history and physical examination, including rectal and neurologic exams, are often sufficient for making the diagnosis
- "Red flags" that may indicate organic disease include: Delayed passage of meconium beyond 24–48 hours after birth, feeding refusal, hematochezia, abdominal distension, failure to thrive, bilious vomiting, failure to improve with typical therapy, or associated neurologic deficit
- Laboratory testing may include thyroid function tests, electrolytes, calcium, magnesium, and lead levels
- Abdominal X-rays can demonstrate stool, but it is unclear how reliable they are in defining constipation
  - Significant fecal loading with associated dilated small intestine suggests true fecal impaction
- Consider celiac screening (serum anti-tissue transglutaminase IgA) in any patient with constipation, especially if there is a family history or there is no response to typical therapy
- MRI of lumbosacral spine may be indicated to assess for a tethered cord, especially if there is associated enuresis, and in patients who do not respond to typical therapy
- Anorectal manometry, suction rectal biopsy, and/or barium enema may be indicated if suspect Hirschsprung disease

TREATMENT & MANAGEMENT

- Treat the underlying etiology (eg, thyroid replacement for hypothyroidism, resection of affected bowel for Hirschsprung disease, correction of electrolyte abnormalities)
- Functional constipation requires multiple interventions
  - Parental education and demystification; family support and reassurance
  - Lubricants (eg, mineral oil), stimulants (eg, bisacodyl), and osmotic agents (eg, polyethylene glycol [PEG] 3350, fiber) to aid evacuation
  - Once evacuation has occurred, maintenance of normal bowel habits may be achieved using lubricants, osmotic agents, and dietary and behavioral modification until toilet trained and asymptomatic (on average, at least 6 months to 1 year)
  - Elimination of cow's milk protein for 4 weeks can be tried in children who are unresponsive to standard therapy because many may have milk intolerance
  - Judicious use of enemas, as these may cause further psychological trauma regarding the rectum and stooling
  - Biofeedback to minimize anismus (the incorrect contraction of the external anal sphincter and pelvic floor muscles with attempts to defecate) offers no long-term benefit
  - Prokinetic agents (eg, cisapride) do not seem to add to conventional therapy

PROGNOSIS & COMPLICATIONS

- Several months of treatment are generally required to achieve resolution
- Symptoms may wax and wane over several years; symptoms persist beyond 5 years in 30–40% of patients
- Symptoms tend to recur during times of stress
- 50% recurrence rate within 1 year after discontinuing stool softener therapy
- In severe, chronic cases, some children with functional constipation can develop atonic sections of the colon and may benefit from surgery to remove nonfunctioning portions of the colon
- Placement of a cecostomy tube may rarely be indicated to help with routine, predictable elimination

Hirschsprung Disease

INTRODUCTION

- Hirschsprung disease represents congenital aganglionosis of the colon that occurs secondary to failure of craniocaudal migration of neural crest–derived ganglion cells during fetal development; results in megacolon proximal to the aganglionic segment due to stasis of stool within the normal part of the colon
- Normally, neurocrest cells are in the esophagus by 6 weeks gestation, transverse colon by 8 weeks, and rectum by 12 weeks
- Should be considered as a diagnosis in any newborn who fails to pass meconium within the first 24 hours of life and requires rectal stimulation to pass stool

ETIOLOGY, EPIDEMIOLOGY, & RISK FACTORS

- In the majority of cases, the aganglionic segment involves only the rectosigmoid colon
- 80% of affected individuals have disease limited to the colon distal to the splenic flexure
- 20% have disease that involves colon proximal to the splenic flexure
- In 3–5% of cases, there is total colonic aganglionosis
- Affects approximately 1 in 5000 births
- Males are affected more than females (3:1)
- Positive family history in nearly 10% of cases
- Less than 10% of cases occur in infants born with a birth weight less than 3 kg
- 8–20% are diagnosed after 3 years of age (mean age at diagnosis is 2.6 months)
- Occurs as an isolated trait in 70%; in other cases, may be associated with Down syndrome, Waardenburg syndrome, cartilage-hair hypoplasia, neonatal appendicitis, or multiple endocrine neoplasia type II
- Genetically seen with abnormalities in the RET and endothelium type B receptor pathway

PATIENT PRESENTATION

- Symptoms typically begin during the newborn period
- Failure to pass meconium within the first 24 hours of life
- Bilious vomiting
- Fever and diarrhea, suggesting enterocolitis
- Constipation with infrequent stools
- Failure to thrive
- Abdominal distension
- Palpable stool on abdominal exam but empty rectal vault on rectal exam
- Explosion of stool after withdrawing finger from rectal exam
- Relatively tight anal canal
- Stools are typically not hard and formed
- Overflow encopresis is rare
- Bleeding from anal fissures is rare

DIFFERENTIAL DX

- Neuronal intestinal dysplasia (hyperganglionosis)
- Functional constipation
- Infectious enterocolitis
- Meconium ileus
- Small left colon syndrome
- Malrotation
- Necrotizing enterocolitis
- Anal atresia
- Hypermagnesemia
- Hypokalemia
- Intestinal atresia
- Infantile botulism
- Infantile dyskinesia
- Irritable bowel syndrome
- Normal breastfed pattern of stooling
- Allergic colitis

DIAGNOSTIC EVALUATION

- Perform an unprepped barium enema to define the transition zone between aganglionic bowel and normal colon
  - Diagnostic accuracy in the first month of life varies from 20–95%
  - Avoid doing a rectal exam prior to the study because it may obscure the transition zone
  - The rectum should always be more distensible than the rest of the colon
  - The rectal tube must be placed low in the rectum for the study
- Anorectal manometry will demonstrate a lack of anal sphincter response to balloon inflation in the rectum
  - When the rectal balloon is inflated, there is normally a reflexive relaxation of the internal anal sphincter; this anorectal inhibitory reflex is absent in Hirschsprung disease
  - Sensitivity of 92%, specificity of 96%
  - Positive predictive value of 85%, negative predictive value of 92%
- Suction rectal biopsy showing absence of ganglion cells is diagnostic; it may also demonstrate increased acetylcholinesterase
  - In 10% of cases, a suction biopsy does not provide sufficient submucosa to make the diagnosis; in such cases, a surgical, full-thickness rectal biopsy should provide a diagnostic sample

TREATMENT & MANAGEMENT

- The patient must be stabilized hemodynamically
- Decompress the colon with nasogastric and/or rectal tube, if necessary
- Antibiotics (eg, ampicillin, gentamicin, metronidazole) directed against bowel flora, especially clostridium, in cases of suspected enterocolitis
- Surgical treatment involves resection of the aganglionic segment and reanastomosis of the remaining colon
  - Surgical specimens are sent to the pathologist from the operating room to histologically identify the agangliotic segment from the normal colon
  - Colostomy is then performed proximal to the transition zone with later reanastomosis to the rectum; some surgeons perform a single-stage pull-through without a colostomy in which the innervated bowel is pulled to the level of the rectum
  - An ileal-anal anastomosis is used for variants with entire colonic involvement
- Ultra short–segment disease (aganglionosis of just 2–4 cm of rectum) is treated by myectomy

PROGNOSIS & COMPLICATIONS

- Prognosis has improved over the past century, but the mortality rate is still significant
- With appropriate surgical care, 85% of patients have normal bowel function
- Postsurgical complications include anal stenosis (5–10%), which is treated with dilatations, surgical revision, or intra-anal Botox injections; incontinence (1–3%); rectal prolapse; and enterocolitis (a major cause of morbidity and mortality)
- Constipation occurs in up to 85% of children less than 5 years old after operation but improves with age

Malrotation and Volvulus

INTRODUCTION

- Rotational anomalies occur as a result of an arrest of normal rotation of the embryonic gut
- They can be associated with other gastrointestinal abnormalities, particularly those in which the intestines are located outside the abdominal cavity (eg, gastroschisis)
- Malrotation can present as an acute surgical emergency when it presents with volvulus
- Malrotation may also be asymptomatic and discovered only incidentally without having caused a volvulus

ETIOLOGY, EPIDEMIOLOGY, & RISK FACTORS

- The midgut rotates counterclockwise around the superior mesenteric artery at the 10th week of gestation; the colon then lengthens, and the duodenum and distal midgut fuse to the posterior abdominal wall, anchoring them at the proximal and distal end of the midgut; if rotation is incomplete, malrotation occurs
- Malrotation of the bowel predisposes to volvulus formation
- A complete volvulus for more than 1–2 hours may completely obstruct blood flow to the gut, resulting in necrosis of the involved segment
- 50% of cases present during the first 2 months of life, but in some cases, diagnosis may be delayed even into adulthood
- The exact incidence is unknown because some cases remain asymptomatic throughout life
  - Approximately 1 in 200–500 live births
  - Symptomatic malrotation occurs in 1 in 6000 live births
- 17% of infants with duodenal atresia have associated malrotation
- 33% of children with jejunal atresia have malrotation
- 100% of children with omphalocele, gastroschisis, or diaphragmatic hernia have malrotation

PATIENT PRESENTATION

- May present with signs or symptoms of an acute obstruction (eg, bilious vomiting, abdominal distension, abdominal pain)
- Symptoms may present abruptly in a previously asymptomatic patient
- Others have chronic symptoms of abdominal pain, intermittent vomiting, failure to thrive, constipation, diarrhea with malabsorption, lethargy, and hematochezia
- Mild abdominal distension
- One or two prominent dilated bowel loops may be palpable, resulting in the sensation of fullness on a diffusely tender abdomen
- Signs of peritonitis with or without shock and hypotension may occur in late presenting cases

DIFFERENTIAL DX

Obstructive Causes of Vomiting
- Pyloric stenosis
- Antral web
- Duodenal stenosis
- Incarcerated hernia
- Enteric duplications
- Complicated Meckel diverticulum
- Hirschsprung disease
- Intussusception

Nonobstructive Vomiting
- Gastrointestinal (GERD, allergy, necrotizing enterocolitis)
- Neurologic (hydrocephalus, brain tumor)
- Metabolic (diabetes mellitus, urea cycle disorders)
- Infectious (Norwalk virus)

DIAGNOSTIC EVALUATION

- Prompt diagnosis and treatment is essential; delayed diagnosis places the patient at risk of intestinal vascular compromise, bowel necrosis, perforation, sepsis, and possibly death
- Any child with symptoms suggestive of malrotation should be investigated with flat and upright X-rays
  - Plain film is usually nonspecific and may be normal; typically will reveal a gasless abdomen
  - May show a "double-bubble" sign, characteristic of partial obstruction of the duodenum
  - Bowel loops at the site of the liver suggest malrotation
  - If a complete volvulus has occurred, the film may show dilated loops of bowel, with air-fluid levels proximally and little or no gas distally
- Diagnosis is confirmed by an upper GI series, which is the gold standard
  - Classical findings of malrotation on upper GI series are seen in only 75% of cases
  - In normally rotated bowel, the duodenum crosses from the left to the right of the spine, then back again to the left, and rises to the level of the gastric antrum
  - Duodenal obstruction is seen when a volvulus is present
- Barium enema can be misleading
  - 20% of patients with malrotation have a normally placed cecum in the right lower quadrant
  - Many normal newborns can have a high or poorly fixed cecum
- Ultrasound with Doppler or CT scan may show reversal of the relationship between the superior mesenteric artery and superior mesenteric vein

TREATMENT & MANAGEMENT

- Nasogastric tube placement
- Fluid and electrolyte resuscitation
- IV antibiotics covering the bowel flora (eg, ampicillin, gentamicin, metronidazole)
- Emergency laparotomy and Ladd procedure (mostly open, but some laparoscopic): Bowel is untwisted, the duodenum and upper jejunum are freed of bands, the intestines are positioned to widen the mesentery and prevent future twisting (the colon is placed to the left, and the small bowel is placed on the right), the appendix is generally removed, and nonviable segments are resected
  - In case of frank bowel ischemia, a period of observation may be necessary before closing the abdomen
  - Postoperative adhesions are then helpful in maintaining the widened mesentery and preventing future episodes of volvulus

PROGNOSIS & COMPLICATIONS

- Mortality less than 3%
- Postsurgical complications include:
  - Short gut syndrome if significant amounts of bowel were resected
  - Small bowel obstruction after surgical manipulation of bowel (up to 15% of patients)
  - Risk of volvulus recurrence after Ladd procedure is estimated to be 2–8%

Biliary Atresia

INTRODUCTION

- Biliary atresia is the most common surgically correctable liver disorder in infancy
- It is also the most frequent indication for liver transplantation among infants and children
- Extrahepatic biliary atresia is a medical emergency requiring surgical intervention prior to 8 weeks of life in order to optimize survival and decrease morbidity; it is characterized by the complete obstruction and obliteration of part or all of the extrahepatic biliary tree
- The presence of jaundice lasting beyond 2 weeks of age requires immediate investigation for evidence of conjugated hyperbilirubinemia

ETIOLOGY, EPIDEMIOLOGY, & RISK FACTORS

- The exact etiology remains unknown; biliary atresia may represent a final phenotypic pathway of neonatal liver injury caused by diverse disorders
  - Suspected etiologies include developmental anomalies, vascular and infectious factors, and altered host immune reactivity
  - Research has shown a predominance of type 1 T-helper cells and related upregulation of genes for gamma interferon and osteopontin
  - In some cases, there may be a failure of the intrauterine remodeling process at the hepatic hilum with persistence of fetal ducts poorly supported by mesenchyme
- The classic perinatal form occurs in 65–90% of cases
- 10–20% of affected infants have a fetal form associated with splenic anomalies (asplenia, polysplenia), total or partial situs inversus, mediopositioned liver, intestinal malrotation, or heart defects
- Occurs in 1 in 8000–12,000 live births
- Females are affected more than males (1.2:1)

PATIENT PRESENTATION

- Jaundice beyond 2 weeks of age
- Acholic stools
  - Stools should be examined for yellow or green pigment
- Mild soft hepatomegaly
- Affected infants usually have normal growth and development; 10% have insignificant failure to thrive
- Ascites or signs of chronic liver disease are rare

DIFFERENTIAL DX

- TORCH infections
- α_1-antitrypsin deficiency
- Sepsis
- Cystic fibrosis
- Toxins
- Choledochal cyst
- Cholestasis induced by total parenteral nutrition
- Tyrosinemia
- Alagille syndrome
- Progressive familial intrahepatic cholestasis
- Disorders of bile acid synthesis
- Caroli disease
- Caroli syndrome
- Neonatal hemochromatosis

DIAGNOSTIC EVALUATION

- Tests of liver function are abnormal
  - Elevated conjugated bilirubin (more than 20% of the total bilirubin)
  - Elevated gamma-glutamyl transpeptidase (GGT) and alkaline phosphatase indicating biliary tract involvement
  - Coagulopathy (elevated PT and INR), which is typically responsive to vitamin K administration
- Abdominal ultrasound may reveal complete or partial absence of the gallbladder
  - The triangular cord sign (a triangular or band-like periportal echogenicity cranial to the portal vein) is very sensitive and specific but is operator dependent
- Hepatobiliary scintigraphy will demonstrate lack of bile excretion into the small intestine
  - This study should be done after administration of phenobarbital for several days to increase bile acid excretion
  - Delayed images at 24 hours will demonstrate absence of excretion into gut
- Magnetic resonance cholangiography may be used but is difficult to perform due to small infant size and motion artifact
- ERCP has only limited utility due to technical difficulty in cannulating the biliary tree
- Liver biopsy is diagnostic in 90% of cases
  - The majority of the portal tracts are expanded by edema, and there is bile duct damage and reduplication and increased fibrosis, all of which are diagnostic of large bile duct obstruction
- The gold standard for diagnosis is open laparotomy with intraoperative cholangiography

TREATMENT & MANAGEMENT

- Untreated disease will lead to periportal fibrosis and cirrhosis of the liver
- Kasai portoenterostomy is indicated before 2 months of age: A roux-en-Y loop of jejunum is anastomosed to the hepatic end of transected extravascular portal structures to reestablish bile flow
  - Administer antibiotic prophylaxis for cholangitis after Kasai procedure
  - The use of steroids after Kasai is controversial and not proven
- Liver transplantation may be necessary in cases of progressive hepatic decompensation, refractory growth failure, hepatic synthetic dysfunction, development of coagulopathy, or intractable portal hypertension with recurrent gastrointestinal hemorrhage
- Fat-soluble vitamin supplementation is necessary in cholestatic infants; administer vitamins A, D, E, and K in water-soluble forms
- Ursodeoxycholic acid may help to thin the biliary fluid and promote bile flow

PROGNOSIS & COMPLICATIONS

- Prognosis is significantly poorer when the diagnosis and corrective surgery occur after 2 months of age
- 5-year survival rate for Kasai surgery:
  - If performed before 2 months of age: 70% survival
  - If performed between 71 and 90 days: 34% survival
  - If performed after 90 days: 10% survival
- There is a risk of cholangitis after Kasai procedure, which may lead to further liver injury
- Resolution of jaundice is most significant prognostic factor; there is a 10-year survival of up to 90% if bilirubin returns to normal
- 85% 2-year survival after liver transplantation

Gastroenteritis

INTRODUCTION

- Gastroenteritis is a general term used to refer to any inflammation of the gastrointestinal tract, although usually it relates to an infectious cause
- Viral gastroenteritis is far more common than bacterial disease; indeed, viral gastroenteritis is the second most common illness in the United States after the common cold
- Rotavirus is one of the most common viral causes
- Winter vomiting disease (Norwalk virus) was identified after an outbreak in Norwalk, OH
- *Campylobacter* is the most common bacterial cause in the United States
- Infections must overcome gastrointestinal tract defenses, including gastric acidity, intestinal motility, intestinal mucus, intestinal flora, and the mucosal immune system

ETIOLOGY, EPIDEMIOLOGY, & RISK FACTORS

- Viral etiologies include rotavirus, enteric adenovirus, enteroviruses, astrovirus, calicivirus, and Norwalk virus
- Bacterial etiologies include *Escherichia coli, Campylobacter jejuni, Aeromonas* species, *Shigella, Salmonella, Staphylococcus aureus, Vibrio* species, *Yersinia* species, *Clostridium* species, *Bacillus cereus*, and *Listeria monocytogenes*
  - Bacterial etiologies that may result in grossly bloody diarrhea include *Yersinia, Campylobacter, Shigella, Salmonella, E. coli* O157, and *Clostridium* species, including *C. difficile*
- Parasitic etiologies include *Giardia lamblia, Cryptosporidium*, and *Entamoeba histolytica*
- Gastroenteritis is the second most common cause of unscheduled visits to the pediatrician
- Incidence of 1–2.5 episodes per child per year in the U.S.
- Diarrhea is a major cause of death worldwide, attributed with at least 4 million deaths per year
- Transmission via fecal-oral route, foodborne, or by respiratory droplets
- Bacteria can cause diarrheal disease by invasion, production of cytotoxins that disrupt intestinal cell function, production of enterotoxins that alter cellular salt and water balance, or adherence to the mucosal surface

PATIENT PRESENTATION

- Dehydration, which may present as dry mucus membranes, tachycardia, prolonged capillary refill time, weight loss, or orthostatic hypotension
- Nausea and vomiting
- Diarrhea, which may be watery, mucoid, or bloody
- Constipation may occur in early stages
- Abdominal cramps and tenderness (colonic inflammation typically causes lower quadrant pain)
- Tenesmus
- Fever may or may not be present
- Prostration, malaise, anorexia, and lethargy
- Headache
- Ill contacts can often be identified

DIFFERENTIAL DX

- Inflammatory bowel disease
- Allergic gastroenteropathy
- Intoxication
- Cystic fibrosis
- Intussusception
- Hemolytic-uremic syndrome
- Pyloric stenosis
- Lactose intolerance
- Sucrase-isomaltase deficiency
- Fructose intolerance
- Bacterial overgrowth
- Hirschsprung disease
- Celiac disease
- Toddler's diarrhea
- Antibiotic-associated diarrhea
- Irritable bowel syndrome
- Constipation with overflow encopresis

DIAGNOSTIC EVALUATION

- History and physical examination usually reveal the clinical diagnosis
- Check electrolytes for dehydration and imbalances
- Urine specific gravity may reveal the degree of dehydration
- Fecal leukocytes may be present in invasive bacterial infections (eg, *E. coli*, *Shigella*, *Campylobacter*) but are neither sensitive nor specific for bacterial etiologies
- Stool occult blood is neither sensitive nor specific for bacterial etiologies
- Stool studies (especially if bloody stools or very ill) should be collected with 3 specimens to increase the sensitivity of testing for ova, parasites, and *C. difficile*
  - *C. difficile* testing is based on detection of the bacterial toxins (A or B), not culture; prior antibiotic use within the last 2 months should increase suspicion for *C. difficile*
  - Ova and parasite testing depends on visualization of the organism by microscope
  - Rotavirus is detected via an immunoassay against the group A rotavirus antigen
  - Exposure to reptiles, raw eggs, or chicken should raise suspicion for *Salmonella*
  - Exposure to raw or undercooked ground beef suggests *E. coli* O157:H7
- Imaging studies should be done if there is vomiting without diarrhea; they may reveal obstruction, volvulus, or possibly increased intracranial pressure

TREATMENT & MANAGEMENT

- Initiate contact precautions in hospitalized patients
- Slow, small-volume rehydration is the treatment of choice; IV rehydration is indicated in hemodynamically unstable patients or in settings where observed oral rehydration is not possible (eg, a busy hospital emergency room)
- Avoid overly rapid hydration, which may result in cerebral edema
- Avoid opiates, anticholinergics, or absorbents in children
- Antiemetics or antimotility agents are not generally recommended but may play a role in avoiding hospitalization by allowing for oral rehydration
- Begin appropriate antibiotics in all cases of bacteremia
- Antibiotics are also warranted in cases of *Shigella* infection; salmonellosis in very young, immunocompromised, or systemically ill children (otherwise, antibiotics prolong the carrier state in *Salmonella* infections); and symptomatic *C. difficile* infection (treat with oral metronidazole)
  - *Yersinia* and *E. coli* typically do not require antibiotic treatment
- For infants, continue breastfeeding or full-strength formula
- Consider a lactose-free diet for children with more prolonged symptoms
- Probiotics have been shown to shorten the duration of illness in cases of viral disease

PROGNOSIS & COMPLICATIONS

- Usually a self-limited disease
- If hydration is maintained, spontaneous recovery is the norm
- Dehydration in younger children leads to increased morbidity and mortality
- May result in seizures (especially with *Shigella* and hemorrhagic *E. coli*), hyponatremia, hypernatremia, colonic perforation, or toxic encephalopathy
- Local spread may result in vulvovaginitis or urinary tract infections
- Remote spread may result in bacteremia, endocarditis, arteritis, osteomyelitis, arthritis, meningitis, pneumonia, hepatitis, soft tissue infection, peritonitis, or immune-mediated disease (eg, erythema nodosum, hemolytic anemia, glomerulonephritis)

Appendicitis

INTRODUCTION

- Appendicitis is the most common cause of acute abdomen in children and adolescents
- It is a common and urgent surgical emergency with protean manifestations, generous overlap with other clinical syndromes, and significant morbidity if the diagnosis is delayed
- There is no single sign, symptom, or test that accurately confirms the diagnosis in all cases
- The development of the appendix begins during the eighth week of gestation
- The position of the appendix within the abdomen is variable
- Leonardo da Vinci was the first to describe and illustrate the appendix in 1492
- Claudius Amyand performed the first appendectomy in 1735
- The etiology of appendicitis was first outlined by Wangensteen and Dennis in 1939

ETIOLOGY, EPIDEMIOLOGY, & RISK FACTORS

- Appendicitis is initiated by obstruction of the appendiceal lumen, which inhibits the normal flow of mucosal secretions and leads to increased intraluminal pressure, comprised venous drainage, and ischemic breakdown of the mucosa; subsequently, luminal bacteria proliferate and invade the appendiceal wall
- Obstruction is most often caused by a fecalith; other causes include a swollen lymphoid follicle, pinworm, or carcinoid tumor
- Histologically, there are serosal exudates, and the mucosa is hyperemic and ulcerated
- Increased neutrophils form crypt abscesses
- Submucosal and muscularis inflammation can result in perforation
- Generally occurs during the ages of 5–30
- Incidence of 4 in 1000 in children younger than 16

PATIENT PRESENTATION

- Periumbilical pain migrating to the right lower quadrant (McBurney point)
  - McBurney point is two-thirds of the distance along a line from the umbilicus to the anterior superior iliac spine
- Diffuse tenderness and guarding
- Nausea and vomiting
- Fever (low-grade prior to perforation)
- Anorexia
- Diarrhea in 10% of cases
- Decreased bowel sounds
- Pain with walking
- Tenderness on rectal exam
- **Rovsing sign**: Pain in the right lower quadrant upon palpation of the left lower quadrant
- **Obturator sign**: Pain w/internal rotation of hip
- **Psoas sign**: Pain in the right lower quadrant brought on by extension of the right hip

DIFFERENTIAL DX

- Intestinal obstruction
- Intussusception
- *Yersinia* enterocolitis
- Inflammatory bowel disease
- Mesenteric adenitis
- Pyelonephritis
- Lower lobe pneumonia
- Cholecystitis
- Salpingitis
- Ectopic pregnancy
- Ovarian cyst or torsion
- Constipation
- Pancreatitis
- Henoch-Schönlein purpura
- Renal stone
- Iliopsoas abscess
- Meckel diverticulitis
- Omental torsion

DIAGNOSTIC EVALUATION

- Characteristic history and physical examination
  - The physical examination may be less impressive if the patient is examined during the window of time between appendix perforation and peritoneal dissemination of the infection
- Complete blood count reveals mild to moderate leukocytosis with left shift (20% of patients have a normal WBC count)
- Abdominal CT scan using IV and either oral or rectal contrast is usually diagnostic
  - Sensitivity of 90–100%, specificity of 91–99%
  - Positive predictive value of 92–98%, negative predictive value of 95–100%
  - Can see thickened appendix and periappendiceal inflammation
  - Can also see free air in cases of perforation
  - Can identify other causes of pain mimicking that of acute appendicitis
- Abdominal X-ray may show a fecalith and/or acute scoliosis (due to psoas muscle spasm)
- Ultrasound may show a thickened, noncompressible appendix or abscess
  - The benefit of ultrasound is that it avoids ionizing radiation and can be done at the bedside
  - However, it is highly operator dependent and has lower sensitivity (79–97%) and specificity (80–94%) compared with CT scan
- Sterile pyuria occurs due to genitourinary irritation from the inflamed appendix
- Misdiagnosis occurs in at least 10% of cases

TREATMENT & MANAGEMENT

- Hospital admission and observation is indicated for patients with a suggestive history and laboratory tests, even if the physical examination is not consistent
- Pain control is important; the use of narcotics for pain control has *not* been shown to "mask" the physical findings of acute appendicitis
- Administer triple-antibiotic therapy (ampicillin, gentamicin, and clindamycin) prior to appendectomy for patients with subacute or smoldering appendicitis
- For patients with acute appendicitis, hydration, correction of electrolyte abnormalities, and immediate appendectomy (open or laparoscopic) are indicated
- Patients with a perforated appendicitis with abscess may be treated with IV antibiotics and percutaneous drainage prior to appendectomy
  - If clinically stable, may treat with prolonged antibiotics for 4–6 weeks before appendectomy

PROGNOSIS & COMPLICATIONS

- Prognosis depends on whether appendicitis is uncomplicated or ruptured, or whether complex abscess is present
- Excellent prognosis with prompt diagnosis and treatment of nonperforated appendicitis
- Prognosis is guarded for patients with widespread secondary peritonitis
- Septic shock may be a complication of appendicitis if the diagnosis and treatment is delayed
- 25–30% of cases are perforated
- Wound infection (pain, erythema, fluctuance, and wound drainage) occurs in 3% of uncomplicated appendicitis and 6–8% of perforated appendicitis
- Intra-abdominal abscess forms in up to 20% of perforated appendicitis

Pancreatitis

INTRODUCTION

- Acute pancreatitis is defined as an acute inflammatory process of the pancreas with variable involvement of other regional tissues or remote organ systems
- Pancreatitis presents with severe abdominal pain, vomiting, and symptoms suggestive of obstruction or ileus
- The clinical course can vary considerably from a mild, self-limited, uncomplicated attack to a severe, complicated course that may be fatal
- The true incidence and prevalence in children are not known; we do know that it is not as common in children as in adults

ETIOLOGY, EPIDEMIOLOGY, & RISK FACTORS

- Occurs due to damage to the pancreatic acinar cells by premature activation of cellular digestive enzymes:
  - Trypsinogen is converted to trypsin in amounts surpassing innate protective mechanisms
  - Trypsin in turn activates proenzymes (eg, trypsinogen) and inactive precursors of elastase, carboxypeptidase, and phospholipase A2
  - Intracellular activation of enzymes induces a cellular injury response
  - Substances released from the cells attracts neutrophils, form free radicals, and activate complement and platelets; additional cytokines are also released, including tumor necrosis factor, interleukin-1, nitric oxide and platelet activating factor
- Etiologies include infections (bacteria, viruses, and parasites); abdominal trauma; postsurgical, anatomic, or mechanical defects (eg, pancreatic divisum, choledochal cyst, gallstones); metabolic defects (eg, cystic fibrosis, hypertriglyceridemia); hereditary pancreatitis (eg, trypsinogen gene mutation, SPINK gene mutation); drug related; toxin related (eg, Trinidad scorpion bite); systemic disease (eg, sepsis, collagen vascular disease)
- Idiopathic in up to 25% of cases

PATIENT PRESENTATION

- Abdominal pain, typically located in the epigastric or left upper quadrant regions
  - Pain may radiate to the back
  - Worsens during the initial 24–48 hours
  - Worsens with eating
- Nausea, vomiting
- Anorexia
- Emesis may be bilious
- Low-grade fever
- Decreased or absent bowel sounds
- Grey-Turner sign: Blue discoloration of the flanks
- Cullen sign: Blue discoloration around the umbilicus
- May have mild scleral icterus
- Increased work of breathing or decreased breath sounds on the lower left lobe may occur due to pleural effusion

DIFFERENTIAL DX

- Gastroenteritis
- Appendicitis
- Pyelonephritis
- Ureteropelvic junction obstruction
- Food poisoning
- Diabetic ketoacidosis
- Cholecystitis
- Gastric volvulus
- Intussusception
- Peptic ulcer disease
- Ulcerative esophagitis
- Diaphragmatic hernia

DIAGNOSTIC EVALUATION

- History and physical examination, including careful medication history
- Pancreatic enzymes are often the first tests ordered
  - Amylase levels usually increase within 2–12 hours and peak at 12–72 hours
  - Lipase levels increase 4–8 hours after symptoms, peak at 24 hours, and decrease over 8–14 days
  - Degree of pancreatic enzyme elevation does not correlate with the severity of pancreatitis
- Other laboratory studies include complete blood count (anemia is seen in cases of hemorrhagic pancreatitis), chemistries (evaluate for disease-related electrolyte imbalances and hypercalcemia), triglycerides (hypertriglyceridemia can cause pancreatitis), and liver function tests (to identify biliary causes of disease)
- Abdominal ultrasound to assess for gallstones or dilated biliary ducts
- Magnetic resonance cholangiopancreatography (MRCP) can identify stones and ductal anomalies
- Cystic fibrosis genotype analysis in patients at risk
- Genotyping for hereditary pancreatitis
- Antinuclear antibody (ANA) and IgG4 levels for autoimmune pancreatitis
- Abdominal CT scan to assess for evidence of necrotizing pancreatitis
- Endoscopic retrograde cholangiopancreatography (ERCP) can remove stones and sample biliary fluid for microlithiasis

TREATMENT & MANAGEMENT

- IV rehydration and aggressive fluid and electrolyte management
- Pain relief is paramount; theoretically, meperidine is used because it causes the least increase in enterobiliary pressure (morphine may cause spasm of the sphincter of Oddi, thereby aggravating pancreatitis)
- Nasogastric tube decompression is indicated when there is an associated ileus with persistent vomiting
- Parenteral nutrition may be necessary for pancreatic rest
  - The use of intravenous intralipids does not exacerbate the disease
- Studies suggest that enteral feeding, particularly beyond the ligament of Treitz, is well tolerated and may result in faster resolution of disease
- Antibiotics are rarely required except for associated cholecystitis or infectious processes
- Monitor patients closely for hypoglycemia and hypocalcemia
- Indications for surgery in acute pancreatitis are controversial; consider surgery in patients with infected pancreatic necrosis or traumatic ductal rupture
- Antisecretory agents (eg, octreotide) have not shown a major clinical effect

PROGNOSIS & COMPLICATIONS

- Most cases resolve after 5–7 days
- Mortality is often associated with a severe multisystemic disorder
- 80–100% mortality in cases of hemorrhagic pancreatitis
- Pseudocyst formation may occur; suspect pseudocyst formation when an acute episode fails to resolve, a palpable mass develops, or pancreatitis recurs after initial improvement
  - Most cases resolve without any intervention, especially if less than 4 cm
  - In cases that progress over 4–6 weeks, drain via surgery, CT or ultrasound guidance, or endoscopically (into the stomach)
- Septic shock and multiorgan system failure may occur in severe cases

Intussusception

INTRODUCTION

- Intussusception is the invagination of a proximal segment of bowel into a more distal segment; it is a gastrointestinal emergency
  - The advancing tube of proximal intestine is the intussusceptum
  - The distal recipient intestine is referred to as the intussuscipiens
- Failure to make a timely diagnosis may result in vascular compromise to intestinal tissue, bowel necrosis, sepsis, and possibly death
- Intussusception is the most common abdominal emergency in infancy and the most common cause of intestinal obstruction between 3 months and 6 years of age

ETIOLOGY, EPIDEMIOLOGY, & RISK FACTORS

- As the associated mesentery gets dragged into the telescoped bowel, edema and congestion develop, which may lead to vascular compromise and currant jelly stools
- The cause of most intussusceptions is unknown
- In 10% of cases, there is a pathologic lead point (eg, Meckel diverticulum, lymph tissue, polyp, duplication cyst, ectopic pancreatic or gastric tissue, suture line, foreign body) that is dragged via peristalsis into distal bowel
  - Lead points are found in less than 4% of infants less than 2 years of age
  - In children older than 2, lead points are found in approximately 33% of cases
- Peak incidence occurs at 5–8 months of age; 60% of affected children are younger than 1 year
- Males are affected much more commonly than females
- More common during gastroenteritis season
- May be preceded by a viral infection (which may lead to lymph tissue as a lead point)
- 80% of cases in infants involve invagination of the terminal ileum into the right colon
- Associated with Henoch-Schönlein purpura, cystic fibrosis, and celiac disease

PATIENT PRESENTATION

- The typical patient is a previously healthy infant with sudden onset of severe, intermittent, colicky abdominal pain in 15- to 20-minute interval bouts
- Associated with pallor, straining, inconsolable crying, and drawing up of legs
- Patient may look comfortable between episodes
- Clear or bilious emesis occurs in most cases
- Initially normal stools, followed by red, bloody, mucous stools (currant jelly)
  - Currant jelly stools are a late sign of intussusception
- Distended abdomen with a tender sausage-shaped abdominal mass in the right upper quadrant during a paroxysm (55–65%)
- Right lower quadrant may feel empty to palpation (Dance sign)
- May present with lethargy
- Not all patients have all signs

DIFFERENTIAL DX

- Infectious diarrhea
- Henoch-Schönlein purpura
- Complicated Meckel diverticulum
- Volvulus
- Incarcerated hernia
- Ureteropelvic junction obstruction
- Renal stones
- Appendicitis
- Crohn disease
- Mesenteric adenitis
- Colic
- Gastroesophageal reflux
- Celiac disease
- Ectopic pregnancy
- Pelvic inflammatory disease

DIAGNOSTIC EVALUATION

- Early diagnosis is crucial to avoid necrosis of the bowel leading to perforation, peritonitis, and death
- Abdominal X-rays (erect and recumbent) may reveal an intestinal obstruction pattern, an empty sigmoid or rectum, soft tissue density surrounded by a crescent of gas in the area of intussusception (25–60%), or free air due to perforation
- Ultrasound shows a target-like lesion with one ring of intestine visualized within the other
  - Positive and negative predictive value can approach 100% but are operator dependent
  - Doppler ultrasound can predict the presence of irreversible ischemia
- Pneumatic enema has replaced barium enema for diagnosis and therapy
  - Shows a filling defect or cupping in the area where the contrast cannot be advanced
  - The classic finding on barium enema is the "coil spring" appearance as contrast is trapped in the folds of the bowel
- Diagnosis can also be made by abdominal CT scan

TREATMENT & MANAGEMENT

- Initial management: No oral intake, initiate nasogastric decompression, administer IV fluids to correct dehydration, and consult a surgical team
- Initial laboratory testing includes complete blood count, BUN, creatinine, and electrolytes
- Pneumatic or hydrostatic reduction with normal saline solution under fluoroscopic or ultrasound control has 80–90% success rate
  - Perforation rate is 1–2%
  - Such reduction can only be performed in ileocolic intussusceptions but are ineffective for small bowel lesions
  - Contraindications for conservative reduction are bowel perforation, peritonitis, and hypovolemic shock
  - Success rate is reduced if symptoms have been present longer than 48 hours
- In case of failure, a repeat attempt may be performed or laparotomy may be attempted
- If there is a known pathologic lead point, surgical reduction of the intussusception and removal of the pathologic process are warranted

PROGNOSIS & COMPLICATIONS

- Postreduction fever is often noted
- Intermittent nasogastric suction should be maintained until bowel function is normal and bowel movements have returned
- Feedings should be advanced as tolerated
- Postoperative complications include fever, prolonged ileus, wound infection, intra-abdominal abscess, or small bowel obstruction
- Most patients may be discharged within 24–36 hours
- 5–10% recurrence rate during the initial 24 hours
- If abdominal pain recurs, diagnostic studies should be repeated
- Occasionally, intussusception may recur even months or years later

Crohn Disease

INTRODUCTION

- Crohn disease is a chronic inflammatory disorder that may involve any portion of the gastrointestinal tract, from the mouth to the anus
- First described as "regional ileitis" in 1932 by Dr. Burrill Crohn
- Incidence has risen dramatically during the past 50 years in both developed and developing countries; this may be related to less exposure to enteric pathogens that promote normal development of the mucosal immune system (the "hygiene hypothesis")
- Most pediatric cases occur in midadolescence (peak age, 14–15 years)
- Crohn disease and ulcerative colitis comprise the two major forms of inflammatory bowel disease (IBD)

ETIOLOGY, EPIDEMIOLOGY, & RISK FACTORS

- Ileum and colon involvement is most common (50%), followed by small bowel alone (30%); isolated colonic disease occurs in only 10–20% of cases
- The exact etiology is unknown; the disorder is associated with a complex interplay of genetic predisposition and environmental factors, including commensal bacterial flora; infectious agents have been proposed, but specific organisms have yet to be determined
- Incidence of 3–4 cases per 100,000 individuals
- Whites are affected more often than nonwhites; northern geographic areas are affected more than southern; urban children are affected more than rural; Jewish ethnicities are affected more than non-Jewish
- The greatest risk factor is having an affected first-degree relative, which may increase risk by 30–100 times
- Susceptible genetic loci are being discovered, including NOD-2/Card15 (IBD1 locus on chromosome 16)
- Increased risk may be related to having a prior appendectomy, older maternal age during pregnancy for females, and possibly maternal smoking
- Higher risk is seen with Turner syndrome, Hermansky-Pudlak syndrome, and glycogen storage disease Ib

PATIENT PRESENTATION

- The average time from onset of symptoms to diagnosis is about 1 year
- Abdominal pain (75%)
- Diarrhea with or without blood (65%)
- Nausea and vomiting (25%)
- Growth failure/short stature (25%)
- Weight loss/poor weight gain (65%)
- Fever
- Perirectal fissures, fistulae, and abscesses (25%)
- Delayed puberty
- Lethargy (in part due to anemia)
- Intestinal obstruction
- Extraintestinal manifestations (25%), including oral aphthous ulcers, arthralgias or arthritis of the large joints, erythema nodosum, pyoderma gangrenosum, uveitis, episcleritis or iritis

DIFFERENTIAL DX

- Ulcerative colitis
- Indeterminate colitis
- Infections (eg, *Salmonella, Shigella, E. coli, Yersinia, Campylobacter, C. difficile,* tuberculous enteritis, amebiasis, cytomegalovirus colitis)
- Allergy (eosinophilic gastroenteritis)
- Neoplasm (eg, lymphoma)
- Anorexia nervosa
- Irritable bowel syndrome
- Henoch-Schönlein purpura
- Typhlitis

DIAGNOSTIC EVALUATION

- Serologic testing may reveal iron deficiency anemia (70%); thrombocytosis (60%), often with normal total leukocyte count; hypoalbuminemia (60%); elevated erythrocyte sedimentation rate (80%) and/or C-reactive protein; or anti-*Saccharomyces* antibodies (50–60%), pANCA (15%), or anti-OmpC (38%)
- Stool guaiac testing
- Upper gastrointestinal X-ray series with small bowel follow-through may show classic cobblestoning and thumbprinting, strictures, and fistulas
- Colonoscopy shows patchy inflammation, ulceration, and areas of stricture
- Visualization of the small bowel via esophagogastroduodenoscopy or capsule endoscopy can reveal patchy inflammation, aphthous ulceration, or strictures
- Biopsy of affected mucosa is diagnostic; the presence of aphthous ulcers, transmural inflammation, granulomas, or architectural distortion suggests a chronic process

TREATMENT & MANAGEMENT

- Treatment should focus on medical interventions and nutritional support
- Medical treatments are numerous:
  - Aminosalicylates (eg, mesalamine) are best used in mild-moderate disease
  - Antibiotics (eg, metronidazole, ciprofloxacin, rifaximin) have limited data for usefulness but are anecdotally helpful in patients with colic and perianal disease
  - Corticosteroids (eg, prednisone, budesonide) are excellent for induction of remission but not effective in maintenance of remission
  - Immunomodulators (eg, 6-mercaptopurine, azathioprine, methotrexate) are used for maintenance of remission in moderate to severe disease
  - Biologics, such as anti-TNF antibodies (eg, infliximab, adalimumab) are excellent for induction and maintenance of remission as well as mucosal healing
- Nutrition with elemental or polymeric formulas; an elemental diet is as effective in inducing remission in small bowel disease as steroids
- Psychological support for children with chronic disease
- Surgery is *not* curative because disease tends to recur at surgical sites; indications for surgical interventions include: Localized area of disease that cannot be medically treated, bowel perforation, persistent stricture, abscess, fistula, or recurrent, intractable bleeding

PROGNOSIS & COMPLICATIONS

- 99% of patients will have at least one relapse after diagnosis
- 10–20% of patients may experience prolonged remission after the first presentation
- Patients with ileocolitis have a poorer response to medical treatment
- 70% of patients require surgery within 10–20 years of diagnosis
- Increased risk of colonic adenocarcinoma, depending on duration and extent of disease
- Side effects of medications can limit their use
  - Azathioprine/6-mercaptopurine: Pancreatitis, bone marrow suppression, lymphoma
  - Anti–tumor necrosis antibodies: Sepsis, anaphylactic reaction, activation of tuberculosis
  - Corticosteroids: Cushingoid facies, avascular necrosis of bone, cataracts, hypertension
  - Aminosalicylates: Renal toxicity

Ulcerative Colitis

INTRODUCTION

- Ulcerative colitis is one of the two major types of inflammatory bowel disease; it is distinctly separate from Crohn disease
- Ulcerative colitis involves chronic, relapsing inflammation extending proximally and continuously from the rectum; in contrast, Crohn disease classically does not affect the rectum and has discontinuous, "skip" lesions
- Despite the rising incidence of Crohn disease during the past 30 years, pediatric incidence of ulcerative colitis has remained stable

ETIOLOGY, EPIDEMIOLOGY, & RISK FACTORS

- The etiology is unknown but involves a complex interplay of genetics and environmental factors such as commensal bacterial flora
- In contrast to Crohn disease, ulcerative colitis is associated with diffuse, continuous mucosal inflammation (v. skip lesions in Crohn disease); inflamed areas of bowel do not alternate with uninvolved areas; there is no small bowel involvement (excluding backwash ileitis); there is no granuloma formation; microabscesses are produced; and the disease is limited to the mucosa/submucosa
- Incidence of 3–15 cases per 100,000 (depending on geographic location and genetic pool)
- Males are affected more often than females
- Family history is important; there is 10 times greater risk in first-degree relatives
- Genetic influence is less strong than with Crohn disease; genetic association with HLA-DR2 and MDR1
- Bimodal peak during ages 10–30 and 50–65 but may present as early as 1 year of age
- Higher incidence than Crohn disease
- Higher incidence in Jewish populations; lower incidence in African-Americans
- Cigarette smoking as a protective agent in pediatric ulcerative colitis is unclear

PATIENT PRESENTATION

- Bloody diarrhea (nocturnal diarrhea occurs in half of cases)
- Lower abdominal pain and cramps, which are often relieved by defecation
- Tenesmus with proctitis is common
- Fever and weight loss may occur in severe disease
- Extraintestinal manifestations occur in 15% of cases: Sclerosing cholangitis (3.5%), which can occur even after colectomy; arthralgias (30%); arthritis (typically of the large joints); erythema nodosum, pyoderma gangrenosum; ankylosing spondylitis (with HLA-B27 cases); uveitis; venous thrombosis
- Growth retardation, poor weight gain, and delayed puberty may occur in affected children, but less frequently than in Crohn disease

DIFFERENTIAL DX

- Infectious colitis (eg, *E. coli*, *Campylobacter*, *Shigella*, *Salmonella*, *Yersinia*, amebiasis, *C. difficile*)
- Crohn disease
- Colorectal cancer
- Malabsorption syndromes (eg, celiac disease, bacterial overgrowth)
- Diverticulitis (rare)
- Ischemic colitis
- Irritable bowel syndrome
- Allergic colitis
- Microscopic colitis
- Henoch-Schönlein purpura

DIAGNOSTIC EVALUATION

- Stool cultures to evaluate for infectious colitis
- Colonoscopy with biopsy is indicated if the patient is not severely ill and does not have signs of toxic megacolon; colonoscopy allows for a histopathologic diagnosis, to determine the extent and degree of involvement, and to evaluate for neoplastic changes
  - Proctoscopy if full colonoscopy not appropriate
  - Divide patients by location of disease into proctitis (rectum), left-sided, or pancolitis
  - Can see loss of normal vascular pattern, erythema, friability, and hemorrhage
  - Pathology may reveal friable mucosa, pseudopolyps, microabscesses, normal serosa (no transmural inflammation and no granulomas)
- Upper GI series with small bowel follow-through to document normal small bowel
- Barium enema (contraindicated in cases of toxic megacolon) will show ulceration, pseudopolyps, and "lead pipe" appearance of colon
- Perinuclear antineutrophil cytoplasmic antibodies (pANCA) is positive in 75% of cases
- Liver transaminases are elevated in 3% of cases at initial diagnosis and especially if cholangitis is present
- Microcytic anemia, thrombocytosis, hypoalbuminemia, and increased ESR are common

TREATMENT & MANAGEMENT

- Oral or rectal aminosalicylates (eg, mesalamine, balsalazide) are the mainstay of treatment; they can induce remission and control disease in 50–90% of mild to moderate cases
  - May have an additional protective effect against development of future colon cancer
- Corticosteroids are indicated during flare-ups to induce remission; corticosteroid enemas may be used as maintenance medications
- Immunomodulators (eg, 6-mercaptopurine, azathioprine) are used to maintain remission
- Anti-TNF-α biologic agents (eg, infliximab) can both induce and maintain remission
- Colectomy is curative for ulcerative colitis (but not for Crohn disease)
  - Indications for surgery include: Dysplasia or carcinoma, perforation, fulminant colitis, hemorrhage, intractable disease, or inability to wean off steroids
  - One-third of patients undergo colectomy with eventual ileo-pouch anal anastomosis (IPAA) or ileorectal anastomosis
  - Approximately 50% of patients who have undergone IPAA surgery for ulcerative colitis will develop at least one episode of pouchitis (inflammation of the surgically created pouch)

PROGNOSIS & COMPLICATIONS

- Follows a chronic, relapsing course, but some patients have only one episode
- Complications include toxic megacolon in 10%, which can be life threatening; strictures, obstruction, or perforation; hemorrhage and shock if fulminate colitis occurs; and hypokalemia if fulminate colitis occurs
- Associated with a higher risk of eventual colon cancer compared with Crohn disease
  - Risk is increased with advancing degree of involvement
  - Rule of thumb is 2% risk at 10 years, 1% risk per year thereafter
  - Annual screening colonoscopy should be performed after 8–10 years of disease
  - Proctitis alone carries minimal cancer risk

Recurrent Abdominal Pain

INTRODUCTION

- Recurrent abdominal pain is classified as a functional gastrointestinal disorder
  - The current Rome criteria prefer the term functional abdominal pain because it addresses the cause rather than just a description of the symptoms
  - The key components of a functional GI disorder are a normal physical exam and absence of red flags that may indicate organic disease
- There is a sense that the amount of organic disease causing chronic abdominal pain is inversely proportionate to the amount of school missed
- "Apley's rules" suggest that functional pain typically does not result in weight loss, blood in the stool, persistent vomiting, pain distant from the umbilicus, or waking at night in pain

ETIOLOGY, EPIDEMIOLOGY, & RISK FACTORS

- Recurrent abdominal pain is defined as at least one monthly episode of severe pain for 3 consecutive months; types include:
  - Isolated, paroxysmal pain
  - Nonulcer dyspepsia: Epigastric pain that may be related to eating and associated with early satiety, bloating, belching, nausea or vomiting
  - Infraumbilical: Cramps, bloating, distension, diarrhea/constipation
- Occurs in 10–15% of all school-age children; 20% of middle school and high school students have daily or weekly pain
- Functional pain cannot be explained by a structural or biochemical cause
- Current thoughts on etiology include abnormalities in the brain-gut axis such that affected patients appear to have an altered threshold for intraluminal distention–associated pain
- Comorbid psychiatric diagnosis (eg, depression, anxiety) appears to be a risk factor for development of functional pain
- A family history of functional pain is also a risk factor for such disorders in children
- Abnormal neurotransmitters (eg, serotonin) may be responsible for some cases of pain
- Small bowel bacterial overgrowth may account for some cases (especially postinfectious)
- Food intolerances may account for some of the associated abdominal complaints

PATIENT PRESENTATION

- Most common pain location is periumbilical or midepigastric
- Most episodes begin gradually and last less than 3 hours
- Patients may appear miserable and listless during episodes
- Episodes may be worsened by stress or anxiety
- Characteristics that suggest an organic etiology:
  - Well-localized pain outside the umbilicus
  - Awakens patient from sleep
  - Associated with urinary or joint symptoms
  - Age younger than 5 years
  - Fever
  - Weight loss or growth delay
  - Bloody or bilious vomiting
  - Blood in stools
  - Perianal disease
  - Family history of inflammatory bowel disease

DIFFERENTIAL DX

- Gastrointestinal: Constipation, pancreatitis, cholecystitis, carbohydrate malabsorption, infection (eg, *Giardia*), inflammatory bowel disease, hepatitis, cholecystitis, celiac disease, gastroesophageal reflux disease, peptic ulcer disease
- Urinary tract infection
- Urolithiasis
- Metabolic disease (eg, diabetes mellitus, sickle cell disease, lead poisoning)
- Lower lobe pneumonia
- Pelvic and gynecologic disorders (eg, ovarian cyst, endometriosis)
- Tumors

DIAGNOSTIC EVALUATION

- A clinical diagnosis is based on a thorough history and careful physical examination
- Patients who meet diagnostic criteria do not necessarily need serologic evaluation
- Most laboratory studies are normal; abnormal labs suggest organic cause
- Basic laboratory evaluation includes complete blood count, erythrocyte sedimentation rate, albumin, aminotranferases, urinalysis and urine culture, stool studies for ova and parasites, amylase and lipase, and anti-tissue transglutaminase IgA
- Consider testing for *H. pylori* infection; the majority of evidence suggests that colonization with *H. pylori* without ulcer formation does not correlate with increased risk of pain, although some studies show that a positive relationship may occur more frequently in younger children
- Attempt to relate pain with stressors and daily events
  - The patient and family should keep a diary recording pain episodes, time of day, meal time and content, activities, and stool pattern
  - Stressors can be those things that are perceived as pleasant (eg, party, vacation, sporting events) or unpleasant (eg, tests, school)
- If indicated, consider an abdominal ultrasound to evaluate for cholelithiasis
- If indicated, consider a diagnostic trial off lactose or fructose or a breath hydrogen test for carbohydrate intolerance
- Endoscopic evaluation is of limited use in patients without warning signs

TREATMENT & MANAGEMENT

- Education, reassurance, and support of the patient and family
- Doctor and family should look for stressors that may trigger the pain
- Therapy is intended to restore normal activity and school attendance (only 10% attend school regularly)
- Adding fiber to the diet may be of benefit, especially if the patient is constipated
- Avoidance of foods that the patient identifies as worsening the symptoms
  - Must be done with caution because this may result in a severely limited diet and subsequent weight loss and malnutrition
  - There are no foods that should be universally avoided
- Drugs have a limited role:
  - Peppermint oil (smooth muscle relaxant) has been proven effective in a pediatric controlled study
  - Anticholinergics have limited efficacy (similar to placebo)
  - Low-dose tricyclic antidepressants are effective in adults; there are no pediatric studies
  - Probiotics may be helpful, especially with "gas-related" complaints of bloating
  - Proton pump inhibitors for 1 month are helpful in adults with nonulcerative dyspepsia
- Stress management techniques (eg, guided imagery, acupuncture, therapy, hypnosis) have all been shown to be effective and often provide better long-term outcomes

PROGNOSIS & COMPLICATIONS

- Up to 50% of patients have complete resolution of symptoms
- In 25%, pain continues into adulthood
- Factors associated with better prognosis include: Children younger than 6 years, duration of symptoms less than 6 months, middle- or upper-class families, patients with no history of surgical procedures, and patients without family history of frequent pain episodes

Nephrology/Urology

Urinary Tract Infections

INTRODUCTION

- Urinary tract infections are best defined as significant bacteriuria in a patient with an inflammatory response (eg, pyuria on dipstick or microscopic urinalysis)
- The urinary tract ranks second only to the upper respiratory tract as a source of morbidity from bacterial infections in childhood
- Urinary tract infections may lead to renal scarring, hypertension, and renal insufficiency
- Infection of what should be a sterile urinary tract can occur within the kidneys (pyelonephritis), within the bladder (cystitis), or within the urethra (urethritis)
- Diagnosis is made by urine culture

ETIOLOGY, EPIDEMIOLOGY, & RISK FACTORS

- *E. coli* accounts for approximately 80% of urinary infections in children
- Other bacteria include both gram-negative species (*Klebsiella, Proteus, Enterobacter,* and *Citrobacter*) and gram-positive species (*Staphylococcus saprophyticus, Enterococcus,* and, rarely, *Staphylococcus aureus*)
- In children younger than 2, the overall prevalence of urinary tract infection is 5% in febrile infants but varies widely by race and sex
  - Caucasian children have 2- to 4-fold higher prevalence versus African-American children
  - Females have a 2- to 4-fold higher prevalence than do circumcised males
  - Uncircumcised febrile males have a 4-fold higher prevalence versus circumcised males
  - Caucasian females with a temperature >39°C have a urinary tract infection prevalence of 16%
- Colonization of the periurethral area by uropathogenic enteric pathogens is the first step in the development of urinary tract infections
- Bacterial attachment to the uroepithelial cells is an active process mediated by specific bacterial adhesions and specific receptor sites on the epithelial cells
- Bacteria possessing pili (also called *P fimbriae*) can adhere effectively to the uroepithelium and ascend into the kidney, even in children without vesicoureteral reflux

PATIENT PRESENTATION

- Older children (>5 years):
  - Fever
  - Suprapubic or flank tenderness
  - Dysuria
  - Hematuria
  - Dysfunctional voiding (eg, frequent urination, dribbling, enuresis)
- In infants and young children, symptoms are subtle:
  - Weight loss
  - Irritability
  - Fever
  - Lethargy
- The examination should include blood pressure, temperature, assessment of suprapubic and costovertebral tenderness, and a search for other sources of fever

DIFFERENTIAL DX

- Neonates: Sepsis
- Toddlers and infants: Gastroenteritis, intussusception, bubble bath urethritis
- Older children: Renal stones, obstruction (eg, ureteropelvic junction), infectious urethritis (eg, gonorrhea, *Chlamydia*)
- Idiopathic hypercalciuria
- Dysfunctional voiding
- Diabetes insipidus
- Diabetes mellitus
- Musculoskeletal flank pain
- Contaminated specimen
- Vaginitis

DIAGNOSTIC EVALUATION

- Significant bacteriuria usually refers to 100,000 organisms from a midstream clean catch specimen (older children), 50,000 organisms from a catheterized specimen (younger children), or the presence of any uropathogenic bacteria from a suprapubic aspirate
- Infections should be associated with elevated urinary white blood cells or positive leukocyte esterase on dipstick so as to differentiate from simple bacteriuria
- Collection of urine using an adhesive external collection bag is unreliable: A negative culture is meaningful, but a positive culture could be due to contamination from the rectum, skin, or prepuce and should be repeated with a more accurate method
- Recommendations for radiologic studies (renal ultrasound and voiding cystourethrogram) include: Children younger than 5 years with a febrile urinary tract infection, males of any age with a first urinary tract infection, girls younger than 3 years with a first urinary tract infection, and children with recurrent urinary tract infection
- All young children with persistent fever without a definite source should undergo urine testing (urinalysis and microscopic examination)
- Complete blood count, blood culture, and C-reactive protein are usually not helpful in making the diagnosis of urinary tract infection but may be necessary for evaluation of fever

TREATMENT & MANAGEMENT

- Antibiotics should be chosen based on local resistance patterns; repeat urine culture and sensitivity 24–48 hours after therapy

Pyelonephritis
- Most infants over the age of 2 months with pyelonephritis can be managed with outpatient oral antibiotics as long as close follow-up is assured
- Treat pyelonephritis in neonates with ampicillin plus cefotaxime/gentamicin in neonates
- Treat pyelonephritis in older children with ceftriaxone or cefotaxime until sensitivities return
- Hospitalization is indicated for children less than 2 months, children not responding to therapy, children who are vomiting and cannot tolerate oral medications, and children in whom close follow-up cannot be assured

Cystitis
- Treat lower UTI (cystitis) with trimethoprim/sulfamethoxazole or cefpodoxime
- Phenazopyridine (Pyridium) may be used symptomatically to treat dysuria

- The duration of therapy for young children and for those with fever or recurrent urinary tract infection should be 10 to 14 days
- Prompt recognition and treatment of urinary tract infections may be the most important factor in the prevention of renal scarring

PROGNOSIS & COMPLICATIONS

- Children with urinary tract infections may develop sequelae, but they are difficult to predict; most children have no long-term sequelae
- Culturing the urine at the slightest sign that the child is unwell, especially if there is fever, and treating urinary tract infection promptly may decrease renal scarring
- The long-term significance of scarring, as identified by dimercaptosuccinic acid (DMSA), remains to be determined
- Most children have resolution of fever within 24 hours of treatment
- 10–30% of children with urinary tract infections experience one or more symptomatic reinfections, usually within the initial 6 months after infection

Vesicoureteral Reflux

INTRODUCTION

- Vesicoureteral reflux is the retrograde passage of urine from the bladder into the upper urinary tract
- It is the most common urologic anomaly in children, occurring in approximately 1% of newborns
- Occurs in as many as 30–45% of young children with urinary tract infection
- It is assumed that this mechanism allows for the transport of infected urine retrograde from the bladder to the kidney and, thus, predisposes the patient to pyelonephritis and potential renal scarring

ETIOLOGY, EPIDEMIOLOGY, & RISK FACTORS

- Reflux may be primary or acquired
  - Primary reflux is more common in children and is caused by abnormal position of the ureteral bud on the wolffian duct during development of the urinary tract, resulting in a smaller, tunneled segment of the ureter
  - Secondary reflux occurs as a result of acquired bladder dysfunction
- More common in Caucasian children
- Girls are twice as likely to have reflux as boys
- Young children and infants (younger than 2 years of age) are more likely to have reflux
- There appears to be a genetic predisposition; reflux is detected in two-thirds of children whose parents had reflux
  - Up to 30% of siblings of patients with reflux may be affected
  - Some speculate that the length of the intravesicular ureter may be genetically determined

PATIENT PRESENTATION

- Presentation may begin prenatal (via abnormal fetal ultrasound showing multicystic kidney or hydronephrosis) or postnatal
  - Reflux is present in 10–40% of children with prenatal hydronephrosis
- Postnatally, reflux is usually diagnosed during an evaluation of a febrile illness or for signs and symptoms consistent with urinary tract infections (eg, enuresis, vomiting, abdominal pain, foul-smelling urine, flank pain, or recurrent lower urinary tract symptoms such as dysuria, urgency, or frequency)

DIFFERENTIAL DX

- Ureteropelvic junction obstruction
- Posterior urethral valves
- Urethral strictures
- Neuropathic bladder
- Ureteral duplication

DIAGNOSTIC EVALUATION

- Voiding cystourethrogram (VCUG) is necessary to visualize the urethra, evaluate the degree of reflux, and define anatomic anomalies
  - Grade I: Retrograde flow into a nondilated ureter
  - Grade II: Retrograde flow into a nondilated ureter and intrarenal collecting system
  - Grade III: Retrograde flow into the ureter, renal pelvis, and collecting system with mild dilation of fornices
  - Grade IV: Retrograde flow into ureter, renal pelvis, and collecting system with complete blunting of fornices and pyramids
  - Grade V: Gross dilation and tortuous ureter, pelvis, and collecting system
- Nuclear renography to evaluate for cortical scarring ($Tc_{99m}MAG3$)
- The extent of diagnostic workup for prenatal hydronephrosis is controversial
  - Repeat renal ultrasound after delivery
  - If there is persistent, moderate hydronephrosis or a strong family history of reflux, then proceed to VCUG
  - If there is mild or no disease, then repeat renal ultrasound in 2–3 months
- The screening of unaffected siblings is controversial
- Patients should be screened for dysfunctional voiding; there is a higher rate of surgical failure if this is not treated

TREATMENT & MANAGEMENT

- The recommendations of the American Urology Association guidelines should be followed for medical management or surgical intervention
- Medical therapy is based on the observations that reflux will usually spontaneously resolve and that the use of continuous antibiotics results in sterile urine
  - For low-grade reflux (grade III or less), prophylactic antibiotics do not appear to offer any advantage in preventing future scarring; thus, their use in such patients is controversial
  - Continued reflux of sterile urine does not cause further renal damage
  - Antimicrobial agents include trimethoprim-sulfamethoxazole, trimethoprim alone, or nitro-furantoin in one-half dose daily at night time (amoxicillin is used only in the neonatal period)
- Surgical treatment to correct the failed antirefluxing ureterovesical junction
  - Open surgical reimplantation of the ureters has been highly successful, with reported correction rates of 95%
  - Endoscopic correction via subureteric transurethral injection (the STING procedure) was first introduced in the U.S. in 2001 when the FDA approved dextranomer/hyaluronic acid (Dx/HA) as an acceptable substance for implantation; the success rate ranges from 75–87%

PROGNOSIS & COMPLICATIONS

- Patients who are treated medically need to be monitored with urine cultures when there are symptoms of UTI or unexplained fever, surveillance cultures every 3–4 months, and yearly radionuclear cystogram
- 80% of grades I and II reflux will spontaneous resolve within 5 years
- 70% of unilateral grade III cases resolve within 1–2 years; bilateral grade III reflux only resolves in <20% of cases within 5–10 years
- 60% of unilateral grade IV cases will resolve spontaneously; only 10% of bilateral cases will resolve
- Spontaneous resolution of grade V reflux is rare
- 30–60% of patients at initial diagnosis of reflux already have evidence of renal scarring

Urine Outflow Obstruction

INTRODUCTION

- Urinary tract obstruction, depending on the timing (early or late in gestation), can result in a sequence of events affecting the fetus (Potter sequence) and impairing renal function
- Anatomic abnormalities (eg, urethral valves or stricture, stenosis at the ureterovesical or ureteropelvic junction) account for the majority of cases in children
- The obstruction to urinary flow may be acute or chronic, partial or complete, or unilateral or bilateral, and may occur at any site in the urinary tract
- Any condition resulting in prolonged oligohydramnios can result in Potter sequence, which is associated with low-set ears, prominent infracanthal folds, a flattened beaked nose, micrognathia, creased skin, and varying positional deformities of the limbs

ETIOLOGY, EPIDEMIOLOGY, & RISK FACTORS

- Posterior urethral valves are abnormal congenital leaflets in the prostatic portion of the urethra that result in narrowing of the bladder outlet and obstruction of urine flow
  - Represents the most common cause of severe obstructive uropathy in children
  - Only affects males
  - Affects 1 in 5000–8000 live births
  - Inheritance is sporadic; rare cases of familial occurrence have been reported
- Ureteropelvic junction obstruction results from fibrosis at the junction of the ureter and renal pelvis, which leads to obstructed urine flow
  - Increased pressure behind the obstruction results in proximal dilatation and hydronephrosis
  - The most common cause of antenatally detected hydronephrosis
  - Lesions are more common on the left, but 40% of cases are bilateral
  - Boys are affected more commonly than girls
  - Incidence of fetal hydronephrosis caused by ureteropelvic junction obstruction is nearly 1 in 500

PATIENT PRESENTATION

- Posterior urethral valves in neonates may present with distended bladder, palpable kidney, abdominal distension, vomiting, poor urinary stream, failure to thrive, urinary tract infections, and renal insufficiency
- Posterior urethral valves in older boys may present with voiding problems, poor urinary stream, urinary retention, bladder distension, hematuria, enuresis, and hesitancy
- Ureteropelvic junction obstruction may present with a palpable mass, nausea or vomiting, failure to thrive, abdominal pain, hypertension, renal tubular acidosis (a hyperkalemic metabolic acidosis), and signs or symptoms of a urinary tract infection, pyelonephritis, or sepsis
- Painful distension of the renal pelvis can cause unilateral flank pain with or without vomiting (Diettel crisis)

DIFFERENTIAL DX

- Meatal stenosis
- Midureteral valves
- Ureteral ectopia
- Ureterocele
- Bladder neck obstruction
- Megaureter
- Prune-belly syndrome
- Urolithiasis
- Vesicoureteral reflux
- Neoplasm
- Cystic kidney disease
- Megalourethra
- Megacystis microcolon hypoperistalsis syndrome
- Persistent cloaca

DIAGNOSTIC EVALUATION

- The diagnosis of a newborn with antenatal hydronephrosis includes a renal ultrasound within 48 hours if moderate to severe and at 7 days if mild
- Posterior urethral valves are often diagnosed prior to birth with prenatal ultrasound showing bilateral hydronephrosis, bladder wall thickening, and a widened prostatic urethra
  - Diagnosis of megacystis can be made as early as 10–14 weeks of gestation
  - A voiding cystourethrogram may be used to define anatomy and demonstrate the posterior urethral valves
- Ureteropelvic junction obstruction can also be identified on prenatal ultrasound
  - Renal ultrasound to evaluate for hydronephrosis should ideally be performed during a painful crisis (Diettel crisis)
  - CT scan may demonstrate hydronephrosis without a dilated ureter
  - Dynamic renal scan to evaluate renal excretion and degree of obstruction
  - Voiding cystourethrogram (VCUG) to rule out reflux or posterior urethral valves; 10% of patients have contralateral low-grade vesicoureteral reflux

TREATMENT & MANAGEMENT

- Posterior urethral valves generally require placement of a transurethral catheter to relieve the obstruction
  - Correct electrolyte imbalances, if present
  - Treat infection, if present
  - If renal function is normal, corrective surgery with transurethral ablation of the valves is performed
  - If uncontrollable infection, rising creatinine, or too small urethra are present, vesicostomy is performed
- Ureteropelvic junction obstruction may only require observation if good renal function exists despite hydronephrosis; if there is no improvement in a few years, consider surgery
  - Surgery is necessary if renal function worsens; it is usually well tolerated by neonates and young children
  - Pyeloplasty is the surgery of choice
  - After release of the obstruction (either via catheterization or surgery), there is massive postobstructive diuresis (natriuresis and polyuria); as a result, "ins" and "outs" and electrolytes must be closely monitored and replaced

PROGNOSIS & COMPLICATIONS

- Posterior urethral valves may result in renal insufficiency or dysplasia
  - Creatinine nadir is best predictor of prognosis
  - Creatinine level >1 is more frequently associated with long-term renal insufficiency
- Ureteropelvic junction obstruction results in increased risk of urinary stasis, infection, hematuria, and renal scarring secondary to obstruction
  - May improve over time without treatment
  - Surgery is corrective

Urolithiasis

INTRODUCTION

- Urolithiasis refers to the formation of crystals within the urinary tract
- It classically presents with flank pain and hematuria
- Evaluation to determine the type of stone and the presence of biochemical abnormalities predisposing to stone formation is necessary to guide therapy and prevent recurrence
- In the U.S., stones are uncommon in children; in contrast, in other countries such as Turkey and Thailand, urolithiasis is endemic and bladder stones predominate

ETIOLOGY, EPIDEMIOLOGY, & RISK FACTORS

- Stones may be due to infection, metabolic derangements, increased urinary calcium excretion, or medications (eg, indinavir, acyclovir, sulfadiazine, triamterene, ceftriaxone)
- Calcium phosphate and calcium oxalate stones account for 90% of cases
  - Risk factors for calcium stones include hypercalciuria, hyperuricosuria, and hypocitraturia
- Magnesium ammonium phosphate (struvite), uric acid, xanthine, and cystine comprise the remainder of cases
  - Struvite stones are frequently associated with vesicoureteral reflux or other urologic abnormalities or infections caused by urease-producing organisms (eg, *Proteus*, *Klebsiella*)
- Patients with short bowel syndrome and Crohn disease are at increased risk
- Males are affected more commonly than females (ratio, 2:1)
- The upper urinary tract is affected more often than the lower urinary tract
- There is often a positive family history
- Certain areas of the U.S. have higher incidence (the "stone belts"), including the mid-Atlantic and Southeast regions

PATIENT PRESENTATION

- May be asymptomatic
- Gross or microscopic hematuria usually occurs but may be absent in up to 30% of patients
- Colicky abdominal pain
  - The location of the pain depends on the location of the stone's obstruction: Flank pain occurs when the upper ureter or pelvis is obstructed; pain in the ipsilateral testicle or labia occurs if the lower ureter is obstructed
  - Paroxysms of severe pain typically last 20–60 minutes
- Fever
- Vomiting
- Dysuria
- Urinary urgency
- Passage of stone or gravel-like material

DIFFERENTIAL DX

- Urinary tract infection
- Appendicitis
- Inguinal hernia
- Crohn disease
- Trauma
- Medullary sponge kidney
- Metabolic disorder associated with renal calculi formation
- Ureteropelvic junction obstruction
- Musculoskeletal back pain
- Iliopsoas abscess
- Testicular torsion
- Ovarian torsion
- Renal tumor
- Ectopic pregnancy
- Intestinal obstruction

DIAGNOSTIC EVALUATION

- Urinary calculi may be seen on radiographic imaging studies, including kidney, ureter, bladder (KUB) plain film, spiral CT scan (usually without contrast), or renal ultrasound
  - Calcium and struvite stones are radiopaque
  - Cystine stones are slightly radiopaque
- Stone and debris should be retrieved and evaluated for composition
- Workup is usually necessary to determine the etiology
  - Laboratory testing includes electrolytes, serum calcium, phosphorus, alkaline phosphorylase, creatinine, pH, partial pressure of carbon dioxide (PCO_2), uric acid, and parathyroid hormone level
  - A 2-day collection for 24-hour stone risk profile may be used to evaluate the urinary environment and risk factors for stone formation; this should only be done when the patient is in his or her usual state of health and not receiving intravenous fluids

TREATMENT & MANAGEMENT

- Acute management includes hydration and pain relief
- If a stone obstructs the genitourinary tract or will not pass, surgical intervention or lithotripsy is indicated
- Antibiotics if infection is present
- Nutritional interventions include a low-salt diet (increased salt intake increases calcium excretion at the tubular level), regular calcium intake (unless the patient has hypercalcemia), and increased fluid intake to increase urine volume
- Specific therapy is based on the type of stone:
  - Calcium stones: Treat underlying disorder, and thiazide diuretics for recurrences
  - Struvite stones: Remove the stone to avoid abscess formation
  - Uric acid stones: Treat the underlying disorder, alkalinize the urine to pH 6.5, and consider allopurinol
  - Oxalate stones: Restrict dietary oxalate and reduce oxalate excretion with thiazide diuretics; increase the solubility of oxalate by administering magnesium, phosphate, and citrate salts; and use pyridoxine therapy to reduce oxalate production
  - Cystine stones: Alkalinize the urine and consider a chelator (eg, penicillamine)

PROGNOSIS & COMPLICATIONS

- Generally carries a good prognosis
- There is a high incidence of recurrence (up to 50%), which varies with the underlying disorder and stone type
- Some metabolic disorders (eg, cystinuria) and inherited renal diseases (eg, hyperoxaluria) that are associated with calculi formation may lead to renal failure

Enuresis

INTRODUCTION

- Urinary incontinence is a common problem in children
- Enuresis is defined as involuntary loss of urine in a child older than 5
- At 5 years of age, 15% of children remain partially incontinent of urine
- Most of these children have isolated nocturnal enuresis (monosymptomatic nocturnal enuresis)
- Primary enuresis (most common) involves never having had a prolonged dry period longer than 6 months
- Secondary enuresis (far less common) involves the presence of a dry period of 6 months in duration followed by regular incontinence

ETIOLOGY, EPIDEMIOLOGY, & RISK FACTORS

- Bladder control is generally achieved by the age of 2–3 years
- Enuresis may be due to delayed maturational control, inadequate antidiuretic hormone secretion during sleep, psychologically stressful events, or small bladder capacity
- Nocturnal enuresis is more common than diurnal enuresis
- The prevalence of nocturnal enuresis depends on age: 5 years of age (16%), 6 years (13%), 7 years (10%), 8 years (7%), 10 years (5%), 12–14 years (2–3%), older than 15 (1–2%)
- Nocturnal enuresis is more common in boys; diurnal enuresis is more common in girls
- There is a genetic component to nocturnal enuresis: If neither parent had enuresis, the incidence is 15%; if one parent had enuresis, the incidence is nearly 45%, and if both parents had enuresis, the incidence is more than 75%
    - There is an autosomal dominant form with 90% penetrance
    - Genetic loci include 13q13-q14.3 (Danish), also 22q11 and 12q

PATIENT PRESENTATION

- Enuresis may be only at nighttime or daytime
- History of dribbling, frequency, constipation, or encopresis may be present

DIFFERENTIAL DX

- Urinary tract infection
- Chemical distal urethritis
- Diabetes mellitus
- Diabetes insipidus
- Psychogenic polydipsia
- Lower urinary tract obstruction (eg, posterior urethral valves, urethral cysts, urethral duplication)
- Ectopic ureter
- Occult spinal dysraphism
- Pelvic masses (eg, presacral teratoma, fecal impaction, hydrocolpos)

DIAGNOSTIC EVALUATION

- Primarily a diagnosis of exclusion
- The main purpose of the evaluation is to determine whether the child has complex enuresis or enuresis as a manifestation of an underlying medical problem (eg, posterior urethral valves or other anatomic abnormality, spinal dysraphism, diabetes); additional evaluation may be necessary to exclude these disorders
- A thorough history and physical examination is important in order to exclude secondary causes of bedwetting
    - Include pattern of enuresis, voiding history, constipation, encopresis, dribbling, incontinence, history of prior urinary tract infections, presence of unexplained fevers, and emotional, social, and developmental histories
    - Full back and neurologic examination is indicated; evaluate for the presence of a sacral dimple, hypospadias, cremasteric reflex, and anal wink
    - Evaluate for the presence of palpable kidneys or bladder
    - Evaluate for palpable stool or constipation, which may contribute to the problem
- Urinalysis and urine culture to rule out urinary tract infection and diabetes mellitus
- Consider assessment of urinary stream to rule out obstruction
- Renal ultrasound and bladder ultrasound before and after void for small bladder capacity

TREATMENT & MANAGEMENT

- Behavior modification is important to control bladder emptying
    - Nighttime fluid restriction and late-night voiding
    - An enuresis alarm may be used to wake the child when urination in bed begins
    - Families are encouraged to involve the child in the management of the problem, including reward systems for dry nights and cleaning the bed after wet nights
- Desmopressin acetate (DDAVP) is an antidiuretic hormone agonist
    - Generally not used on a daily basis; rather, it is most often used for occasions when bedwetting is a significant problem, such as sleepovers or camp
    - Monitor for hyponatremia when using this medication
- Tricyclic antidepressants, such as imipramine, may be used to induce urinary retention
- Children who have clinical or radiographic findings suggestive of renal or urologic abnormalities or bladder instability should be referred to a pediatric nephrologist or urologist for further evaluation

PROGNOSIS & COMPLICATIONS

- Spontaneous cure rate is 15% per year
- Generally resolves by age 12

Acute Renal Failure

INTRODUCTION

- Acute renal failure (ARF) is defined by a rapid decline in glomerular filtration rate, resulting in impairment of excretion of nitrogenous waste products and loss of water, electrolyte, and acid-base regulation
- ARF is an important contributing factor to the morbidity and mortality of critically ill infants and children
- The causes of ARF can be categorized as prerenal, renal, or postrenal
- The incidence of renal failure in children is rising with increased availability of advanced pediatric medical technology including bone marrow, hepatic, and cardiac transplantation; congenital heart disease surgery; and advances in care of very low birth weight infants

ETIOLOGY, EPIDEMIOLOGY, & RISK FACTORS

- The causes of ARF can be categorized as prerenal, renal (intrinsic), or postrenal
  - Prerenal failure results from volume depletion (hypovolemia), decreased effective arterial pressure (shock), or decreased effective circulating volume (heart failure)
  - Intrinsic renal failure includes disorders that involve the renal vasculature (eg, arterial or venous thrombosis), glomerulus (eg, glomerulonephritis), renal tubules (eg, acute tubular necrosis), or renal interstitium
  - Postrenal failure is usually due to bilateral urinary tract obstruction (unless there is a solitary kidney)
- Hemolytic uremic syndrome is the most common form of ARF requiring intervention
- Postinfectious glomerulonephritis (eg, poststreptococcal) is the most common form of ARF leading to renal dysfunction without a need for acute intervention
- Drugs may also cause renal failure (eg, contrast dye, antibiotics, lead, mercury, antihypertensives)
- The precise incidence and prevalence of ARF has been difficult to ascertain but has been estimated as a yearly incidence of about 0.8 cases per 100,000 children

PATIENT PRESENTATION

- History and physical exam can detect signs or symptoms favoring an underlying diagnosis
- History of volume losses: GI losses (vomiting, diarrhea), bleeding or trauma, urine losses (eg, diabetes insipidus)
- Gross hematuria
- Oliguria (usually due to acute glomerulonephritis; evaluate for hypertension and rashes)
- Abdominal pain, mass, or hematuria suggests a stone, hydronephrosis with obstruction, or a renal mass
- Edema (may be insidious); tends to occur periorbitally in the morning and pretibially at night
- Headache may be related to hypertension
- Respiratory difficulty due to pulmonary edema
- Tachypnea due to metabolic acidosis

DIFFERENTIAL DX

- Prerenal failure: Dehydration (vomiting, diarrhea, hemorrhage), septic shock, perinatal asphyxia, CHF
- Intrinsic renal failure: Acute tubular necrosis (antibiotics, radiocontrast, nephrolithiasis), glomerulonephritis, vasculitis (Wegener syndrome, Goodpasture syndrome, SLE), interstitial nephritis
- Postrenal failure: Obstructions, cystic disease, calculi, tumor, renal vein thrombosis

DIAGNOSTIC EVALUATION

- Serum analysis includes evaluation of electrolytes, BUN, creatinine, calcium, uric acid, and phosphorus
- Urinalysis with microscopy; use the urine osmolality (U_{osm}) and sodium (U_{Na}) to calculate fractional excretion of sodium (FE_{Na})
  - $FE_{Na} = (U_{Na} \times P_{Cr})/(P_{Na} \times U_{Cr}) \times 100\%$
  - $FE_{Na} < 1\%$, $U_{Na} < 10$ mEq/L, and $U_{osm} > 500$ mOsm/L suggest tubular and glomerular function are intact; therefore, evaluate for a prerenal etiology
  - $FE_{Na} > 2\%$, $U_{Na} > 50$ mEq/L, and $U_{osm} < 300$ mOsm/L suggest tubular dysfunction and decreased glomerular filtration rate; therefore, evaluate for an intrinsic renal etiology
- Other serologies to assess include ANA, C3, and C4 for systemic lupus erythematosus; ANCA for Wegener syndrome; and ASO for poststreptococcal glomerulonephritis
- Renal ultrasound to assess the renal structure and rule out obstruction
- If postrenal and prerenal causes have been ruled out, consider a renal biopsy to assess for an intrinsic renal cause
- If the patient has a history of concurrent diarrhea, consider testing for *E. coli* O157:H7 or other bacterial pathogens linked to hemolytic uremic syndrome

TREATMENT & MANAGEMENT

- The goal of treatment is to provide anticipatory management and prevent the development of secondary complications
- Ensure appropriate water and sodium balance
  - In isonatremic patients, correct for insensible water loss (400 mL/m^2) plus urine output
  - In hyponatremic patients, fluid restriction is usually indicated
  - Sodium should not be given because the patient has already accumulated sodium and has positive extracellular fluid volume
- Monitor volume assessment and management via strict ins and outs, daily weights, and electrolyte monitoring
- Discontinue nephrotoxic drugs, if indicated
- Adjust medication dosage for decreased glomerular filtration rate
- Indications for dialysis include hyperkalemia, volume overload with pulmonary edema or hypertension, metabolic acidosis with pH <7.2, azotemia (BUN >150 or rapidly rising), symptomatic uremia, or calcium/phosphate imbalance
- Dialysis options include peritoneal dialysis, intermittent hemodialysis, and continuous arteriovenous or venovenous hemofiltration (CAVH, CVVH)
- Ensure appropriate nutrition to maintain adequate caloric intake

PROGNOSIS & COMPLICATIONS

- Prognosis depends on the underlying disease process
- Complications of acute renal failure include hyperkalemia; metabolic acidosis due to retention of hydrogen, sulfate, and phosphate ions; hypertension; and malnutrition
- Mortality increases with the presence of sepsis or multiorgan failure
- The oliguric period tends to last about 10 days
- It may take up to 8 weeks for renal function to recover in cases of acute tubular necrosis
- Prolonged oliguria or anuria (>3 weeks) is indicative of poor prognosis

Chronic Kidney Disease

INTRODUCTION

- Chronic kidney disease (CKD) is defined as irreversible deterioration of renal function
- The kidneys can compensate for decreased renal function until the glomerular filtration rate (GFR) becomes less than 15 mL/min/1.73 m^2
- Incidence of up to 20 new cases per 1 million children less than 15 years old
- 1.5–3 children per million develop end-stage renal disease
- Complications of CKD can be prevented or delayed through early detection and treatment

ETIOLOGY, EPIDEMIOLOGY, & RISK FACTORS

- The K/DOQI workgroup developed a formal staging system for stratification of CKD based on the level of kidney function, independent of the primary renal diagnosis:
  - Stage 1: normal GFR ($\geq$ 90 mL/min/1.73 m^2)
  - Stage 2: GFR of 60–89 mL/min/1.73 m^2
  - Stage 3: GFR of 30–59 mL/min/1.73 m^2
  - Stage 4: GFR of 15–29 mL/min/1.73 m^2
  - Stage 5: GFR of less than 15 mL/min/1.73 m^2 or end-stage renal disease
- Children in stages 1 and 2 are usually asymptomatic and should be closely followed for deterioration of kidney function; this period should be used to educate the child and family about CKD, highlighting awareness of risk factors that aggravate renal failure and measures that may slow the progression of renal failure
- The early clinical symptoms and most of the laboratory abnormalities related to progressive CKD begin to appear in stage 3 disease
- May be congenital or acquired
- Obstructive uropathy is the most common etiology, accounting for 50% of pediatric cases
- Smoking and hypertension tend to increase the rate of progression of renal failure, independent of the renal disease

PATIENT PRESENTATION

- Growth failure
- Unexplained dehydration
- Salt craving
- Hypertension
- Edema
- Nocturia
- Polyuria
- Lethargy, reduced exercise tolerance
- Encephalopathy
- Gross hematuria or abnormal urinalysis
- Renal osteodystrophy
- Normochromic anemia
- Pruritus
- Nausea/vomiting
- Abnormal tooth development
- Peripheral neuropathy

DIFFERENTIAL DX

Congenital CKD
- Potter's syndrome
- Hypoplasia or dysplasia
- Polycystic kidney disease
- Posterior urethral valves
- Prune belly
- Ureteropelvic junction obstruction
- Alport syndrome
- Cystinosis
- Urethral atresia

Acquired CKD
- Hemodynamic catastrophe
- Steroid-resistant nephrotic syndrome (eg, FSGS)
- Rapidly progressive glomerulonephritis
- Systemic lupus erythematosus
- Vesicoureteral reflux

DIAGNOSTIC EVALUATION

- Laboratory evaluation includes serum chemistries (electrolytes, BUN, creatinine to estimate GFR according to the Schwartz formula, serum phosphorus, albumin), serum cholesterol, and urinalysis with microscopy
  - The presence of proteinuria is the best predictor of progressive renal damage
- Serologies for disease activity (eg, falling levels of C4 in cases of SLE)
- Imaging to assess kidney structure, cystic kidney disease, and hydronephrosis
- Renal biopsy to delineate the histopathology
- Assess risks factors for worsening GFR (eg, smoking, hypertension)
- In cases of active renal disease, the underlying primary disease should be treated promptly to prevent the development of renal scars from pyelonephritis
- Optimize blood sugar control in diabetic patients
  - Polycystic kidney disease and glomerular diseases tend to progress faster to end-stage renal failure than tubular or interstitial diseases

TREATMENT & MANAGEMENT

- The goal of treatment is to prevent further loss of renal function and avoid associated complications
- Diet modification to provide adequate caloric intake, low phosphorus intake, and low potassium intake
- Calcium carbonate is used as a calcium supplement and phosphate binder
- Vitamin D (1,25-dihydroxycholecalciferol) is used to manage renal osteodystrophy
- Iron supplement and erythropoietin for anemia
- Sodium restriction and antihypertensive drugs for hypertension
- Sodium bicarbonate or citrate supplement to correct metabolic acidosis
- Growth hormone supplementation to manage growth failure
- Dialysis may be necessary
  - Indications for dialysis may include volume overload with pulmonary edema; hypertension refractory to pharmacologic therapy; hyperkalemia with potassium levels >6.5 mEq/L despite ion exchange therapy; EKG changes due to hyperkalemia (eg, peaked T waves); metabolic acidosis with pH <7.2 or bicarbonate level <10; BUN level >150 (or less if rapidly rising); calcium/phosphorus imbalance; and neurologic symptoms due to uremia or electrolyte imbalance
- Renal transplantation is ultimately necessary in progressive cases

PROGNOSIS & COMPLICATIONS

- Complications include decreased exercise tolerance, poor oral intake, short stature, delay in sexual maturation, and emotional problems related to the extent of complications and the chronic nature of the disease and treatments
- Electrolyte abnormalities may lead to cardiac arrhythmias, which can be life threatening
- Hypertension can rarely cause seizures
- Outcomes have improved steadily over the last few years
- Prompt referral to a pediatric nephrologist can help prevent many of the complications

Nephrotic Syndrome

INTRODUCTION

- Nephrotic syndrome is characterized by proteinuria, edema, and hypercholesterolemia
- The most common cause in preschool and school-aged children is minimal change disease
- Very young (<1 year old) and adolescent children usually have other causes, including infantile nephrotic syndrome or congenital nephrotic syndrome in infants and focal segmental glomerulosclerosis (FSGS) or membranous glomerulonephritis (GN) in adolescents

ETIOLOGY, EPIDEMIOLOGY, & RISK FACTORS

- Increased permeability of the glomerular wall leads to abnormal protein excretion and loss of albumin
- As a result of protein loss in the urine, edema occurs as fluid shifts from the intravascular to the interstitial space due to decreased oncotic pressure; this shift causes decreased renal perfusion, increased salt and water retention, and worsening edema
- Nephrotic syndrome often follows a flu-like syndrome
- Mild proteinuria is found in 3% of children; however, proteinuria is persistent in less than 0.5% of children
- Nephrotic syndrome has an incidence of 2–7 cases per 100,000 children per year
- Most commonly occurs in children 2–6 years old but can occur at any age
- Males are affected more than females (ratio, 3:2)
- Minimal change disease is the most common cause of nephrotic syndrome (80% of cases) in children
  - Light microscopy shows relatively normal glomeruli
  - Electron microscopy shows diffuse foot process fusion
  - Immunofluorescence shows no immunoglobulin or complement deposition

PATIENT PRESENTATION

- Mild proteinuria may be asymptomatic and is often found during a routine urinalysis
- Foamy urine indicates significant proteinuria
- Periorbital edema
- Ascites
- Pitting edema
- Anasarca
- Weight gain
- Malaise
- Pleural effusions
- May have hypertension (25%)

DIFFERENTIAL DX

Primary Nephrotic Syndrome
- Minimal change disease
- FSGS
- Membranous nephropathy
- Membranoproliferative GN

Secondary Nephrotic Syndrome
- HIV nephropathy
- SLE
- Malignancy (eg, lymphoma)
- Sickle cell nephropathy
- Diabetic nephropathy
- Drug or heavy metal toxicity

Children Under 1 Year
- Diffuse mesangial sclerosis
- Deny-Drash syndrome
- Congenital nephrotic syndrome (Finnish)

DIAGNOSTIC EVALUATION

- Proteinuria greater than 1+ on dipstick correlates with >150 mg/day
  - Proteinuria can be defined as: Urine protein-to-urine creatinine ratio >0.2; or >4 mg/m2/hr of protein on 24-hour urine collection
- Nephrotic range proteinuria is 3–4+ on dipstick, or >1000 mg/day
  - Urine protein-to-urine creatinine ratio >2.0
  - >40 mg/m2/hr of protein on 24-hour urine collection
- Lipiduria and microscopic hematuria occurs in 25% of cases
- Significant hematuria with proteinuria indicates nephritis
- Serologic evaluation reveals elevated cholesterol and triglycerides, decreased albumin (<2.5 mg/dL), and normal C3 and creatinine
- Renal biopsy should be performed in steroid-dependent cases needing alternative therapy (eg, tacrolimus), steroid-resistant cases, unusual presentations (eg, hematuria, GFR impairment, hypertension), and extremes of age (younger than 1 year and older than 8 years)

TREATMENT & MANAGEMENT

- Upon initial diagnosis, patients should be promptly evaluated by a nephrologist for education, dietary restriction (salt and water), diuretic therapy, and initiation of steroids
- Corticosteroids are the first-line therapy
  - Prednisone (60 mg/m^2) daily for 6 weeks, followed by 40 mg/m^2/day for another 6 weeks
  - Document negative PPD prior to initiation of steroids
  - Proteinuria should resolve within 2–3 weeks in cases of minimal change disease
  - Test the first morning urine for proteinuria on a daily basis to monitor progress
  - Avoid live virus immunizations while on steroids
- Diuretics (albumin/furosemide combination) are rarely used to increase delivery of furosemide to the kidneys in cases of massive ascites resulting in respiratory distress or severe edema
- Immunosuppressive agents (eg, alkylating agents, mycophenolate mofetil, tacrolimus) are used as second-line therapy, depending on the results of biopsy; may also be used as steroid-sparing therapy
- Calcineurin inhibitors (cyclosporine/tacrolimus) are used in steroid-resistant cases

PROGNOSIS & COMPLICATIONS

- Complications include infections, especially with pneumococcal and gram-negative organisms (pneumococcal vaccine should be given); steroid-induced cataracts; and hypertension, obesity, infections, osteoporosis, growth retardation, mood changes, and thromboembolism (arterial and venous, due to decreased antithrombin III protein)
- Relapse occurs in 80% of cases, usually during steroid taper
- Good prognosis for minimal change disease; more than 90% of children respond to prednisone therapy, but 40% will suffer a relapse

Postinfectious Glomerulonephritis

INTRODUCTION

- Poststreptococcal glomerulonephritis is the most common cause of glomerulonephritis in children
- However, other bacterial or viral infections can cause an identical syndrome; thus, it is most often called postinfectious glomerulonephritis
- Spontaneous recovery occurs in almost all patients
- Irreversible renal failure probably occurs in less than 1% of cases

ETIOLOGY, EPIDEMIOLOGY, & RISK FACTORS

- Acute inflammation of glomeruli as a result of immune complex–mediated renal injury
  - Immune deposits in the subendothelial space result in complement activation
  - The local influx of inflammatory cells leads to a proliferative glomerulonephritis, an active urine sediment, and a variable decline in glomerular filtration rate
  - The deposits are cleared rapidly by the inflammatory cells, accounting for the resolution of hematuria and renal insufficiency
  - Deposits may not be seen on renal biopsy unless performed early in the course of disease
- Most commonly associated with a recent streptococcal (group A, β-hemolytic) pharyngitis, but also seen following other respiratory or cutaneous infections (eg, impetigo)
  - Nephritogenic strains of *Streptococcus* include types 12 and 49
- Renal symptoms usually develop 2–6 weeks after infection
- During epidemics, 5–10% of cases occur due to a postpharyngitis source of *Streptococcus* and 25% of cases are due to a streptococcal skin infection
- Highest incidence occurs in preschool and elementary school children (average age, 7 years)
- Males are affected more commonly than females
- Treatment of the prodromal infection does not prevent the nephritis

PATIENT PRESENTATION

- Symptoms range from asymptomatic to severe
- Manifestations of acute renal failure occur
- Hematuria is the hallmark of disease
- 30–50% of children present with gross hematuria, described as "smoky" or "tea-colored" urine
- Edema occurs due to salt and water retention
  - Periorbital edema
  - Pulmonary edema, resulting in dyspnea, orthopnea, cough, rales, and gallop
- Hypertension
- Oliguria

DIFFERENTIAL DX

Infectious Causes
- Streptococci
- Staphylococci
- Viruses
- Fungal
- Parasites

Other Glomerular Diseases
- IgA nephropathy
- Henoch-Schönlein purpura nephritis
- Lupus nephritis
- Hereditary nephritis
- Membranoproliferative glomerulonephritis
- Alport nephritis
- Wegener granulomatosis

DIAGNOSTIC EVALUATION

- Suspected in a child presenting with the appropriate history and physical findings, including history of recent infection
- Serologic confirmation for streptococcal infection via ASO and anti-DNAase B titers
- Serum C3 levels are decreased at presentation secondary to activation of the alternate complement pathway and generally return to normal within 8 weeks; C4 may also be decreased
- Laboratory evaluation includes chemistries (BUN, serum creatinine, serum albumin, cholesterol), urinalysis (typically reveals high specific gravity, low pH, hematuria, RBC casts, leukocyte casts, hyaline casts, granular casts, and proteinuria)
- Renal biopsy is rarely needed for diagnosis

TREATMENT & MANAGEMENT

- Usually self-limiting
- Supportive therapy includes loop diuretics, fluid restriction, and low-sodium diet to control the edema and antihypertensive medications (eg, diuretics, vasodilators)
- Antibiotic therapy should be instituted if there is evidence of ongoing infection
- Follow-up with repeat serum C3 levels in 6–8 weeks after the onset of nephritis
  - C3 typically returns to normal within 10 days to 8 weeks after onset
  - If C3 levels continue to be low, consider alternate diagnosis of membranoproliferative glomerulonephritis or lupus nephritis and reevaluate via renal biopsy

PROGNOSIS & COMPLICATIONS

- Excellent prognosis; full recovery occurs in 98% of cases
- Gross hematuria and hypertension resolve within 3 weeks
- Proteinuria resolves in a month
- Microscopic hematuria may persist for many months to years
- May have mild, late sequelae (10–20 years) of hypertension, proteinuria, hematuria, or decrease in renal function

Rapidly Progressive Glomerulonephritis

INTRODUCTION

- Rapidly progressive glomerulonephritis (RPGN) is characterized morphologically by extensive glomerular crescent formation and clinically by progression to end-stage renal disease in most untreated patients within a period of weeks to months
- The severity of the disease is in part related to the degree of crescent formation
- Patients with circumferential crescents in more than 80% of glomeruli tend to present with advanced renal failure and may not respond well to therapy
- Patients with crescents in less than 50% of the glomeruli, particularly if the crescents are noncircumferential, typically follow a more indolent course

ETIOLOGY, EPIDEMIOLOGY, & RISK FACTORS

- Multiple diseases can lead to severe glomerular basement membrane (GBM) injury with gaps and crescent development
- The disorder is termed idiopathic RPGN when no other primary glomerular disease can be diagnosed and when crescents are identified in 50% or more of the sampled glomeruli
- Subtypes of idiopathic RPGN are classified based on the type of GBM injury:
  - Type I (anti-GBM antibody disease): Antibodies to GBM antigens are formed secondary to an unknown stimulus, leading to linear IgG along the GBM; most affected patients have measurable circulating anti-GBM antibody
  - Type II (immune complex RPGN): Circulating immune complexes of unknown etiology are deposited in the mesangium and subendothelial portions of the GBM; these deposits are recognized as a granular pattern of IgG or IgM by immunofluorescence staining or electron-dense deposits by electron microscopy; may be associated with underlying disease (eg, postinfectious glomerulonephritis, lupus nephritis, mixed cryoglobulinemia)
  - Type III (pauci-immune): Characterized by minimal or absent immune deposits in the glomeruli; this type may represent a renally limited necrotizing vasculitis
- 80% of patients are ANCA positive; ANCA may participate in the pathogenesis of the lesion by activating neutrophils and monocytes within the glomerular capillaries

PATIENT PRESENTATION

- Symptoms of acute nephritis
- Gross hematuria
- Edema
- Hypertension
- Oliguria/anuria
- Symptoms of underlying disorder
- Goodpasture syndrome presents with hemoptysis due to pulmonary hemorrhage
- Wegener granulomatosis presents with hemoptysis due to pulmonary hemorrhage, sinusitis, serous otitis media, epistaxis, and saddle nose (loss of height of the nose due to collapse of the bridge)
- Henoch-Schönlein purpura presents with a palpable, purpuric rash typically on the legs and buttocks

DIFFERENTIAL DX

- Membranoproliferative glomerulonephritis
- Membranous glomerulonephritis
- SLE nephritis
- Goodpasture syndrome
- Wegener granulomatosis
- Henoch-Schönlein purpura nephritis
- Hepatitis B or C nephritis
- Postinfectious glomerulonephritis
- IgA nephropathy
- Hereditary nephritis

DIAGNOSTIC EVALUATION

- An accurate and urgent diagnosis is required to limit glomerular injury and prevent end-stage renal disease
- Serum electrolytes, serum albumin, serum cholesterol, coagulation studies (PT, PTT, INR), and urinalysis with microscopy are indicated in anticipation of renal biopsy
- Patients should undergo renal biopsy and appropriate serologic assays to determine the etiology
  - Testing for ANCA, anti-GBM antibodies, antinuclear antibodies, and others may be indicated depending on the biopsy results
  - Serum ANCA is positive in cases of pauci-immune necrotizing crescentic glomerulonephritis
  - Cytoplasmic (cANCA) is positive in Wegener granulomatosis
  - pANCA and cANCA are positive in pauci-immune polyarteritis nodosa
- Serum C3 levels vary depending on the etiology
  - Normal in microscopic polyarteritis nodosa, Wegener granulomatosis, Henoch-Schönlein purpura, and IgA nephropathy
  - Decreased in systemic lupus erythematosus nephritis, membranoproliferative glomerulonephritis (MPGN), and membranous glomerulonephritis (MGN)

TREATMENT & MANAGEMENT

- The goal of treatment is to prevent further glomerular injury and additional loss of renal function
- High-dose corticosteroids with cytotoxic agents and plasmapheresis may be used, depending on underlying disorder; they should be considered for patients with anti-GBM disorders or ANCA-associated vasculitis (eg, Wegener granulomatosis, SLE nephritis), especially in the presence of pulmonary hemorrhage
  - Empiric pulse steroid therapy may be initiated until biopsy results are available
  - The usual first line of management is pulse steroids followed by maintenance steroids and cyclophosphamide
- Renal replacement therapy via dialysis or renal transplantation may be necessary

PROGNOSIS & COMPLICATIONS

- Most patients require dialysis and ultimately develop hypertension
- Recurrence rate in the transplanted kidney is 10–30%

Polycystic Kidney Disease

INTRODUCTION

- Renal cysts occur in a wide variety of renal diseases in children
- The term polycystic kidney disease should be reserved to describe two hereditary diseases: Autosomal recessive polycystic kidney disease (ARPKD) and autosomal dominant polycystic kidney disease (ADPKD)
- ADPKD is the more common form, affecting 1 in 1000 children
- ARPKD is rare, occurring in 1 in 10,000 live births

ETIOLOGY, EPIDEMIOLOGY, & RISK FACTORS

- ADPKD is inherited in an autosomal dominant fashion, with 50% of offspring affected
  - PKD1, located at 16p13.3, accounts for 85% of cases
  - PKD2, located at 4q13-p23, accounts for 10–15% of cases
  - PKD3 is responsible for a small group of patients; gene location is unknown
- ARPKD is inherited in an autosomal recessive pattern, with 25% of offspring affected
  - PKHD1, located at 6p21, encodes a gene for the proteins fibrocystin or polyductin
  - The cause of cyst formation is unknown, but theories include papillary hyperplasia of the tubular epithelium with secondary tubular obstruction, delayed tubular canalization, structural alterations in the tubular basement membrane, and changes secondary to toxic metabolites
  - In ARPKD, the parenchyma is filled with dilated renal collecting tubules that appear as small radial cysts; the collecting system (renal pelvis, pedicle, and ureter) is normal

PATIENT PRESENTATION

- May be asymptomatic
- Both forms have enlarged kidneys that may be palpable as a mass
- Hypertension may be present
- Increased incidence of urinary tract infections
- Both forms may lead to end-stage renal disease
- ADPKD may present with flank pain or hematuria; it is also associated with berry aneurysms and cysts in other organs, including the liver, pancreas, and ovaries
- ARPKD is associated with congenital hepatic fibrosis (Caroli syndrome)
  - Younger children have more renal and less hepatic involvement
  - Oliguric fetuses may have oligohydramnios and subsequent lung hypoplasia, and pulmonary insufficiency leading to death in the newborn

DIFFERENTIAL DX

- Multicystic dysplastic kidney disease
- Simple cysts
- Renal dysplasia
- Medullary cystic kidney disease
- Other causes of a palpable renal mass (eg, ureteropelvic junction obstruction, Wilms tumor, renal cell carcinoma)
- Other causes of hematuria (eg, nephrolithiasis, urinary tract infection, glomerulonephritis)

DIAGNOSTIC EVALUATION

- ADPKD should be suspected if a family history is present
  - Renal ultrasound confirms cysts but may be normal early in life
  - The cysts are almost always bilateral
  - Genetic testing for the two common mutations is available
- ARPKD should be suspected prenatally if ultrasound shows large, echogenic kidneys or postnatally if bilateral palpable renal masses are present
  - Intravenous urography shows radial streaking of the dilated collecting tubules persisting more than 24 hours after injection
  - Abdominal CT scan and MRI may show the cysts better than ultrasound
  - No commercially available genetic test is available at this time
  - Investigations to detect portal hypertension include ultrasound with Doppler; esophageal varices can be detected via endoscopy or with capsule endoscopy designed to visualize the esophagus

TREATMENT & MANAGEMENT

- There is no specific treatment for either form of PKD
- Monitor blood pressure, renal function, and urine
- Treat hypertension, infections, pain, and/or renal insufficiency as necessary
- For those with poor renal function, dialysis or transplantation may be necessary
  - The disease does not recur in the transplanted kidney
- For those with portal hypertension, prophylactic management of esophageal varices may prevent future bleeding
  - Varices can be ablated using endoscopic sclerosis or banding
  - Portal pressure can be lowered using β-blockers (eg, propranolol)
- In ADPKD, there is in vitro evidence that intracellular cAMP plays a role in cystogenesis
  - Selective vasopressin V2 receptor antagonists in animal models can prevent renal enlargement and dysfunction and inhibit cyst formation
  - Cyst drainage can help with painful cysts but has no effect on disease progression
  - There is only limited evidence that protein restriction is helpful in aiding renal function
  - Controlling hypertension may also reduce the risk of bleeding from cerebral aneurysm

PROGNOSIS & COMPLICATIONS

- Most patients with ARPKD will develop end-stage renal disease during adolescence
  - Several patients survive into their 30s with preserved renal function
  - Prognosis is related to age at diagnosis; those detected at birth have a worse outcome
  - Death is often related to complications of the liver disease
- ADPKD has a variable course, with some patients developing end-stage renal disease early, while others live with normal renal function
  - Most affected children have few or no symptoms during childhood and present as adults
  - Children frequently have markedly high glomerular filtration rates

Renal Vein Thrombosis

INTRODUCTION

- The newborn's kidney appears to be at risk for the development of thrombosis
- Renal vein thrombosis accounts for approximately 10% of cases of venous thrombosis in newborns
- Renal vein thrombosis is the most common form of venous thrombosis other than vascular catheter-associated thrombosis
- The classic triad of flank mass, hematuria, and thrombocytopenia is not often seen clinically (13%)

ETIOLOGY, EPIDEMIOLOGY, & RISK FACTORS

- Tends to occur in neonates who suffer from hypovolemic shock, hemoconcentration, or polycythemia
- The increased risk in neonates is due to small vessel size, low renal blood flow, high vascular resistance, and immature clotting system
- Comorbid conditions include perinatal asphyxia, prenatal or postnatal stress, septicemia, congenital renal anomalies, congenital nephrosis, severe pyelonephritis, and maternal diabetes
- May also occur iatrogenically during umbilical vein catheterization
- Up to 80% of cases occur in children less than 1 month old
- Males are affected more often than females
- Unilateral thrombosis is more common than bilateral thrombosis
- Commonly preceded by diarrhea or use of radiocontrast materials
- Thrombosis after infancy is usually associated with nephritic syndrome or cyanotic congenital heart disease

PATIENT PRESENTATION

- Sudden enlargement of one or both kidneys detected as a flank or abdominal mass (60%)
- Hematuria (gross or microscopic)
- Pallor
- Tachypnea
- Vomiting
- Abdominal distension
- Shock
- Fever
- Oliguria/anuria
- Hypertension is uncommon

DIFFERENTIAL DX

- Hemolytic uremic syndrome
- Disseminated intravascular coagulation
- Perirenal hematoma
- Perirenal abscess
- Hydronephrosis
- Renal tumor
- Cystic kidney disease
- Glomerular disease (specifically membranoproliferative glomerulonephritis)

DIAGNOSTIC EVALUATION

- Ultrasound with Doppler is typically diagnostic
  - Echogenic streaks appear in a peripheral focal segment of the affected kidney within the first few days
  - In the first week, the kidney appears swollen and echogenic, with prominent and less echogenic medullary pyramids
  - The kidney appears heterogeneous with loss of corticomedullary differentiation as the swelling decreases
  - The kidney may subsequently atrophy with focal scarring or recover
  - Color Doppler ultrasound may show absent intrarenal and renal venous flow in the early stages of renal vein thrombosis
- Complete blood count to investigate for polycythemia and thrombocytopenia
- Increased BUN can reflect a state of dehydration
- Peripheral blood smear shows evidence of microangiopathic hemolytic anemia
- Other laboratory testing includes fibrin degradation products (increased), fibrinogen (decreased), factor V, and plasminogen
- Urinalysis reveals proteinuria
- IV urography is contraindicated; selective venography will define the location of thrombosis but is highly risky
- Workup for hypercoagulable states (eg, factor V Leiden, protein C and S deficiency, mutation of methylenetetrahydrofolate reductase) may be indicated

TREATMENT & MANAGEMENT

- Initial treatment is conservative and supportive
- Correct the underlying pathophysiologic abnormalities
- Anticoagulation with heparin should be considered if there is ongoing evidence of intravascular coagulation; however, efficacy has not been proven in controlled studies
- If oliguric or anuric, manage the patient as if in acute renal failure:
  - Fluid restriction to insensible losses and urine output
  - Correct electrolyte abnormalities
  - Adjust medication doses for reduced glomerular filtration rate
  - Consider dialysis
- Surgery is rarely indicated during the acute period

PROGNOSIS & COMPLICATIONS

- Complications include extension of thrombosis into the inferior vena cava and pulmonary emboli
- Mortality generally reflects the underlying disease process
- With unilateral thrombosis, adequate renal function is usually present
- Chronic renal failure or tubular dysfunction can develop in patients with bilateral disease
- The affected kidney may atrophy and scar, resulting in hypertension
- Neonates have increased morbidity and may develop end-stage renal disease requiring transplantation

Pediatric Hypertension

INTRODUCTION

- The National High Blood Pressure Education Program Working Group (NHBPEP) established guidelines for the definition of normal and elevated blood pressures in children
- Blood pressure percentiles are based on gender, age, and height based on measurements on three separate occasions
- Evidence suggests that essential hypertension begins in childhood as blood pressure in childhood predicts blood pressure in adulthood
- In children and adolescents with hypertension, 40–45% have left ventricular hypertrophy
- In pediatric autopsy series, elevations of blood pressure in children have been correlated with early development of fatty streaks and fibrous plaques in the aorta and coronary arteries

ETIOLOGY, EPIDEMIOLOGY, & RISK FACTORS

- Hypertension occurs in 1–3% of the pediatric population
- Essential, or primary, hypertension is unusual in infants, but incidence increases throughout childhood
- Most younger children with hypertension have a secondary cause
  - Renal-induced secondary hypertension accounts for 80% of cases in younger children and is related to abnormal activity of the renin-angiotensin-aldosterone system
  - The most common renal cause is vascular (eg, renal artery stenosis, fibromuscular dysplasia, abdominal coarctation of the aorta, Marfan syndrome), which occurs due to a disturbance in the circulation to one or both kidneys resulting in increased renin secretion
- Stage 1 hypertension: Systolic and/or diastolic blood pressure between the 95th percentile and 5 mmHg above the 99th percentile
- Stage 2 hypertension: Systolic and/or diastolic blood pressure greater than 99th percentile plus 5 mmHg
- Body size is the most important determinant of blood pressure in children and adolescents
  - Blood pressures among children and adolescents in the U.S. increased by an average of 1.4 mmHg and 3.3 mmHg, respectively, between 1988–1994 and 1999–2000, in part because of the increased prevalence of overweight and obese children

PATIENT PRESENTATION

- Usually asymptomatic; hypertension is found incidentally on routine exam
- Depending on the etiology, may present with failure to thrive, headache, unexplained seizures, unexplained congestive heart failure, palpitations, chest pain, sweating, flushing, weight gain or loss, stroke, or nephritis
- Renovascular hypertension may present with abrupt, progressive onset of severe hypertension, unilateral small kidney, abdominal bruit, and/or retinopathy and other signs of end-organ damage

DIFFERENTIAL DX

- Renal: Renovascular, glomerulonephritis, polycystic kidney disease, obstructive renal disease, infections, reflux nephropathy
- Cardiovascular: Arteriovenous malformation, coarctation of the aorta, arteritis
- Endocrine: Thyroid disease, congenital adrenal hyperplasia, hyperaldosteronism, corticosteroid excess, catecholamine excess, 17-hydroxylase deficiency
- Others (eg, drug exposure, fracture immobilization, burns, increased intracranial pressure, dysautonomia, obesity)

DIAGNOSTIC EVALUATION

- History should focus on:
  - Family history of hypertension, diabetes, obesity, sleep disorders, hyperlipidemia, stroke, myocardial infarction, and renal and endocrine diseases
  - Comorbid risk factors for cardiovascular disease, such as obesity and abnormal sleep patterns (eg, snoring, sleep apnea)
  - Drug history, including over-the-counter, prescription, or illicit drugs, smoking, and alcohol
- Diagnosis is based on elevated blood pressure for age, height, or weight on three separate occasions (taken with appropriate size cuff in a sitting position)
  - The cuff size should have a bladder width approximately 40% of the circumference of the upper arm midway between the olecranon and the acromion
  - The cuff bladder should cover 80–100% of the circumference of the upper arm
  - The bladder width-to-length ratio should be at least 1:2
- Assess for evidence of end-organ damage (eg, ophthalmologic exam for retinopathy, EKG or echocardiogram for left ventricular hypertrophy)
- Laboratory evaluation includes complete blood count, electrolytes, BUN, creatinine, fasting plasma glucose and lipids, peripheral renin activity, thyroid function, cortisol level, aldosterone level, urinalysis, and urine catecholamines
- Renal ultrasound is a useful screening for kidney size, architecture, and location
- Renal angiography or MRA if suspect renal artery stenosis

TREATMENT & MANAGEMENT

- Control blood pressure to prevent end-organ damage and further loss of renal function
- Nonpharmacologic therapy is recommended in children with stage 1 hypertension or prehypertension, particularly for essential hypertension: Weight control, exercise, sodium restriction, and avoidance of alcohol, tobacco, and illicit drugs
- Pharmacologic therapy is indicated for:
  - Symptomatic hypertension (HTN)
  - Stage 2 HTN or stage 1 HTN that persists despite nonpharmacologic therapy
  - Hypertensive target-organ damage, most often left ventricular hypertrophy
  - Stage 1 hypertension in patients with diabetes mellitus
  - Consider in those with dyslipidemia or cigarette smoking
- Antihypertensive medication is based on known or suspected etiology of hypertension:
  - ACE inhibitors for renin-mediated etiologies (never initiate ACE inhibitors without first ruling out bilateral renal artery stenosis; severe renal ischemia and damage may occur)
  - β-blockers are contraindicated in patients with asthma or heart block and should be used with caution in patients with diabetes
  - Calcium channel blockers are contraindicated in patients with sick sinus syndrome but may be the desired class in patients with asthma

PROGNOSIS & COMPLICATIONS

- Good prognosis if blood pressure is brought under control
- Long-term effects of uncontrolled hypertension have been studied in adults but have not been well studied in children; effects in adults include increased cardiovascular risk, stroke, retinopathy, and renal insufficiency
- Surgery offers cure in selected cases with low rates of recurrence
- Closely monitor kidney function during ACE inhibitor use; if deterioration in kidney function occurs, consider surgery

IgA Nephropathy

INTRODUCTION

- IgA nephropathy (Berger disease) is the most common cause of primary glomerulonephritis
- The most common worldwide cause of glomerular disease
- Patients may present at any age, but there is a peak incidence in the second and third decades of life

ETIOLOGY, EPIDEMIOLOGY, & RISK FACTORS

- IgA nephropathy results in IgA deposition in the mesangium and immune-mediated injury of the glomeruli
- The etiology is unknown; a combination of polyclonal stimulation of IgA plus structural anomalies of IgA may lead to mesangial deposition and glomerular injury
- Males are affected more commonly than females (ratio, 3:1)
- Mean age at presentation is 9 years
- Associated with HLA-BW35, HLA-B27, HLA-DR1, and HLA-DR4
- IgA nephropathy occurs with greatest frequency in Asians, Caucasians, and Native-Americans in the Southwestern U.S.
- Relatively rare in blacks

PATIENT PRESENTATION

- Hematuria occurs in nearly all patients
  - Microscopic hematuria in 100% of patients; macroscopic in 85%
  - Gross hematuria occurs episodically in conjunction with febrile illness
- Fever, malaise, and abdominal pain with episodic gross hematuria
- Most patients with IgA nephropathy present with either gross hematuria (single or recurrent), usually following an upper respiratory infection, or microscopic hematuria with or without mild proteinuria that is incidentally detected on a routine examination
- Rarely, patients may develop acute renal failure with or without oliguria; this is due to either crescentic IgA nephropathy or to gross hematuria causing tubular occlusion and/or damage by red blood cells
- Hypertension may be present

DIFFERENTIAL DX

- Acute poststreptococcal glomerulonephritis or other postinfectious glomerulonephritis disorders
- Hereditary nephritis
- Membranoproliferative glomerulonephritis
- Henoch-Schönlein purpura nephritis
- Benign hematuria
- Idiopathic hypercalciuria
- Urinary tract infection
- Renal trauma
- Urolithiasis

DIAGNOSTIC EVALUATION

- Urinalysis reveals hematuria and proteinuria (or just hematuria)
- Laboratory evaluation should include complete blood count, chemistries, BUN, serum creatinine, serum albumin, and serum cholesterol
- Serum IgA levels are often increased
- Serum C3, IgM, and IgG levels are generally normal
- Definitive diagnosis is established by kidney biopsy
  - The pathognomic finding is observed on immunofluorescence microscopy, which demonstrates prominent, globular deposits of IgA (often accompanied by C3 and IgG) in the mesangium and to a lesser degree along the glomerular capillary wall
  - Histologic findings in IgA nephropathy are indistinguishable from Henoch-Schönlein purpura

TREATMENT & MANAGEMENT

- No specific therapy exists
- Steroids and/or cytotoxic drugs are used if there is nephrotic-range proteinuria or if the patient presents with crescentic glomerulonephritis
- Fish oil supplementation has been found to delay progression in some studies
- Antihypertensive agents to control hypertension
- General interventions to slow progression of disease (not specific to IgA nephropathy) include blood pressure control, angiotensin-converting enzyme (ACE) inhibitors and/or angiotensin II receptor blockers (ARBs) in patients with proteinuria, and statin therapy in patients with chronic kidney disease and elevated cholesterol levels

PROGNOSIS & COMPLICATIONS

- Episodic gross hematuria persists for only a few days
- Progresses to chronic renal failure during adulthood in 50% of cases
- The remaining patients enter a sustained clinical remission or have persistent low-grade hematuria or proteinuria
- Children with moderate to severe proteinuria, hypertension, and renal biopsy showing crescents or sclerosis are at increased risk for renal insufficiency and have a poorer prognosis

Endocrinology

Congenital Hypothyroidism

INTRODUCTION

- Hypothyroidism is defined as a state in which the thyroid gland fails to secrete sufficient quantities of thyroid hormone
- Primary hypothyroidism results from a problem inherent to the gland
- Secondary or central hypothyroidism results from failure of pituitary stimulation of the thyroid gland
- Primary and central hypothyroidism can be either congenital or acquired

ETIOLOGY, EPIDEMIOLOGY, & RISK FACTORS

- 85% of cases are sporadic and occur due to thyroid dysgenesis (ectopic thyroid tissue is more common than thyroid aplasia or hypoplasia)
  - Rare cases of thyroid dysgenesis have been linked to loss of function mutations in the PAX-8 and TTF-2 (thyroid transcription factor) genes and transcription factor NKX2.1
- 15% of cases are due to hereditary defects in thyroid hormone synthesis, all of which are autosomal recessive disorders; the most common defect is in thyroid peroxidase activity
- Transient hypothyroidism of the newborn (as many as 40% of cases) may be due to maternal thyroid-blocking antibodies that cross the placenta, maternal use of antithyroid drugs, or iodine exposure (most commonly via betadine, which is used in surgical procedures, including Caesarian section deliveries)
  - More common in Europe
- Overall incidence of 1 in 4000 live births
- Girls are affected twice as often as boys
- There is some ethnic variability; Hispanics are affected more often than Caucasians; African-Americans are less commonly affected

PATIENT PRESENTATION

- Signs and symptoms may be attributed to other disorders because they tend to be nonspecific and may be minimal or absent in the newborn period (95% have few if any clinical manifestations)
- Open fontanel and widely open sutures
- Umbilical hernia in large infants
- Prolonged, unconjugated jaundice (over 7 days)
- Constipation
- Hypotonia
- Hoarse cry
- Feeding and sucking difficulties
- Excessive sleepiness
- Dry skin
- Birth weight and length are typically normal
- Absence of knee epiphysis (more common in males than females)

DIFFERENTIAL DX

- Congenital infections
- Intrauterine drug exposure
- Intestinal obstruction
- Physiologic jaundice
- CNS damage
- Congenital myopathies
- Dysmorphogenetic chromo-somal syndromes

DIAGNOSTIC EVALUATION

- The majority of cases are diagnosed through mandated state screening programs
  - Screening programs occur in all 50 United States, Canada, Israel, Japan, Australia, and New Zealand
  - Screening is usually with T_4; if abnormally low, TSH level is measured
- Thyroid function studies may be diagnostic
  - Low T_4 with high TSH is diagnostic of primary hypothyroidism
  - TSH elevation is absent in secondary (central) hypothyroidism and total T_4 may still be within the normal range; thus, free T_4 is better screen for those infants
  - The normal range for newborns is greater than for nonneonates
- Imaging includes thyroid ultrasound and radionuclide scanning with ^{99}Tc to assess thyroid location (ie, looking for ectopic thyroid tissue)
  - Radionuclide scanning with ^{123}I and perchlorate washout can also provide functional information (may identify some types of dyshormonogenesis)
- Initial evaluation should be completed within 2–5 days of birth to avoid long-term sequelae
- In children with central hypothyroidism, tests to evaluate the remainder of the pituitary axis are warranted (eg, growth hormone testing, MRI imaging of the pituitary)

TREATMENT & MANAGEMENT

- Treat with synthetic thyroid replacement (L-thyroxine)
  - Begin treatment as soon as diagnosis is confirmed and raise thyroid hormone concentration rapidly; delay in treatment may increase mental damage
  - Dose is 10–15 μg/kg/day (this is about 5 times the adult dose)
- Monitor for response to therapy
  - Check T_4 and TSH at 4–6 weeks after any dose change to see if further correction is needed
  - Otherwise, monitor T_4 and TSH every 3 months during the first 2 years of life and every 6 months thereafter
  - Keep serum T_4 concentration in the upper half of the normal range and TSH in the normal range
  - Maintain normal growth and development, but avoid overtreatment
  - If hypothyroidism is presumed to be transient, wait until 2 years of age (when brain growth is done) to attempt weaning from medication

PROGNOSIS & COMPLICATIONS

- Neurologic sequelae will occur in the absence of early replacement therapy, including mental retardation, poor motor coordination, muscular hypotonia, and ataxia
- Mental retardation is usually avoided with early hormone replacement
- The earlier the replacement therapy is initiated, the better the prognosis
- Even with treatment, subtler psychomotor dysfunction, such as learning disabilities, may still occur
- Cretinism is an older term used to describe untreated patients

Acquired Hypothyroidism

INTRODUCTION

- Hypothyroidism is defined as a state in which the thyroid gland fails to secrete sufficient quantities of thyroid hormone to meet the body's demands
  - Primary hypothyroidism results from a problem inherent to the gland
  - Secondary or central hypothyroidism results from failure of pituitary stimulation to the thyroid gland
- Primary and central hypothyroidism can be either congenital or acquired
  - Acquired hypothyroidism appears after the newborn period
  - Certain types of congenital and acquired hypothyroidism are familial

ETIOLOGY, EPIDEMIOLOGY, & RISK FACTORS

- In the U.S., hypothyroidism is most commonly due to autoimmune destruction of the thyroid, known as Hashimoto thyroiditis (also called chronic lymphocytic thyroiditis); occurs due to a defect in cell-mediated immunity resulting in lymphocytic infiltration of the thyroid gland
- Other causes of acquired hypothyroidism include iodine deficiency (the most common cause worldwide), iatrogenic (eg, neck irradiation, surgical thyroidectomy, some medications such as lithium and amiodarone), and subacute thyroiditis (postviral)
- Central hypothyroidism is due to deficiencies of TSH or TRH and may be caused by CNS cancer or irradiation, congenital malformations, or trauma; it is frequently associated with other pituitary hormone deficiencies
- Prevalence is estimated at 0.1–0.2% of schoolchildren in the U.S.
- Antithyroid antibodies are found in 1% of schoolchildren, although this does not always lead to abnormal thyroid function tests
- Hashimoto thyroiditis is 5–10 times more common in girls than boys
- Hashimoto thyroiditis occurs more often in patients with chromosomal or genetic syndromes (eg, Down syndrome, Turner syndrome) and autoimmune diseases (eg, type 1 diabetes mellitus, polyglandular autoimmune syndrome)

PATIENT PRESENTATION

- Fatigue (naps, voluntary early bedtimes), decreased energy, decreased activity
- Decreased linear growth velocity with delayed skeletal maturation: delayed dental age/eruption, delayed onset of puberty (although severe cases can cause central precocious puberty)
- Increased weight gain, although generally not morbid obesity
- Cold intolerance
- Constipation
- Coarse hair, dry skin
- Dull facial expression
- Delayed relaxation of deep tendon reflexes
- Poor school performance
- Goiter may or may not be present
- Irregular menses in adolescent girls
- Bradycardia
- May present with symptoms of thyrotoxicosis

DIFFERENTIAL DX

- Mononucleosis
- Depression
- Panhypopituitarism (central hypothyroidism)
- Illicit drug use
- Thyroid cancer
- Thyroglossal duct cyst
- Anemia
- Celiac disease
- Hepatitis
- Inflammatory bowel disease

DIAGNOSTIC EVALUATION

- Thyroid function studies reveal elevated thyroid-stimulating hormone (TSH) with low T_4 (in central hypothyroidism, free T_4 is low, total T_4 may still be normal, and TSH elevation cannot be mounted)
- Presence of antithyroglobulin and antimicrosomal antibodies suggests autoimmune thyroiditis (present in more than 80% of cases of Hashimoto disease)
- Autoimmune thyroiditis can be associated with autoimmune polyglandular syndrome; assess for signs of candidiasis, Addison disease, and diabetes mellitus
- Radionuclide imaging with ^{123}I can be helpful to distinguish between the differential diagnoses:
  - Can be used to locate areas of absent or ectopic thyroid gland
  - Can be used in infants with a small goiter in whom an enzymatic defect in thyroid hormone synthesis is suspected
  - The presence of reduced radionuclide uptake in normally located thyroid tissue of newborns supports a diagnosis of transient hypothyroidism, perhaps because of maternal antithyroid drug therapy
  - Benign thyroid nodules appear as "cold" areas with decreased uptake
- Fine-needle aspirate may be used to confirm the diagnosis and/or rule out thyroid cancer
- MRI of the hypothalamic and pituitary regions if suspect central hypothyroidism
- Laboratory testing may reveal anemia, elevated CPK, elevated cholesterol, and elevated triglycerides

TREATMENT & MANAGEMENT

- Thyroid hormone replacement with synthetic thyroid hormone (L-thyroxine)
  - Per kilogram body weight dosing is highest in infants and decreases during childhood to adulthood
- Monitor serum thyroxine concentrations and TSH every 6 months for adequacy of dosage and compliance
- Many children may experience school and behavior problems with increased energy and decreased attention when they become euthyroid

PROGNOSIS & COMPLICATIONS

- If the condition presents after 2–3 years of age, there is little risk of permanent intellectual impairment
- 20% of patients with autoimmune hypothyroidism may revert to normal
- The presence of antithyroid antibodies does not necessarily mean that clinical hypothyroidism will occur (antithyroid antibodies are found in 1% of school-age children, but only 0.1% manifest clinical hypothyroidism)
- Children with primary hypothyroidism and serum TSH >20 mU/L on two occasions will rarely recover normal thyroid function
- Hypothyroidism requires special attention in females who become pregnant to protect fetal neurodevelopment

Hyperthyroidism

INTRODUCTION

- Hyperthyroidism occurs due to excessive amounts of circulating thyroid hormone
- The synthesis of thyroid hormone is regulated through a central biological feedback system: Under the stimulation of hypothalamic thyrotropin-releasing hormone (TRH), the pituitary thyrotrophs secrete thyroid-stimulating hormone (TSH), which enters the circulation and binds to receptors on the thyroid gland to stimulate secretion of thyroid hormone (T_4); thyroid hormone then feeds back to the pituitary and hypothalamus to regulate TSH secretion
- The clinical manifestation of hyperthyroidism is called thyrotoxicosis

ETIOLOGY, EPIDEMIOLOGY, & RISK FACTORS

- May be congenital or acquired
- Autoimmune hyperthyroidism (Graves disease) is the most common etiology in children and newborns; it occurs due to autoantibodies directed against the TSH receptor
  - In newborns, the antibodies are maternal
- Other causes of hyperthyroidism include any cause of excessive hormone release, including acute or subacute thyroiditis, iodine overdose, the toxic thyroiditis stage of Hashimoto thyroiditis (antibody destruction of the gland leads initially to excessive release of thyroid hormones, followed by hypothyroidism), genetic activating mutations of the TSH receptor signaling (eg, McCune-Albright syndrome), and hyperfunctioning autonomous thyroid nodules
- Up to 60% of Graves disease patients have a positive family history of autoimmune thyroid disease (hyperthyroidism or hypothyroidism)
- Associated with HLA-DR; identical twin concordance is 40%
- The incidence increases in childhood and adolescence
- Increased incidence in females compared with males (ratio, 4:1)

PATIENT PRESENTATION

- A goiter is present in 98% of cases
- Poor school performance (hyperactivity, mood swings, poor attention span)
- Heat intolerance
- Nervousness
- Tremors
- Insomnia and daytime fatigue
- Increased appetite despite weight loss
- Menstrual irregularities
- Gastrointestinal hypermotility (occasional diarrhea)
- Exophthalmos, lid lag
- Bruit over thyroid
- Tachycardia and palpitations
- Increased pulse pressure
- Decreased exercise tolerance
- Hyperreflexia

DIFFERENTIAL DX

- Attention deficit hyperactivity disorder
- Stimulant use, including β-agonists
- Anxiety disorder
- Ingestion of exogenous thyroid hormone (ie, for weight loss purposes)
- Lymphoma
- Thyroglossal duct cyst
- Inflammatory bowel disease
- Manic disorder
- Carcinoid syndrome
- VIPoma
- Tachyarrhythmia

DIAGNOSTIC EVALUATION

- Thyroid function tests show increased circulating levels of free T_4, total T_4, and T_3
- In cases of primary hyperthyroidism, TSH is suppressed (abnormally low)
- In cases of secondary hyperthyroidism, T_4 is normal or increased, and TSH is increased
- Radionucleotide thyroid scan may be indicated to evaluate the etiology
  - Low uptake (less than 5%) suggests that hyperthyroidism is due to damage to thyroid or exogenous thyroid hormone ingestion
  - Increased uptake suggests Graves disease
  - Focal increased uptake indicates a hyperfunctioning nodule
- Antimicrosomal (thyroid peroxidase) and antithyroglobulin antibodies are present in autoimmune thyroid disease (Graves disease or lymphocytic thyroiditis)
  - Thyroid-stimulating immunoglobulins are more specific for Graves disease

TREATMENT & MANAGEMENT

- The treatment plan depends on age and severity of disease
- First-line treatment is antithyroid drugs (propylthiouracil or methimazole)
  - Toxic side effects of antithyroid drugs include granulopenia, dermatitis, arthritis, hepatitis, and vasculitis
- β-blockers are used temporarily to decrease adrenergic symptoms until thyroid function is stabilized
- Radioiodine ablation should be considered if antithyroid drugs are not tolerated or homeostasis cannot be achieved after 2 years of drug therapy
- Surgery to remove thyroid tissue may be indicated for thyroid cancer or as an alternative to radioactive iodine
- Neonatal Graves disease is treated with propylthiouracil and steroids

PROGNOSIS & COMPLICATIONS

- 30% of cases of Graves disease remit within 2 years; thus, medical management is preferred to surgery
- Therapeutic hypothyroidism (induced by surgery or radioactive iodine treatments) requires lifelong exogenous hormone replacement and monitoring of thyroxine levels
- Thyroid storm (abrupt onset of severe hyperthyroidism) is an endocrine emergency
  - May be produced by surgery or radioactive iodine treatment
  - Results in hyperthermia, high output cardiac failure, and altered mental status
  - Treat with iodide (Lugol solution), steroids, and propranolol
  - Associated with 40–60% mortality

Diabetes Mellitus

INTRODUCTION

- Type 1 (insulin-dependent) diabetes mellitus is a common, serious disease of childhood and adolescence
- Developments since the 1980s have made the attainment of metabolic control a technical possibility, but management is stressful to the family and compliance may be poor; psychological and behavioral issues interfere with the goal of metabolic control
- The prevalence of type 1 diabetes in U.S. children is 1.2–1.9 cases per 1000 children; worldwide variations exist, with the U.S. having an intermediate incidence
- Insulin is the body's major anabolic hormone; in the fed state, it stimulates energy storage as glycogen, protein, and fat

ETIOLOGY, EPIDEMIOLOGY, & RISK FACTORS

- Glucose is toxic to nerve cells (resulting in neuropathy), blood vessels (resulting in heart disease, kidney disease, peripheral vascular disease, hypertension, impotence in adult men), retinal cells (blindness), and many other cell types
- Insulin is required to shuttle glucose into cells, thereby lowering blood glucose levels and limiting the toxic effects of glucose
- Type 1 diabetes is caused by autoimmune destruction of the insulin-producing beta-cells of the pancreas, resulting in significant insulin deficiency; patients require insulin
  - The majority of childhood cases are type 1, with peak incidences at ages 5–7 and puberty
  - More new cases occur during the winter months
  - 5–15% have family history; 40% identical twin concordance
- Type 2 diabetes is due to impaired insulin secretion ("burnout" of beta-cells), insulin resistance (at the level of peripheral insulin receptors), and increased hepatic glucose production; patients may or may not require insulin
  - Type 2 diabetes is increasing in adolescents and preadolescents due to obesity, sedentary lifestyles, and poor diets; 2–3 times higher prevalence in minority groups
  - 80% have a family history
- Other etiologies of diabetes include cystic fibrosis and certain medications (eg, steroids)

PATIENT PRESENTATION

Type 1 Diabetes
- Polyuria and polydipsia are generally the first symptoms
- New-onset nocturia or enuresis
- Polyphagia or anorexia, weight loss
- Dehydration
- Abdominal pain and vomiting
- Vaginitis secondary to glucosuria
- Intermittent blurry vision
- Diabetic ketoacidosis (DKA), a metabolic hyperosmolar acidosis with ketonuria, may occur

Type 2 Diabetes
- Obesity
- Acanthosis nigricans
- Polyuria, polydipsia
- Vaginitis
- Intermittent blurry vision

DIFFERENTIAL DX

- Hyperglycemia due to stress (eg, trauma, infection)
- Benign glucosuria
- Iatrogenic (eg, corticosteroid use, excessive administration of dextrose in IV fluids)
- Urinary tract infection
- Acute abdomen (when abdominal pain is present)
- Maturity-onset diabetes of youth (MODY) syndromes

DIAGNOSTIC EVALUATION

- Diagnosed based on characteristic symptoms plus abnormal serum glucose values
  - Diabetes is defined by a random blood glucose >200 mg/dL or fasting blood glucose (8-hour fast) >126 mg/dL
  - Impaired glucose tolerance ("prediabetes") is defined by fasting glucose of 100–125 mg/dL or postprandial glucose of 140–200 mg/dL
- Diabetic ketoacidosis is diagnosed by the presence of hyperglycemia with serum or urine ketones and metabolic acidosis
  - Associated with total-body potassium and phosphorus depletion
  - Determine acid-base status by arterial pH, respiratory rate, and anion gap
  - Assess volume status by change in weight, skin turgor, and moistness of mucus membranes
- Although not yet used for diagnosis, 80% of type 1 diabetes patients have positive antibodies to glutamic acid decarboxylase (GAD65) or autoantibodies against insulin or islet cells
- Type 2 diabetics may have initial hyperinsulinemia; eventual "burnout" of pancreatic beta-cells will occur, resulting in hypoinsulinemia
- C peptide levels may be indicated to differentiate type 1 from type 2 diabetes
- Hemoglobin A_{1c} is a measure of average blood glucose levels over the past 3 months

TREATMENT & MANAGEMENT

- Type 1 diabetes is treated with exogenous insulin (injections or pump infusion)
  - Rapid-acting, short duration: Regular insulin or Lispro
  - Intermediate-acting, medium duration: NPH or Lente
  - Long-acting: Ultralente or glargine
  - Combinations: 70/30 (70% NPH/30% regular), 75/25 (75% NPH/25% Lispro)
  - Insulin dose is determined by weight, caloric intake, and blood glucose levels throughout the day
  - Diet and exercise should be encouraged to increase insulin sensitivity
  - Annual eye exam and urine microalbumin levels should be checked
- Diabetic ketoacidosis is treated with fluids, insulin, and electrolyte replacement
  - Fluid replacement: assume 7–10% dehydration for moderate to severe cases; use isotonic solution and replace gradually, unless the patient is hypotensive
  - Insulin is typically given as continuous infusion (start at 0.1 unit/kg/hr); delay the insulin infusion for 1 hour after starting fluid replacement to prevent cerebral edema
  - Replace total-body phosphorus, potassium and sodium
- Type 2 diabetes is treated with weight loss (caloric restriction and regular exercise), oral hypoglycemic medications, and insulin in advanced cases

PROGNOSIS & COMPLICATIONS

- Glycemic control should be measured by Hb_{A1c} levels every 3 months
- Patients with good glycemic control have much better prognosis (Hb_{A1c} less than 8%)
- Poor glycemic control may result in end-organ complications (eg, retinopathy, nephropathy, neuropathy)
- Patients receiving insulin are at risk for hypoglycemia and should be educated about symptoms (sweating, dizziness, pallor, hunger, change in mental status) and treatment
- Hyperglycemia and ketonuria may lead to dehydration and ketoacidosis; each episode is acutely life threatening
- Type 1 patients at risk for other autoimmune diseases (eg, celiac disease, hypothyroidism)
- Type 2 can be associated with depression and other psychiatric morbidities

Hypoglycemia

INTRODUCTION

- Hypoglycemia is a common and treatable cause of encephalopathy in children
- Glucose is a critical substrate for energy production in the brain; when glucose availability is interrupted, significant central nervous system dysfunction results and may be permanent
- The goal of diagnosis and treatment is the prevention of acute and chronic episodes of hypoglycemia

ETIOLOGY, EPIDEMIOLOGY, & RISK FACTORS

- Etiologies include transient neonatal hypoglycemia (due to immaturity of glucose homeostasis), exogenous hyperinsulinemia (eg, overadministration of insulin with therapeutic intent, factitious insulin administration), endogenous hyperinsulinemia (eg, infant of diabetic mother, congenital hyperinsulinism, insulin-secreting tumor, islet cell tumor), inborn errors of metabolism, hormone deficiencies (eg, cortisol, growth hormone), toxins (eg, alcohol, aspirin, plant or drug ingestion), sepsis (especially due to malaria), asphyxia or anoxia, severe liver dysfunction, malabsorption, post-transfusion, and prolonged fasting
- Persistent neonatal hypoglycemia is most often caused by congenital hyperinsulinism, which occurs due to genetic defects in the regulation of insulin secretion
- Neonatal hypoglycemia occurs in 4 out of 1000 live births
- Persistent hypoglycemia occurs in 4 out of 10,000 live births
- There has been a decrease in iatrogenic hypoglycemia over the last 3 decades due to early neonatal feeding and advances in the treatment of childhood diarrhea

PATIENT PRESENTATION

- Symptoms due to excess catecholamines:
  - Nonapocrine sweating (eg, upper lip, hands)
  - Shakiness
  - Tachycardia
  - Anxiety
  - Weakness
  - Hunger, nausea
- Symptoms due to low cerebral glucose:
  - Headache
  - Visual disturbances
  - Mental confusion, speech difficulty, poor concentration,
  - Lethargy, irritability
  - Seizures, coma, death
- Newborns and infants:
  - Apnea, cyanotic episodes, somnolence
  - Brief myoclonic jerks, convulsions
  - Sweating

DIFFERENTIAL DX

- Deficits of glucose production:
  - Glycogen storage diseases
  - Amino acid metabolism defects
  - Glucose synthesis defect
  - Fatty acid oxidation defects
- Beckwith-Wiedemann syndrome
- Panhypopituitarism

DIAGNOSTIC EVALUATION

- Defined as serum glucose <60 mg/dL
- In-patient fasting study is gold standard diagnostic test
- Serum studies (when symptoms are present or at end of fasting study) include testing for insulin, ketones, alcohol, growth hormone, cortisol, lactate, and free fatty acids; C peptide levels may be measured to rule out factitious insulin use
- Urine should be examined for ketones, toxins, and drugs; if no ketones are present, suspect hyperinsulinemia or a defect in fatty acid oxidation
- Glucagon stimulation test may be done at the time of documented hypoglycemia; an increased glucose response suggests hyperinsulinism
- Pyruvate, amino acids, ammonia, and genetic testing are indicated if an inborn error of metabolism is suspected

TREATMENT & MANAGEMENT

- Initial treatment is IV dextrose solution
  - Administer a mini-bolus of IV dextrose
  - Continue IV infusion until glucose is stable; then slowly wean
  - Avoid high concentrations to prevent hyperglycemia
  - Intramuscular glucagon may be used in an emergency if there is no IV access; this is only helpful if hypoglycemia is due to excessive insulin of any cause
- Subsequent treatment depends on the diagnosis:
  - Congenital hyperinsulinism: Diazoxide, octreotide, or subtotal pancreatectomy
  - Diabetes: Insulin adjustment and patient education
  - Hormonal deficiency: Specific hormone replacement
  - Metabolic conditions: Avoid prolonged fasting, night feedings may be required, uncooked cornstarch in feeds may allow for prolonged release of usable dietary sugars

PROGNOSIS & COMPLICATIONS

- Recurrent or severe hypoglycemia may result in repeated seizures, and long-term neuro-logic sequelae may occur
- Recurrent hypoglycemia can lead to loss of symptoms, such that episodes occur silently; however, asymptomatic hypoglycemic episodes remain just as dangerous as when symptomatic
- Immature glucose homeostasis may result in hypoglycemia
  - In neonates, spontaneous resolution occurs within 48 hours
  - Ketotic hypoglycemia resolves by age 9 years

Diabetes Insipidus

INTRODUCTION

- Diabetes insipidus (DI) is the result of decreased secretion or ineffective action of antidiuretic hormone, resulting in the inability to reabsorb water in the renal collecting ducts
- Antidiuretic hormone (known as ADH or vasopressin) is released from the posterior pituitary by neurons originating in the hypothalamic supraoptic and periventricular nuclei
- ADH release is mediated through osmoreceptors and baroreceptors; secretion increases in response to hypovolemia and hyperosmolarity
- ADH acts by increasing water reabsorption in the kidneys
- Water resorption results in decreased urine volume and increased urine osmolarity

ETIOLOGY, EPIDEMIOLOGY, & RISK FACTORS

- Central diabetes insipidus is due to decreased secretion of ADH from the pituitary gland
  - 30–50% of cases are idiopathic; other causes include neurosurgery, trauma, primary or secondary tumors, or infiltrative diseases (eg, Langerhans cell histiocytosis)
  - Rare causes include postsupraventricular tachycardia, anorexia nervosa, and Wolfram syndrome (characterized by diabetes insipidus, type 1 diabetes mellitus, optic atrophy, and deafness)
- Nephrogenic diabetes insipidus is due to decreased ADH action due to insensitivity at the renal tubules
  - Most cases are hereditary: X-linked disease may occur due to mutations in the AVPR2 gene; autosomal recessive and dominant diseases may occur due to mutations in the aquaporin-2 gene
  - May also be caused by chronic lithium use and hypercalcemia
- Secondary diabetes insipidus may occur due to "wash out" of the renal concentration gradient by excessive intake of fluids or other disease process
- A rare disease in children

PATIENT PRESENTATION

- Infants: Failure to thrive, fever, vomiting, and constipation
- Children: Excessive drinking, nocturia, polyuria, and nocturnal enuresis
- Central diabetes insipidus: Headache, ocular signs (eg, diminished visual fields, optic atrophy, strabismus, nystagmus), and may also present with symptoms related to deficiency of other pituitary hormones (eg, hypoglycemia, short stature)

DIFFERENTIAL DX

Central DI
- Trauma, infection, hypoxia/ischemia, CNS tumors
- Post-CNS surgery
- Wolfram syndrome
- ADH gene defect or congenital CNS malformations

Nephrogenic DI
- Drugs
- Genetic

Secondary/Syndromic Disease
- Polydipsia
- Diabetes mellitus
- Hypercalcemia/hypokalemia
- Sickle cell disease
- Renal disease and postobstructive diuresis

DIAGNOSTIC EVALUATION

- Screening includes serum and urine osmolality; urinalysis; and serum sodium, potassium, calcium, glucose, and BUN
  - Serum hypertonicity with inappropriate urine hypotonicity is diagnostic
  - Serum osmolality >300 mOsm with urine osmolality <300 mOsm is suggestive of the diagnosis
- Water deprivation test may be used when serum osmolality is <300 mOsm; the test is done by restricting water and then injecting ADH
  - Normal response is increased urine concentration and maintenance of normal serum osmolality during water restriction with no response to the injected ADH (because maximum concentration has already been achieved by endogenous ADH)
  - In central diabetes insipidus, there is no increase in urine concentration despite rising serum osmolality during water restriction; there is a positive response to the ADH injection (ie, urine concentration increases)
  - In nephrogenic diabetes insipidus, there is no increase in urine concentration during water restriction and no response to the ADH injection
- For patients with central diabetes insipidus, an MRI of the brain may be indicated to visualize the posterior pituitary and rule out tumors

TREATMENT & MANAGEMENT

- Central diabetes insipidus is treated with a long-acting vasopressin analog (desmopressin), which may be administered intranasally (spray) or orally (tablet), and diuresis of excessive free water
  - Avoid desmopressin treatment in infants until they can eat solids; instead, treat with free water replacement
  - Salt and free water must be carefully titrated
- Nephrogenic diabetes insipidus is treated with a low-salt diet, thiazide diuretics, and amiloride (a potassium-sparing diuretic that has an additive effect with thiazides)
- After CNS surgeries, careful hourly balance of inputs and outputs must be maintained to assess for the development of diabetes insipidus
  - Beware of a triphasic response in patients with craniopharyngioma or other tumors: First, diabetes insipidus; followed by SIADH due to hormone leakage in the injured and dying posterior pituitary cells; ultimately resulting in diabetes insipidus when the pituitary cells have died

PROGNOSIS & COMPLICATIONS

- Central diabetes insipidus associated with neurosurgery can be transient
- Diabetes insipidus generally does not result in significant morbidity or mortality if thirst mechanism is intact and sufficient water is available
- Infants are difficult to treat because their diet is liquid, so hunger and thirst drives can lead to inappropriate water or caloric intake
- Children without intact thirst mechanisms are much more challenging because they cannot self-regulate (ie, they do not know to drink more water in times of increased losses, as occurs during illness)
- Dilutional hyponatremia and seizures may result from exogenous vasopressin administration

Syndrome of Inappropriate ADH

INTRODUCTION

- Antidiuretic hormone (ADH) plays an important role in responding to changes in extracellular volume by altering renal clearance of free water to maintain appropriate serum tonicity
- ADH release from the posterior pituitary gland is influenced by changes in plasma osmolarity and effective circulating blood volume
- Hypothalamic osmoreceptors maintain osmolarity over a narrow range
- Alterations of 1–2% signal ADH secretion
- Response to volume changes in the carotid body or left atrium is less sensitive

ETIOLOGY, EPIDEMIOLOGY, & RISK FACTORS

- Syndrome of inappropriate ADH (SIADH) occurs when there is interference in the osmotic suppression of ADH, resulting in unchecked water reabsorption
- Normal sodium excretion and retained water results in serum hyponatremia and highly concentrated urine
- Etiologies include:
  - Cerebral trauma, cerebrovascular accident, hemorrhage, infection, or tumor
  - Ectopic secretion of ADH (eg, small-cell carcinoma of the lung, cancer of the duodenum or pancreas, or olfactory neuroblastoma), which is rare in children
  - Psychiatric disease (eg, psychosis)
  - Pneumonia: Viral (eg, respiratory syncytial virus), bacterial, or tuberculous
  - Drugs (eg, chlorpropamide, vincristine, imipramine, phenothiazines, ciprofloxacin)
  - Iatrogenic (excess administration of ADH)
  - Major abdominal or thoracic surgery (increased ADH meditated through pain afferents)
- 15% of children with CNS injury or infection have SIADH

PATIENT PRESENTATION

- Seizures and coma
- Confusion
- Nausea
- Headaches
- Malaise
- Lethargy
- Anorexia
- Typically edema is not seen
- Symptoms do not necessarily depend on the concentration of serum sodium but instead on its rate of change; gradual development of hyponatremia may be asymptomatic

DIFFERENTIAL DX

- Inappropriate atrial natriuretic peptide (IANP) (cerebral salt wasting)
- NaCl losses (eg, vomiting, diarrhea, advanced renal failure, thiazide drugs)
- Postoperative hyponatremia
- Adrenal insufficiency
- Polydipsia
- Congestive heart failure
- Cirrhosis
- Nephrotic syndrome
- Severe burns
- Lung disease (eg, pneumonia, cystic fibrosis, bronchopulmonary dysplasia, asthma)
- Dehydration

DIAGNOSTIC EVALUATION

- Normovolemic, hyponatremia (sodium <135 mmol/L) is the hallmark of SIADH
  - Tears are present, normal mucus membranes, no tachycardia signifies normovolemia
- Hypo-osmolality
- Inappropriately high urine sodium
- Improvement with fluid restriction is required for diagnosis
- Increased serum ADH (vasopressin)
- Frequently confused with inappropriate atrial natriuretic peptide (cerebral salt wasting)
  - These two conditions differ in serum volemia and urine output
  - SIADH is euvolemic or hypervolemic; treat with fluid restriction
  - Inappropriate atrial natriuretic peptide is hypovolemic; treat with fluid replacement

TREATMENT & MANAGEMENT

- Treat the underlying disease process
- Slow correction of hyponatremia (10% increase in sodium per 24 hours) is essential; acute treatment of hyponatremia is only indicated if cerebral dysfunction is present
- Fluid restriction is the mainstay of therapy: Restrict intake to less than urinary output plus insensible losses; insensible losses are 800–1000 mL/m^2/day
- Hypertonic saline solution (3% NaCl) may be used in cases of severe hyponatremia or hyponatremia resistant to correction by fluid restriction
- Demeclocycline (an ADH antagonist) may be used to induce a nephrogenic diabetes insipidus to balance fluid
- Furosemide may be given simultaneously to ensure diuresis and excretion of dilute urine

PROGNOSIS & COMPLICATIONS

- Severe hyponatremia may be fatal
- Overly rapid correction of hyponatremia may be fatal or may result in central pontine myelinolysis (CPM)
- CPM is characterized by spastic quadriparesis, ataxia, abnormal extraocular movements, swallowing dysfunction, and mutism
- Young children under chronic fluid restriction may not consume adequate calories for growth; consider nutrition consult and/or alternate therapies

Congenital Adrenal Hyperplasia

INTRODUCTION

- Congenital adrenal hyperplasia (CAH) is a family of diseases caused by an inherited deficiency of any of the enzymes needed in cortisol biosynthesis
- These enzymes, except 3-beta-hydroxysteroid dehydrogenase, are members of the cytochrome P450 family; the cytochromes are microsomal and mitochondrial terminal oxidases involved in electron transport and require NAD and flavoproteins as cofactors

ETIOLOGY, EPIDEMIOLOGY, & RISK FACTORS

- CAH occurs due to defects in the synthesis of cortisol from cholesterol precursors
- 90% of cases are due to 21-hydroxylase deficiency, which is responsible for conversion of 17-hydroxyprogesterone to 11-deoxycortisol
- Cortisol deficiency causes ACTH hypersecretion, which results in adrenal hyperplasia, overproduction of precursors, and increased steroids in alternative pathways
- Three types of CAH exist: Classic salt-losing disease (complete enzyme deficiency), classic simple virilizing/non–salt-losing disease (partial enzyme deficiency), and nonclassic form (mild disease, late onset)
- Worldwide incidence of classic disease is 1 in 15,000
- Inherited as autosomal recessive transmission

PATIENT PRESENTATION

Classic Salt-Losing Disease (Severe)
- Virilization of newborn females (ambiguous genitalia)
- Hyperpigmentation of areolar and scrotal area in males with nondescended testes
- Adrenal crisis occurs at 7–10 days post delivery: Progressive lethargy, emesis, seizures, metabolic acidosis, hyponatremia, hyperkalemia, hypoglycemia, hypotension or shock, death

Classic Simple (Non–Salt-Losing) Disease
- Rapid growth and advanced bone age
- Virilization
- Early adrenarche
- Enlarged phallus

Nonclassic Disease
- Precocious adrenarche or hirsutism
- Acne and menstrual irregularity

DIFFERENTIAL DX

Neonatal Ambiguous Genitalia
- Congenital adrenal hyperplasia
- Adrenal hypoplasia
- Gonadal dysgenesis
- Pituitary/CNS defects (present with micropenis more than ambiguity of genitalia)
- Prenatal drug or androgen exposure
- Androgen insensitivity

Adolescent Onset
- Polycystic ovarian syndrome
- Idiopathic hirsutism
- Virilizing tumors

DIAGNOSTIC EVALUATION

- Prenatal/newborn diagnosis is possible via chorionic villous sampling and molecular genetic analysis by 8 weeks after conception; 17-hydroxyprogesterone has become part of newborn screening panels

Classic Diseases
- Elevated serum 17-OH-progesterone and androstenedione are diagnostic of 21-hydroxylase deficiency
- Elevated urinary 17-ketosteroids is an older test that is no longer performed
- Elevated ACTH and plasma renin activity despite low cortisol and aldosterone indicate defects in glucocorticoid and mineralocortico pathways, respectively
- Other subtypes are characterized by specific patterns of adrenal precursors and products

Nonclassic Diseases
- Basal 17-OH-progesterone may be normal
- ACTH stimulation test may bring out an abnormally high 17-OH-progesterone response

TREATMENT & MANAGEMENT

Classic Diseases
- Hydrocortisone (glucocorticoid) and fludrocortisone (mineralocorticoid) replacement
- Monitor for adequate growth and further virilization via 17-OH progesterone, androstene-dione, and testosterone levels and bone age to monitor growth acceleration
- Monitor mineralocorticoid action with electrolytes and plasma renin activity
- Ambiguous genitalia may require surgery; sex determination is made by multidisciplinary team evaluation of potential for normal sexual function

Nonclassic Disease
- The severity of symptoms determines whether treatment is necessary.
- Glucocorticoid replacement with prednisone or hydrocortisone
- Antiandrogens (eg, spironolactone) can be used to slow bone maturation in children and treat hirsutism in adult women with nonclassic disease
- If diagnosed prenatally, administer oral dexamethasone to the mother (must monitor for steroid-induced diabetes and hypertension) to prevent virilization of the genitalia of female fetuses (applies to both classic and nonclassic forms)

PROGNOSIS & COMPLICATIONS

- In classic disease, there may be difficulty in adjusting medications, which may result in poorly treated hyperandrogenism and/or iatrogenic hypercortisolism
  - Short stature and infertility may result; men may develop testicular and adrenal tumors
  - Psychological effects of excess testosterone may occur
  - Adequately treated patients should have no fertility or pregnancy issues
- In nonclassic disease, abrupt cessation of corticosteroid replacement may result in adrenal crisis
  - Long-term corticosteroid therapy (classic or nonclassic) suppresses ACTH; increased (stress) dosing is required to prevent adrenal crisis during intercurrent illness or surgery

Addison Disease

INTRODUCTION

- Addison's disease is defined as primary adrenal failure
- The adrenal glands produce 3 classes of steroid hormones: glucocorticoids (cortisol), mineralocorticoids (aldosterone), and androgens
  - Primary adrenal failure affects all three hormone lines
  - Secondary (central) adrenal failure principally involves the glucocorticoids
- In most cases, symptoms of the deficiencies develop slowly
- ACTH is a proteolytic cleavage product of the anterior pituitary prohormone, propiomelanocortin; other cleavage products include beta-endorphin and melanocyte stimulating hormone (MSH)
  - The loss of negative feedback leading to ACTH elevation also leads to increased MSH and skin hyperpigmentation, an important clinical clue for Addison's disease

ETIOLOGY, EPIDEMIOLOGY, & RISK FACTORS

- Adrenal insufficiency (cortisol and aldosterone deficiency) occurs due to destruction or hypoplasia of adrenal cortex tissue
- May be congenital or acquired
- Primary adrenal insufficiency is most commonly due to an autoimmune process
- Other causes include genetic (eg, congenital hypoplasia, adrenoleukodystrophy), ACTH insensitivity, infections (eg, meningococcemia, HIV, tuberculosis), perinatal trauma, infections, or tumors
- Secondary adrenal insufficiency is caused by inadequate ACTH stimulation of the adrenal cortex and may be caused by hypopituitarism, cessation of steroid treatment, removal of a cortisol-producing tumor, and infants born to steroid-treated mothers
- Rare in children; equal incidence in males and females
- May result from mutations of the autoimmune regulator gene, which causes APECED (autoimmune polyglandular syndrome type 1)
- The disease appears to be HLA-DR related

PATIENT PRESENTATION

- Fatigue and weakness
- Weight loss
- Anorexia
- Nausea/vomiting
- Dehydration
- Salt craving
- Hyperpigmentation of skin and mucous membranes (eg, lip borders and buccal mucosa, palm and scrotal creases, nipples, absence of "tan lines" over the buttocks/genitals)
- Delayed or decreased pubic and axillary hair (adrenarche is controlled by the adrenals)
- Patient may present in "adrenal crisis" with hypotension and shock or death

DIFFERENTIAL DX

- APECED (autoimmune polyendocrinopathy, candidiasis, and ectodermal dystrophy)
- Withdrawal of long-term systemic corticosteroid therapy
- Hypothalamic/pituitary defect (eg, craniopharyngioma, radiation injury)
- Infection
  - Meningococcemia (Waterhouse-Friderichsen syndrome)
  - Tuberculosis
  - Fungal infections

DIAGNOSTIC EVALUATION

- Low plasma cortisol level despite elevated ACTH is diagnostic (check in the morning or when symptomatic)
- ACTH stimulation test is diagnostic
  - Measures cortisol release from the adrenal cortex 1 hour after cosyntropin (synthetic ACTH) administration
  - Normal response: Increased cortisol levels
  - Addison response: Cortisol levels do not increase sufficiently
  - Similarly, mineralocorticoid deficiency is characterized by low aldosterone but high plasma renin activity
- Antiadrenal autoantibodies may be elevated
- CT scan or MRI of the adrenals may show calcifications following hemorrhage
- Rule out other infections (tuberculosis, HIV)
- Rule out metabolic disease of very long–chain fatty acids (adrenoleukodystrophy)
- Adrenal crisis may result in hypotension or shock following minor injury or illness
  - Hyperkalemia, hyponatremia, hypoglycemia, metabolic acidosis, eosinophilia, and increased plasma renin may be present during the crisis

TREATMENT & MANAGEMENT

- Hormone replacement, including glucocorticoids (hydrocortisone) and mineralocorticoids (fludrocortisone)
  - Monitor clinical improvement and electrolytes, ACTH, and renin levels for adequacy of treatment
- Patients must have stress doses of steroids (3–4 times higher concentration than the maintenance dose) in situations of stress (eg, infection, trauma, surgery)
- For adrenal crisis, obtain blood for diagnosis, and empirically treat shock and hypotension emergently with normal saline, dextrose, and hydrocortisone intravenously (do not wait for hormone results)
- Medical alert identifier should be worn at all times

PROGNOSIS & COMPLICATIONS

- Adrenal crisis (Addisonian crisis) is an acute exacerbation of adrenal insufficiency due to stresses that necessitate increased levels of cortisol
  - Typical causes include infection, fever, shock, surgery, trauma, gastrointestinal upset (vomiting, diarrhea), and strenuous physical exertion (eg, running a marathon)
  - Symptoms include nausea, vomiting, severe abdominal pain, lethargy, somnolence, dehydration, unresponsiveness, and hypotension; may rarely present as sudden death
  - Treatment includes immediate IV glucocorticoid infusion and rapid replacement of sodium, glucose, and water deficits
- With appropriate treatment, long-term prognosis is good

Amenorrhea

INTRODUCTION

- Menstrual disorders are common during adolescence
- Amenorrhea is defined as the complete absence of menses
- Regulation of menstrual function is a complex and delicate process and perturbations at any point can result in amenorrhea; the organs most responsible for normal menstrual flow are the hypothalamus, pituitary, ovaries, uterus, and vagina
- Thyroid and adrenal dysfunction can also create menstrual irregularities

ETIOLOGY, EPIDEMIOLOGY, & RISK FACTORS

- Primary amenorrhea is defined as absence of menarche by age 16
- Because menarche normally occurs within a set sequence of pubertal progression, amenorrhea should be evaluated according to the extent of sexual development:
  - Full secondary sex characteristics versus partial or incomplete sexual development
  - Estrogen-influenced (breast) versus androgen-influenced (pubic and axillary hair, acne, hirsutism) sexual development
- Secondary amenorrhea is defined as cessation of menses for at least 6 months during or beyond the third postmenarchal year
- Pregnancy is the most common etiology of amenorrhea
- Turner syndrome is the most common pathologic etiology (1 in 3000)
- Congenital absence of the vagina and absent/rudimentary uterus occurs in 1 in 5,000 newborn girls (Mayer-Rokitansky-Kuster-Hauser syndrome)
- Constitutional delay in puberty is a common reason for primary amenorrhea; assess for family history of late puberty
- Any chronic illness, particularly those that affect growth and nutrition, can affect the hypothalamic-pituitary axis and cause amenorrhea (eg, inflammatory bowel disease, cystic fibrosis, chronic renal failure, eating disorders, stress, strenuous exercise)

PATIENT PRESENTATION

- Presentation varies based on etiology
- Imperforate hymen: Urinary difficulties, cyclic abdominal pain
- Turner syndrome: Short stature, webbed neck, wide nipples, shield chest, increased arm-carrying angle, increased nevi; 5–10% will menstruate spontaneously
- Androgen insensitivity syndrome (46,XY): Normal breast development and absence of androgen-mediated hair growth occur in complete disease; tanner I breasts, hirsutism, and clitoromegaly occur in incomplete disease
- Adrenal disease: Hirsutism, clitoral growth, fatigue, and weakness
- Polycystic ovarian syndrome: Obesity, hirsutism, and other symptoms
- Prolactinoma: Galactorrhea, headache

DIFFERENTIAL DX

Primary Amenorrhea
- Turner syndrome
- Imperforate hymen
- Müllerian anomalies

Androgen Insensitivity Syndrome
- "Late bloomer"
- Pregnancy
- Excessive exercise
- Stress, drugs, diet, or illness
- Eating disorders
- Polycystic ovarian syndrome
- Hypothyroidism
- Hypogonadotropism
- Primary ovarian failure

DIAGNOSTIC EVALUATION

- History and physical examination to assess diet, lifestyle, exercise, sexual activity, and family history
- Pregnancy test
- Laboratory tests may include serum FSH/LH (high levels indicate gonadal failure), prolactin (high levels suggest pituitary adenoma or prolactinoma), estradiol and testosterone (total and free), complete blood count, chemistries, erythrocyte sedimentation rate, thyroid hormones, and karyotype analysis
  - Cortisol and androgen levels may be indicated if suspect adrenal disease
  - GnRH stimulation test is indicated if there are low levels of FSH or LH
- Bone age (a measure of skeletal maturity) is obtained by assessing the appearance and shape of the bones of the left hand and wrist from an X-ray and comparing them to age-specific norms found in the Greulich and Pyle Atlas
- Pelvic ultrasound to assess uterine size and development, ovarian size, cysts or tumors, and vaginal development
- Abdominal ultrasound or CT scan of the adrenals and kidneys may be indicated because adrenal hyperplasia, tumors, and renal abnormalities are associated with Turner syndrome
- MRI of the brain is indicated if prolactin level is elevated or if there are CNS-related symptoms

TREATMENT & MANAGEMENT

- Delayed puberty: Reassurance is sufficient
- Exercise-induced amenorrhea: Estrogen replacement to protect bone mass, nutritional and emotional counseling
- Eating disorders (anorexia nervosa): Nutritional and psychiatric counseling
- Turner syndrome: Hormone replacement with estrogen/progesterone and growth hormone
- Imperforate hymen and Müllerian abnormalities: Surgical repair/reconstruction
- Polycystic ovarian syndrome: Weight loss (diet modification and regular exercise), metformin, and/or oral contraceptive pills
- Congenital hypogonadotropic hypogonadism: Estrogen/progesterone for sexual development; in adults who desire fertility, ovulation can be induced with pulsatile GnRH administration
- Prolactinoma: Bromocriptine or cabergoline; surgery is reserved for macroadenomas or refractory cases

PROGNOSIS & COMPLICATIONS

- Prognosis and fertility depend on the underlying cause
- Counseling may be needed to reduce stress and/or modify lifestyle
- If a Y chromosome is found in a patient with a female phenotype, gonads should be removed due to malignant potential

Precocious Puberty

INTRODUCTION

- Precocious puberty is defined as the appearance of secondary sexual characteristics before age 7 years in girls (before 6 in black girls) or before age 9 in boys
- In most girls, puberty begins between 8–13 years of age and is completed on average in 4.2 years (range, 1.5–6 years); the time from onset of breast buds to menarche is 2.3 years $\pm$ 1 year
- In boys, puberty begins between 9–14 years of age and is completed on average within 3.5 years (range, 2–4.5 years)
- The majority of cases occurs in girls
- 80% of cases are idiopathic

ETIOLOGY, EPIDEMIOLOGY, & RISK FACTORS

- Puberty is initiated by changes in the sensitive negative-feedback system between the gonads, the hypothalamus, and the pituitary in the prepubital child
- Puberty involves an increase in gonadal steroid production (gonadarchy) and an increase in adrenal steroid production (adrenarche)
- Gonadotropin-releasing hormone (GnRH)–dependent (central) etiologies include: CNS tumors, head trauma or injury, CNS malformations, untreated hypothyroidism, congenital adrenal hyperplasia, or idiopathic
- Gonadotropin-releasing hormone (GnRH)–independent etiologies include: Adrenal, ovarian, and Leydig cell tumors; other hormone-producing tumors; polycystic ovarian syndrome; and exposure to exogenous sex steroids
- McCune-Albright syndrome is a genetic disorder characterized by precocious puberty, skeletal dysplasia, café-au-lait spots, and other endocrine abnormalities
- In boys, the most likely etiology is a gonadotropin-producing or sex steroid–producing tumor

PATIENT PRESENTATION

- GnRH-dependent precocious puberty follows the normal sequence of pubertal events
  - In girls, premature thelarche is followed by the appearance of pubic and axillary hair and menstruation
  - In boys, enlargement of the testes and phallus occurs, accompanied by pubic hair, voice change, and acne
- GnRH-independent disease results in a less pre-dictable pubertal course
- Accelerated linear growth and skeletal matura-tion occur in both sexes
- Adult body odor may be present
- Virilization may appear in girls
- Focal neurologic signs may be present if a CNS tumor is present

DIFFERENTIAL DX

- Isolated premature thelarche (usually benign)
- Premature adrenarche
  - Neurologic problems
  - Mild 21-hydroxylase deficiency
  - Polycystic ovarian syndrome

DIAGNOSTIC EVALUATION

- Assess serum levels of luteinizing hormone (LH), follicle-stimulating hormone (FSH), estradiol, testosterone, dehydroepiandrosterone sulfate (DHEA-S), and thyroid function tests
- Gonadotropin-releasing hormone (GnRH) stimulation test: LH is measured prior to stimulation with GnRH, which allows differentiation of central (GnRH-dependent) from peripheral (GnRH-independent) disorders
  - In GnRH-independent precocious puberty, LH and FSH levels are low at baseline and do not increase with GnRH stimulation
  - In GnRH-dependent disorders, basal levels of LH and FSH are often at pubertal levels and will increase upon GnRH stimulation
- Further testing depending on clinical suspicions include 17-OH-progesterone level to rule out congenital adrenal hyperplasia, beta-hCG if suspect a testicular tumor, pelvic or testicular ultrasound, MRI of the brain with special cuts of the pituitary gland, and adrenal, hepatic, or abdominal ultrasounds
- X-ray of the hand and wrist to determine bone age (skeletal development is advanced by circulating sex steroids)
- Skeletal survey may show osseous lesions of McCune-Albright syndrome

TREATMENT & MANAGEMENT

- Administration of a GnRH analog (only effective in GnRH-dependent etiologies) will suppress endogenous GnRH pulse generator, causing arrest of pubertal development, decrease in secondary sexual characteristics, deceleration of linear growth, and prevention of premature closure of growth plates
- Treat the underlying disease as necessary (eg, thyroxine administration for hypothyroidism, corticosteroids for congenital adrenal hyperplasia, surgical excision of tumors)
- Estrogen inhibitors, including estrogen receptor antagonists (eg, tamoxifen) and aromatase inhibitors (eg, arimidex), are experimental approaches to treating peripheral precocity

PROGNOSIS & COMPLICATIONS

- Final adult height is generally decreased in these patients
- GnRH analog therapy will often increase final adult height; it is most effective if initiated before 5–8 years of age
- If puberty advances sufficiently in congenital adrenal hyperplasia, it may not be reversible with corticosteroid therapy alone

Gynecomastia

INTRODUCTION

- Defined as the presence of excessive breast tissue in boys
- Young men usually first become aware of the breast masses because they are tender
- Occurs in 40–50% of boys during puberty, depending on ethnicity and nutritional status
- Breast enlargement in young men may cause them to question their masculine identity

ETIOLOGY, EPIDEMIOLOGY, & RISK FACTORS

- Defined as Tanner stages II–V breasts in males of any age
- Pubertal gynecomastia: During puberty, the low ratio of testosterone to estrogen may lead to benign gynecomastia that regresses with age
- Obesity can lead to true gynecomastia or pseudogynecomastia
  - True gynecomastia: Adipose tissue converts adrenal precursors to estrogens, thereby increasing estrogen stimulation of the breast tissue
  - Pseudogynecomastia: Fat deposition occurs in breast area without glandular development
- Neonates may have benign breast development lasting up to 6 months due to transfer of maternal hormones
- Pubertal gynecomastia has onset at ages 10–12 and peaks at ages 13–14
- Klinefelter syndrome is the most common sex chromosome abnormality resulting in gynecomastia; prevalence of 0.2% (1 in 500 males)
- Gynecomastia may occur due to testicular neoplasms
  - Germ cell tumors account for 95% of testicular neoplasms; up to 6% of affected patients have gynecomastia at the time of presentation
  - Leydig cell tumors and large-cell calcifying Sertoli cell (sex-cord) tumors of the testes are also associated with gynecomastia
- Premature thelarche: Thelarche in girls younger than 6–7 years

PATIENT PRESENTATION

- Gynecomastia can be unilateral or bilateral, symmetric or asymmetric
- Benign gynecomastia has an otherwise normal physical examination
- Pubertal gynecomastia manifests as Tanner stage II or greater breasts in males
  - Timing is key to the diagnosis
- Signs and symptoms of underlying disease may be present
  - Klinefelter syndrome (46, XXY) presents with small testes, tall and thin body habitus, and long limbs

DIFFERENTIAL DX

- Pubertal gynecomastia
- Neonatal gynecomastia
- Pseudogynecomastia
- Estrogen excess (endogenous or endogenous)
- Genetic syndromes (eg, Klinefelter syndrome, testosterone biosynthesis defects, androgen insensitivity)
- Drugs (eg, androgens, anabolic steroids, ketoconazole, other cytochrome P450 inhibitors, CNS drugs, marijuana)
- Tumors (testicular, adrenal, liver, breast)
- Cirrhosis

DIAGNOSTIC EVALUATION

- Pubertal gynecomastia should be differentiated from true gynecomastia by careful examination of the breast adipose tissue
  - If examination is consistent with pubertal gynecomastia and there are no abnormalities in history and physical exam, provide reassurance and reexamine in 6 months
  - Bone age will aid in assessment of sex steroid activity
- Gynecomastia with other findings or prolonged course may prompt the need for karyotype analysis, particularly in patients with testicular volumes less than expected for their pubertal stage
- Testicular ultrasound is indicated if suspect a testicular germ cell tumor (eg, testicular mass with high serum hCG level)
- CT scan or MRI of adrenals to detect adrenal tumor may be indicated
- Hormonal analyses (including androgen, estrogen, and gonadotropin levels) may be indicated

TREATMENT & MANAGEMENT

- Reassurance is sufficient in most cases
- Exercise and nutritional counseling for weight loss in obesity-related gynecomastia
- Medical therapy may be indicated for specific diseases:
  - Antiestrogens (tamoxifen) may cause regression of glandular tissue
  - Aromatase inhibitors have been tried with variable success
  - Androgens for Klinefelter syndrome
- Medical therapy is controversial for patients with pubertal gynecomastia; may be used for patients who are severely socially affected
- Surgical breast reduction should be deferred until after puberty for patients who have persistent, distressing gynecomastia
- Underlying diseases should be treated as required

PROGNOSIS & COMPLICATIONS

- Pubertal gynecomastia usually regresses after 1–2 years and is generally resolved by age 16–17
- Neonatal gynecomastia usually resolves by 2–3 weeks; however, it may persist as long as 6 months
- In germ cell tumors, gynecomastia is a poor prognostic sign

Rickets

INTRODUCTION

- Normal bone growth and mineralization require adequate availability of calcium and phosphate, the two major constituents of the crystalline component of bone
- Deficient mineralization can result in rickets and/or osteomalacia
  - Rickets refers to the changes caused by deficient mineralization of growing bones
  - Osteomalacia refers to impaired mineralization of the bone matrix
- Rickets and osteomalacia usually occur together as long as the growth plates are open; only osteomalacia occurs after the growth plates have fused
- Most cases in the U.S. occur in dark-skinned children, strict vegans, and ethnic groups who completely cover the skin

ETIOLOGY, EPIDEMIOLOGY, & RISK FACTORS

- Nutritional rickets may be caused by inadequate vitamin D intake, prolonged exclusive breast-feeding without vitamin D supplementation, and inadequate sunlight exposure
- Malnutrition and calcium deficiency are frequent causes
- Malabsorption of fat-soluble vitamins (A, D, E, and K) may occur in cases of pancreatic insufficiency, cholestatic liver disease, and intestinal villous atrophy
- Rickets of prematurity may be caused by lack of third-trimester bone mineralization, furosemide or corticosteroid therapies, or high nutritional needs (esp. parenteral feeding)
- Genetic rickets (vitamin D resistant) may be due to X-linked hypophosphatemia (defect in renal reabsorption of phosphate) or renal alpha-hydroxylase deficiency (decreased conversion of 25-OH-vitamin D to 1,25-[OH]$_2$-vitamin D)
- End-organ vitamin D resistance (eg, X-linked hypophosphatemia, the most common form of hereditary rickets) is caused by reduced activity of the renal membrane sodium-phosphate cotransporter in the proximal tubule and abnormal regulation of renal 1-α-hydroxylase activity, resulting in inappropriately low serum levels of 1,25-dihydroxyvitamin D relative to the degree of hypophosphatemia
- Rickets is three times more common in boys than in girls, except in ethnic societies in which there is total-body coverage of girls

PATIENT PRESENTATION

- Failure to thrive
- Slow growth
- Delayed walking
- Frontal cranial bossing
- Craniotabes (softening of the skull)
- Rachitic rosary (enlarged costochondral junctions of the ribs)
- Widened wrists or ankles
- Bowed legs (only develops after the child starts weight-bearing)
- Muscle weakness
- Near the equator, rickets occur in half of children with pneumonia

DIFFERENTIAL DX

- Intestinal osteodystrophy (malabsorption syndromes)
- Liver disease
- Renal disease
- Physiologic bowed legs
- Blount disease
- Severe anemia
- Juvenile arthritis
- Metabolic bone disease of epileptic drug therapy
- Schmidt metaphyseal dysplasia

DIAGNOSTIC EVALUATION

- Rickets is a radiologic diagnosis via bone X-rays that show rachitic bone features; generalized osteopenia; and widening, cupping, and fraying of the metaphyses
- Laboratory studies include 25-OH-vitamin D (low); 1,25-(OH)$_2$-vitamin D (may be normal or elevated); maternal 25-OH-vitamin D level if breastfeeding (low); parathyroid hormone and alkaline phosphatase (high); calcium (low in advanced disease); and phosphate (low)
- Screening may be indicated for related nutritional deficiencies (eg, iron deficiency anemia, vitamin A deficiency, vitamin E deficiency, abnormal coagulation studies) or failure to thrive

TREATMENT & MANAGEMENT

- Treat nutritional rickets with vitamin D supplementation (400 IU/day; some clinicians use higher doses)
- Treat vitamin D–resistant rickets with sunlight exposure, weight-bearing exercise, and phosphate and vitamin D supplementation
  - Phosphopenic rickets: Administer phosphate and high-dose vitamin D
  - α-Hydroxylase deficiency: Administer 1,25-(OH)$_2$-vitamin D
  - Vitamin D supplementation and adequate phosphate and calories will prevent rickets of prematurity

PROGNOSIS & COMPLICATIONS

- The bone deformities of nutritional rickets usually resolve with nutritional (vitamin D) therapy alone
- Phosphopenic rickets may have long-term complications, including short stature, renal stones, joint deformities, and dental crowding or malformations
- Rickets of prematurity usually completely resolves
- Hungry bone syndrome may complicate the acute management of severe rickets; "vigorous calcium deposition in bones (stimulated by the rickets therapy) may cause hypocalcemia"

Short Stature

INTRODUCTION

- Problems related to growth are common in pediatric practice
- Growth failure is the single most sensitive sign that something is amiss with a child
- A single measurement of height is not as helpful as following the height velocity over time
- Using standard growth curves, the length of a child can be plotted against normal values from birth to 3 years of age
- The standing height of a child can be measured and compared to age-related norms beginning at 2 years
- Short stature with a low weight for height often reflects a nutritional or gastrointestinal disorder, whereas an elevated weight-for-height often reflects an endocrine disorder

ETIOLOGY, EPIDEMIOLOGY, & RISK FACTORS

- Short stature is defined as height less than 3% of normal on a growth curve, height abnormally small relative to the parents' heights (genetic potential), or falling across major percentiles on the growth curve (ie, you do not have to wait—and should not wait—until it falls below 3%)
- Normal growth velocity is 5 cm/yr between 3 years of age and puberty
- Disease states that cause short stature include: Growth hormone deficiency, intrauterine growth retardation (IUGR), chronic infection or illness, neglect, nutritional deficiencies and malabsorption syndromes, other endocrine disorders (eg, hypothyroidism, Cushing syndrome), chromosome abnormalities, and bone dysplasias
- Benign causes of short stature, including genetic/familial short stature and constitutional growth delay, are most common in the U.S.
- Worldwide, nutritional deficiencies are the most common cause
- In the U.S., the prevalence of growth hormone deficiency is estimated at 1 in 3500

PATIENT PRESENTATION

- Constitutional delay is characterized by:
  - Retarded linear growth in the first 3 years of life
  - Parallel growth curve throughout prepuberty
  - Delayed pubertal onset
  - Catch-up growth later in adolescence
- Intrauterine drug exposure or infections and genetic syndromes are often associated with multiple anomalies
- Signs or symptoms of systemic diseases may be present
- In cases of growth hormone deficiency, birth size is usually normal, and growth failure begins postnatally
  - Presentation includes infantile facies with chubby cheeks, open fontanelle, delayed bone age, fine hair, truncal obesity, micropenis, and hypoglycemia

DIFFERENTIAL DX

- Normal variants
- Low birth weight (eg, prematurity, IUGR, small for gestational age)
- Fetal drug exposure (eg, alcohol, nicotine)
- Bone and cartilage dysplasia
- Chronic disease (eg, poorly controlled diabetes, cystic fibrosis, inflammatory bowel disease, celiac disease, asthma)
- Chronic infections (eg, HIV, tuberculosis, chronic respiratory infections)
- Genetic syndromes (eg, Turner, Seckel, Noonan, Down, Prader-Willi syndromes)
- Nutritional insufficiency
- Psychosocial deprivation

DIAGNOSTIC EVALUATION

- Birth and past medical histories, family history, review of systems, and thorough physical and neurologic exams will indicate priorities for the diagnostic evaluation
- Growth curve pattern is fundamental to diagnosis
- Midparental height indicates genetic potential
  - Girls: 13 cm is subtracted from the father's height and averaged with the mother's height
  - Boys: 13 cm is added to the mother's height and averaged with the father's height
  - 8.5 cm on either side of this calculated value (target height) represents the 3rd to 97th percentiles for anticipated adult height
- Initial screening tests include CBC, electrolytes, BUN/creatinine, liver function tests (ALT, AST, alkaline phosphatase, bilirubin, albumin), erythrocyte sedimentation rate, and thyroid studies (TSH and free T_4)
- X-ray of left hand and wrist to determine bone age
- Tissue transglutaminase IgA or antiendomysial IgA to rule out celiac disease
- Karyotype in females to rule out Turner syndrome
- MRI of brain to assess midbrain and pituitary abnormalities
- IGF-1 or IGFBP-3 may reflect growth hormone status (low levels suggest deficiency)
- Growth hormone stimulation test will definitively diagnose growth hormone deficiency
- Return visits to monitor growth velocity (and pubertal development, if age appropriate) are often helpful in distinguishing normal variants from pathologic growth

TREATMENT & MANAGEMENT

- Treat growth hormone deficiency with daily supplementation of recombinant growth hormone; other conditions approved for treatment with growth hormone include chronic renal failure, Turner syndrome, Prader-Willi syndrome, small for gestational age, idiopathic short stature, and SHOX deficiency
- Treating non–GH-deficient (ie, idiopathic) short stature with growth hormone is still controversial
- No treatment is required for constitutional delay; adolescent males may be given testosterone for psychological problems of short stature and delayed puberty, but it does not improve final height
- Treat the underlying cause whenever possible
  - Treat panhypopituitarism with replacement of all deficient hormones except gonadal steroids, which are reserved until puberty
  - Systemic diseases need to be appropriately managed
  - Nutritional deficiencies must be corrected
  - Psychosocial deprivation may warrant removal from the harmful home environment

PROGNOSIS & COMPLICATIONS

- In patients treated with growth hormone, the maximum benefit in height occurs during the first year of treatment
- Growth hormone–deficient patients achieve normal heights in up to 85% of cases
- Side effects of growth hormone therapy include pseudotumor cerebri, slipped capital femoral epiphysis, scoliosis, and potential to stimulate growth of cancer; some boys will develop reversible gynecomastia
- Psychosocial support for all children with short stature and their families
- Cost of growth hormone treatment for idiopathic short stature was calculated at approximately $100,000 for a 2-inch gain in height
- Growth hormone and illicit GHRH analogs are drugs of abuse in athletes

Neurology

Hydrocephalus

INTRODUCTION

- Hydrocephalus results from overproduction or impaired absorption of cerebrospinal fluid
- The majority of cerebrospinal fluid is produced in the choroid plexuses in the lateral ventricles
- From the lateral ventricles, cerebrospinal fluid flows through the foramen of Monro, the third ventricle, and the aqueduct of Sylvius into the fourth ventricle
- Cerebrospinal fluid leaves the fourth ventricle via the foramen of Luschka and Magendie and drains into posterior fossa and basal cisterns
- From the cisterns, most of the cerebrospinal fluid is directed over the hemispheres towards the superior sagittal sinus, where it is resorbed into the blood through the arachnoid villi

ETIOLOGY, EPIDEMIOLOGY, & RISK FACTORS

- **Noncommunicating (obstructive) hydrocephalus** is due to obstruction of CSF
  - In infants, stenosis of the aqueduct of Sylvius is the most common cause
  - In children, tumors are more common (primitive neuroectodermal tumor [PNET], ependymoma, astrocytoma)
- **Communicating hydrocephalus** results from obliteration of the subarachnoid cisterns or malfunctioning of the arachnoid villi
  - Etiologies include infections (eg, meningitis), subarachnoid or intraventricular hemorrhage, leukemic infiltrates, and aneurysm or abscess of the vein of Galen
  - Communicating hydrocephalus can also occur due to increased production of cerebrospinal fluid from a choroid plexus papilloma
- Hydrocephalus is relatively common in pediatric populations
  - There are approximately 125,000 individuals with shunts secondary to hydrocephalus
  - Children born prematurely who develop intraventricular hemorrhages are at increased risk for hydrocephalus

PATIENT PRESENTATION

- In infants, the presentation includes rapid head enlargement, irritability, vomiting, decreased upward vertical gaze
- In children, headache, lethargy, and vomiting
- Delayed closure of anterior fontanel (normal closure occurs by 18 months), frontal bossing, occipital prominence, and/or widely split cranial sutures may occur
- Papilledema due to increased intracranial pressure is an important sign
- Assess for signs of herniation (eg, change in respiratory pattern, unilateral dilation of a pupil, ptosis, decreased heart rate, increased BP)
- Chronic hydrocephalus may be associated with optic nerve atrophy; "sunsetting" of eyes may occur due to pressure on superior colliculus, causing eyes to rotate downward
- Hyperreflexia, spasticity, and poor head control

DIFFERENTIAL DX

- Congenital malformations (Arnold-Chiari malformation, aqueductal stenosis)
- Infection (meningitis/abscess)
- Neoplasms (ependymoma, PNET, astrocytoma)
- Genetic (achondroplasia)
- Hemorrhage: Intraventricular, subarachnoid, subdural hematoma, epidural hematoma
- Vascular malformations (vein of Galen aneurysm)
- Benign subdural effusion
- Causes of macrocephaly:
  - Megalencephaly (familial, Canavan, Alexander diseases)
  - Ventriculomegaly
  - Bony overgrowth of skull (thalassemia, osteopetrosis)

DIAGNOSTIC EVALUATION

- Evaluate and secure the airway, breathing, and circulation
- History and physical examination
  - History should include questions about trauma, seizures, vomiting, double or blurry vision, birth history, fever, neck stiffness, headache, and antibiotic use
  - Physical examination should assess vital signs, temperature, pattern of breathing (Cheyne-Stokes, apneustic, ataxic), retinal hemorrhages, otorrhea, spinal fluid rhinorrhea, cardiac exam, and meningismus
  - Neurologic exam should assess for responses to voice and noxious stimulation, papilledema, pupillary size and light reflex, eye movements (spontaneous, doll's eye, calorics), corneals, gag, motor response to pain, decerebrate or decorticate posturing, muscle tone, deep tendon reflexes, and Babinski
- The diagnosis is often made clinically and then confirmed by radiologic studies
- Ultrasound, CT scan, or MRI can be used to evaluate hydrocephalus depending on the child's age and urgency of symptoms; imaging reveals enlarged ventricles; may also identify associated congenital anomalies (eg, Dandy-Walker syndrome, Arnold-Chiari malformation)
- Increased intracranial pressure is often diagnosed clinically and then confirmed by an elevated opening pressure while placing a shunt, drain, or lumbar puncture
- Aqueductal stenosis results in markedly enlarged lateral and third ventricles, as well as the cephalic portion of the aqueduct

TREATMENT & MANAGEMENT

- Because highly elevated intracranial pressure can be rapidly fatal, prompt recognition and treatment are essential
  - Evaluate the airway, breathing, and circulation, and obtain intravenous access
  - Assess for signs of herniation (eg, change in respiratory pattern, unilateral dilation of a pupil, ptosis, decreased heart rate, increased blood pressure)
- Keep the head of the bed at 15–30 degrees, intubate and hyperventilate, and consider administration of mannitol with or without furosemide
- Shunting should be considered soon after the discovery of hydrocephalus
- Neuroimaging should be performed immediately
- Lumbar puncture may be contraindicated if there are signs of herniation or mass lesion
  - If there are no such signs and meningitis or subarachnoid hemorrhage is possible, lumbar puncture should be performed
- Surgical shunting may be necessary to bypass the obstruction and decrease intracranial pressure, thereby protecting the brain from further damage
  - The most common shunt is the ventriculoperitoneal (VP) shunt, which has pressure control devices to help prevent overdrainage
  - Ventriculostomy is an option in patients with aqueductal stenosis

PROGNOSIS & COMPLICATIONS

- Associated with increased risk of developmental disabilities
- Problems with memory, visual function, and visual acuity may result
- Many children will have behavior problems
- Children who have hydrocephalus due to congenital causes may have a better developmental outcome than acquired cases
- Complications of shunting include infection, mechanical malfunction, ascites, peritonitis, meningitis, and subdural hematoma

Neural Tube Defects

INTRODUCTION

- The neural tube is the embryologic origin of the brain and spinal cord
- Failure of closure of the embryonic neural tube creates an area of anatomic and functional defect; neural tube defects, also known as spinal dysraphism, represent a developmental structural abnormality of the nervous system
- Neural tube defects are second only to cardiac malformations as the most prevalent congenital anomaly in the U.S.
- Myelomeningocele is the most common form and can affect both the central and peripheral nervous system; other forms of neural tube defects include diastematomyelia, lipomeningocele, and lipomyelomeningocele

ETIOLOGY, EPIDEMIOLOGY, & RISK FACTORS

- Myelomeningocele is the most common neural tube defect; it represents a restricted failure of posterior neural tube closure, which results in a saclike casing filled with cerebrospinal fluid, spinal cord, and nerve roots that have herniated through a defect in the vertebra and dura
- Anencephaly is the most severe neural tube defect; it occurs due to failure of anterior neural tube closure
- Lipomeningocele consists of a lipomatous mass that herniates through the bony defect and attaches to the spinal cord, thereby tethering the cord and often the associated nerve roots
- Diastematomyelia or split cord refers to abnormal congenital division of the spinal cord by a bony spicule or fibrous band protruding from a vertebra or two, with each half surrounded by a dural sac
- Neural tube defects are associated with folic acid deficiency, chromosomal defects (eg, trisomy 13 and 18), gestational diabetes, and numerous teratogens (eg, radiation, valproic acid, carbamazepine)
- Increased risk in families with one affected child and females
- Incidence can be significantly decreased by folic acid supplementation prior to conception and during pregnancy, especially during the first trimester

PATIENT PRESENTATION

- Myelomeningocele is seen as a neuronal lesion at birth
  - 80% of cases involve the lumbar vertebrae
  - The majority of patients have hydrocephalus due to aqueductal stenosis or a Chiari malformation
- Affected patients may have defects of the overlying skin, commonly at the lower lumbar region (eg, dimple, sinus, skin tag, tuft of hair)
- Slowly progressive weakness or sensory loss in the legs and feet
- Gait disturbance and foot deformities
- Bowel and bladder dysfunction (eg, decreased rectal tone on exam)
- Decreased deep tendon reflexes due to pressure on nerve roots
- Babinski sign due to spinal cord compression
- Recurrent meningitis may occur due to external contamination of CSF near the site of the defect

DIFFERENTIAL DX

- Tethered spinal cord
- Caudal regression syndrome
- Cysts or tumors of the spinal cord
- Diastematomyelia

DIAGNOSTIC EVALUATION

Prenatal Diagnosis
- Elevated alpha-fetoprotein in the second trimester suggests a neural tube defect
- Prenatal ultrasound often detects most of the larger defects and may help determine the best method of delivery to prevent further damage

Postnatal Diagnosis
- Ultrasound of sacral dimples or tracts will verify defects
- MRI provides details of anatomic defects, especially the level of spinal involvement
- Imaging of the brain will help assess for the presence of hydrocephalus, Chiari malformation, and cortical malformations (eg, cerebral cortical dysplasia, cerebellar dysplasia, hypoplasia or aplasia of cranial nerve nuclei, fusion of the thalami, agenesis of the corpus callosum, complete or partial agenesis of the olfactory tract and bulb)
- Neurophysiologic monitoring, including brainstem and somatosensory potentials
- Assess for difficulties with feeding, swallowing, gastroesophageal reflux, sleep apnea
- Assess for fractures of the lower extremities, which occur in 30% of cases
- Baseline renal ultrasound and voiding cystourethrogram to assess for patients who have upper tract deterioration in addition to a neurogenic bladder

TREATMENT & MANAGEMENT

- Maternal folic acid supplementation before conception and during early pregnancy
- Sterile nonlatex gloves should be used during all surgical interventions and delivery to minimize the risk of latex sensitization
- Delivery is typically by Caesarian section
- Surgical treatment within 48 hours of delivery is necessary to close meningoceles and myelomeningoceles
- Progressive hydrocephalus should be treated by insertion of a ventriculoperitoneal shunt
- Surgical release of the tethered cord may be indicated for symptomatic neural tube defects
- Orthopedic intervention for hip subluxation and release of tendon contractures
- Intermittent catheterization for patients with bladder dysfunction to prevent infection
  - Patients with vesicoureteral reflux should receive antibiotic prophylaxis and anticholinergic medication to lower detrusor filling and voiding pressures
  - Surgical augmentation of the bladder, vesicostomy, or ureteral reimplantation may be needed for neurogenic bladder
- Treat constipation with laxatives; severe cases may require cecostomy
- Rehabilitation to optimize independence and mobility, splinting to prevent deformities, and ambulatory devices to maximize function

PROGNOSIS & COMPLICATIONS

- Prompt medical attention and selective surgical intervention has improved outcomes
- 5-year survival rate of 75–95%, depending on the level of the lesion (the higher the lesion, the greater the morbidity)
- Myelomeningocele is associated with higher mortality rates due to infection; it requires lifelong, multidisciplinary treatment
- Children with sacral and lower lumbar defects are usually able to walk; some with upper lumbar and thoracic lesions may walk
- Hydrocephalus often requires shunting to relieve increased intracranial pressure
- Renal complications may occur due to frequent urinary tract infections
- Many children (up to 33%) develop latex allergies due to multiple surgeries

Cerebral Palsy

INTRODUCTION

- Cerebral palsy is a static, nonprogressive disorder of movement and posture that occurs due to pre-, peri-, or postnatal brain injury
- The disorder is divided into four types: Spastic hemiplegia, spastic diplegia, spastic quadriplegia, and athetoid
- Clinically, children present with spasticity (60%), dyskinesia (20%), ataxia (1%), or mixed findings
- Many infants with mild clinical impairments will improve to develop similarly to unaffected children

ETIOLOGY, EPIDEMIOLOGY, & RISK FACTORS

- Incidence of 2 cases per 1000 births; the rate is much higher in preterm (vs. full-term) children and increases with decreasing birth weight and gestational age
- The etiology is multifactorial; known causes account for only a minority of cases
  - Although neonatal asphyxia/hypoxia is often thought to be causative, it likely accounts for just a small percentage of cases
  - Cerebral palsy has been associated with trauma, anoxic insult, prematurity and low birth weight, prenatal infections (eg, TORCH organisms), perinatal illness, brain malformations, intraventricular hemorrhage, genetic disorders, metabolic disorders, and toxic exposures (eg, mercury)
  - Up to 20% of cases are acquired after the neonatal period; acquired etiologies include kernicterus, near-drowning, meningitis, stroke, and trauma
- Incidence has not changed despite better obstetrical care; this may be explained by the increased survival of premature and low birth weight infants
- Magnesium sulfate may have a neuroprotective effect in reducing the incidence of cerebral palsy

PATIENT PRESENTATION

Spastic Hemiplegia
- Hand dominance before 1 year of age
- Delayed motor milestones
- Growth arrest of the affected extremity
- Upper motor neuron signs

Spastic Diplegia
- Bilateral spasticity
- Toe-walking
- Upper motor neuron signs

Spastic Quadriplegia
- Motor delays
- Spasticity
- Bulbar dysfunction

Athetoid
- Initial hypotonia
- Writhing, erratic quality of movement
- Dystonia uncommon

DIFFERENTIAL DX

- Muscle weakness: Metachromatic leukodystrophy, pontocerebellar atrophies
- Diplegia or quadriplegia: Arginase deficiency, holocarboxylase synthetase deficiency
- Dystonia or choreoathetosis: Glutaric aciduria type 1, dopa-responsive dystonia, Lesch-Nyhan disease, pyruvate dehydrogenase complex deficiency, Rett syndrome
- Ataxia: Ataxia telangiectasia, Niemann-Pick disease
- Opercular syndrome

DIAGNOSTIC EVALUATION

- A clinical diagnosis is based on history and physical examination; no laboratory tests are diagnostic
  - Confirm that the history does not suggest a progressive or degenerative CNS disorder (eg, Rett syndrome, mitochondrial disease)
- MRI is necessary for radiologic confirmation of central nervous system changes that can account for clinical findings
  - Periventricular leukomalacia results in spastic diplegia
  - Focal ischemic changes in a cerebral vascular territory may be associated with spastic hemiplegia; this finding may necessitate an investigation for coagulopathy or sources of emboli
- Baseline tests of hearing, vision, or EEG may be useful for functional assessment
- Consider metabolic or genetic testing if there is a family history of cerebral palsy or if there is evidence of deterioration or episodes of decompensation
- Close monitoring for early identification of learning and developmental problems is important
- EEG is indicated if there is clinical suspicion of seizures

TREATMENT & MANAGEMENT

- Early intervention is necessary to optimize functioning and prevent secondary problems
- Intensive occupational and physical therapy
- Speech therapy for swallowing and speech dysfunction
- Oromotor dysfunction can lead to drooling, which can be treated with behavioral techniques, anticholinergic agents (glycopyrrolate), salivary gland botulinum toxin, or surgery
- Close ophthalmology follow-up for strabismus and other ocular dysfunction
- Behavioral intervention and treatment of learning disabilities
- Spasticity can be treated with oral medications, muscle relaxants (eg, diazepam, dantrolene, baclofen), botulinum toxin injections into selected muscles, or surgery (eg, selective dorsal rhizotomy, intrathecal baclofen pump, release or recession of limb muscles and tendons [muscle-tendon surgery] to reduce restricted joint motion or malalignment)
- Orthopedic intervention may be necessary to treat scoliosis, hip dislocation or degeneration, or other orthopedic complications
- Electrical stimulation of muscles to improve strength has not demonstrated a consistent benefit

PROGNOSIS & COMPLICATIONS

- The majority of children with cerebral palsy survive into adulthood
- Prognosis varies depending on the etiology and type of cerebral palsy, degree of motor delay, persistence of pathologic reflexes, and degree of associated cognitive involvement
- Some patients may require the use of leg braces to walk
- Visual field deficits due to involvement of optic nerve radiations may affect learning
- Significant truncal hypotonia precludes acquisition of sitting and standing skills
- Bulbar dysfunction requires placement of feeding tubes

Encephalopathy

INTRODUCTION

- Encephalopathy refers to diffuse disease of the brain that alters brain function or structure
- The hallmark of encephalopathy is an altered mental state
- Depending on the severity of encephalopathy, symptoms range from subtle personality changes and inability to concentrate to lethargy and coma
- Changes in level of consciousness can occur due to bilateral dysfunction of the cerebral cortex, dysfunction of the reticular activating system in the brainstem, or both combined
- Encephalitis is a term that is typically used to denote an infectious cause
- Static encephalopathy is a disorder of motor function against a background of nonprogressive brain injury usually from a prenatal or perinatal event

ETIOLOGY, EPIDEMIOLOGY, & RISK FACTORS

- Etiologies are numerous and include:
  - Trauma (eg, concussion, diffuse axonal injury)
  - Increased intracranial pressure (eg, tumor, abscess, hydrocephalus)
  - Vascular: Intracranial hemorrhage, stroke, hypoxic ischemic injury (cardiac arrest, arrhythmia, near-drowning, hypotension), vasculitis
  - Metabolic disorders: Mitochondrial, hypoglycemia, acidosis, hyperammonemia, uremia, electrolyte abnormalities (hyponatremia, hypernatremia, hypomagnesemia), Reye syndrome, mitochondrial diseases
  - Oxygen, substrate, or cofactor deprivation: Pulmonary disease, alveolar hypoventilation, carbon monoxide poisoning, methemoglobinemia, anemia
  - Vitamin or cofactor deficiency: Thiamin, niacin, pyridoxine, vitamin B_{12}, folate
  - Toxins: Uremia, ethanol, atropine, opiates, lead, substance abuse
  - Hepatic encephalopathy due to liver dysfunction
  - Infections: Meningitis/encephalitis (bacteria, virus, fungi, spirochete)
  - Postinfectious: Acute disseminated encephalomyelitis (ADEM)
  - Seizures: Nonconvulsive status epilepticus, postconvulsive state
  - Endocrine disorders: Adrenal insufficiency, thyroid disorders

PATIENT PRESENTATION

- Some or all of the following signs and symptoms may be associated with encephalopathy:
- Increased intracranial pressure
- The presence of Cushing triad (bradycardia, hypertension, and Cheyne-Stokes respirations) suggests increased intracranial pressure
- Reactive pupils imply an intact midbrain
  - A unilaterally dilated and unreactive pupil results from uncal herniation and compression of the 3rd cranial nerve
  - Small reactive pupils indicate opiate use or pontine damage (stroke)
- Abnormal extraocular movements
- Asterixis can be seen in hepatic encephalopathy
- Decerebrate posturing occurs with upper brainstem damage
- Cognitive defects common in early stages
- Fine tremors or myoclonus may be present
- Primitive reflexes may be elicited

DIFFERENTIAL DX

- Psychogenic unresponsiveness
- "Locked-in" syndrome
- Severe neuromuscular weakness (eg, botulism, Guillain-Barré syndrome)
- Postictal state
- Intussusception

DIAGNOSTIC EVALUATION

- General physical and neurologic examination, including survey for trauma, abuse, rashes, and toxic exposures
  - Physical examination should include vital signs, temperature, pattern of breathing (eg, Cheyne-Stokes, apneustic, ataxic), and assessment for retinal hemorrhages, otorrhea, spinal fluid rhinorrhea, thyroid, cardiac arrhythmia or murmur, skin lesions (eg, cyanosis, petechia, splinter hemorrhages, ecchymoses), hepatosplenomegaly, and meningismus
  - Neurologic exam should assess response to voice and noxious stimulation, papilledema, pupillary size and light reflex, eye movements (spontaneous, doll's eyes, calorics), corneal reflex, gag reflex, motor response to pain, decerebrate or decorticate posturing, muscle tone, deep tendon reflexes, and Babinski
- Initial laboratory testing includes glucose levels, basic chemistries, complete blood count, liver function tests, ammonia level, workup for infection and toxic ingestions, and other metabolic tests, as indicated
- Imaging should be considered to rule out structural causes
- Lumbar puncture (only after herniation has been ruled out by head CT scan) if subarachnoid hemorrhage or infection is suspected
- EEG to rule out nonconvulsive status epilepticus or to give clues to a metabolic process (eg, triphasic waves)

TREATMENT & MANAGEMENT

- In patients with an acute change in level of consciousness, assess "ABCD": airway, breathing, circulation, and dextrose (glucose) levels
- Glasgow Coma Scale should be assessed serially to evaluate consciousness and guide treatment
- Consider specific antidotes (eg, naloxone for opiate overdose, flumazenil for benzodiazepine overdose)
- Assess and treat increased intracranial pressure with intubation, hyperventilation, sedation, use of diuretics (eg, mannitol or furosemide), and corticosteroids if suspect mass effect due to a tumor
- Treat seizures with appropriate antiepileptic medications; treat suspected underlying causes of seizures (eg, infection, acid-base disturbances, electrolyte abnormalities), as necessary
- Treat fever with antipyretics
- Manage agitation, which may exacerbate increased intracranial pressure

PROGNOSIS & COMPLICATIONS

- Pediatric outcomes of coma (traumatic or nontraumatic) are somewhat better than adults
- Severity of coma, motor patterns, blood pressure, and seizure type at the time of illness correlate with neurologic outcome
- Neuropsychiatric testing is indicated after recovery from an encephalopathic state
- Mortality is highest in children younger than 1 year old
- Higher mortality is correlated with inability to maintain body temperature and absent papillary responses or extraocular movements
- Children in a persistent vegetative state have a shorter life expectancy than other children
- Only a small minority of children are completely normal at follow-up

Seizure Disorders

INTRODUCTION

- A seizure represents the clinical expression of abnormal, excessive, synchronous discharges of neurons that primarily reside in the cerebral cortex
- Epilepsy is defined as having two or more unprovoked seizures
- Each year, between 25,000 and 40,000 children in the U.S. have a first, unprovoked, afebrile seizure; however, most of these children will not have a second seizure and do not require prophylactic treatment
- The neurologic exam and the EEG help guide the evaluation and treatment
- The International Classification of Epileptic Seizures is used by most epileptologists to classify seizure types into partial or generalized based on EEG and clinical data

ETIOLOGY, EPIDEMIOLOGY, & RISK FACTORS

- Most cases of seizures are of idiopathic/cryptogenic etiology
- Other etiologies include vascular, traumatic, developmental (conditions manifested by mental retardation and/or cerebral palsy), infectious, neoplastic, and degenerative causes
- Localized seizures are due to distinct brain pathology, such as a stroke, neoplastic lesion, developmental problem (eg, cortical dysplasia, lissencephaly), or genetic syndrome (eg, tuberous sclerosis)
- Idiopathic seizures may be age related (eg, "fifth-day fits," juvenile myoclonic epilepsy, childhood absence seizures, infantile spasms, Lennox-Gastaut syndrome)
- Febrile seizures are provoked seizures; they may be recurrent but are not defined as epilepsy
- Seizures can arise from any site in the brain but typically are localized to the neocortical gray matter and the limbic system, particularly the hippocampus and amygdala
- Overall incidence of childhood epilepsy from birth to 16 years is approximately 40 cases per 100,000 children per year
- 1% of children will have at least one afebrile seizure by age 14
- Generalized tonic-clonic or partial seizures account for 75% of cases
- Absence seizures account for 15% of cases

PATIENT PRESENTATION

- Generalized tonic-clonic seizures: Alternating stiffening/shaking, tongue biting, incontinence, loss of consciousness, and postictal recovery phase
- Partial seizures: Brief, tonic-clonic movements of the face, neck, and extremities; head turning; eye deviations
- Complex partial seizures: Impairment of consciousness; children may pick at things, blink, and stare
- Absence seizures: Brief loss of consciousness (rarely longer than 30 seconds) *without* loss of postural tone
- Myoclonic seizures: Brief, often symmetric, jerking of the body causing loss of body tone and forward falling
- Infantile spasms: Symmetric contractions of head, neck, and extremities

DIFFERENTIAL DX

- Generalized tonic-clonic seizures: Syncope, breath-holding spells, cardiac arrhythmia, cataplexy
- Generalized absence seizures: Behavioral staring, complex partial seizures, tic disorder
- Complex partial seizures: Sleepwalking, night terrors, benign paroxysmal vertigo, migraine disorders, self-stimulatory behavior
- Epileptic myoclonus: Physiologic in sleep, startle myoclonus
- Conversion disorder

DIAGNOSTIC EVALUATION

- The history, including eyewitness accounts, will often define the type of seizure and narrow the differential
  - Detailed description of the spell, loss of consciousness, eye deviation, time of onset, other suspicious spells (jerking, staring, daydreaming)
  - Birth and developmental history, previous history of head trauma, encephalitis, febrile seizures, medications at home, recent infections
- Physical examination may reveal genetic syndromes that predispose to seizures (eg, hypopigmented areas and shagreen patches seen in tuberous sclerosis complex)
- EEG may clarify the type of seizure:
  - 3-Hz generalized spike and wave activity occurs during hyperventilation in absence seizures
  - Centrotemporal spikes seen in the drowsy state in patients with benign Rolandic epilepsy
  - Hypsarrhythmia pattern seen in infantile spasms
- MRI or other imaging will reveal the etiology (eg, focal cortical dysgenesis, prior stroke, neoplasm) in 40–60% of cases
- Response to pyridoxine administration is diagnostic for pyridoxine-dependent seizures, which is a cause of refractory infantile seizures

TREATMENT & MANAGEMENT

- Keep the patient in a safe environment during the seizure to avoid injury
- Avoid placing objects in the child's mouth
- If vomiting occurs, turn the patient to the side to avoid aspiration
- Treat underlying systemic causes, if possible, and avoid substances (eg, medications) that provoke seizures
- Treat with appropriate anticonvulsant medication, as necessary:
  - Status epilepticus: Benzodiazepines, phenobarbital or phenytoin bolus, or induce pentobarbital coma
  - Partial seizures: Carbamazepine, valproic acid, lamotrigine, phenytoin
  - Generalized seizures: Valproic acid, lamotrigine
  - Absence seizures: Ethosuximide, valproic acid
  - Infantile spasms: ACTH, vigabatrin, valproic acid, benzodiazepines
- A ketogenic diet (high in fat and low in carbohydrates and protein) may be of value in treating some types of refractory seizures
- Epilepsy surgery (eg, cortical resection, corpus callosotomy, vagal nerve stimulators) may be useful in refractory cases

PROGNOSIS & COMPLICATIONS

- Prognosis depends on the etiology
- Some seizure types (eg, infantile spasms, Ohtahara syndrome) are associated with poor developmental outcome
- Status epilepticus, a prolonged seizure activity greater than 30 minutes, is a life-threatening emergency
- Less than half of first-time seizures will have a recurrence
- After a second seizure, nearly 75% of cases will develop epilepsy
- Seizures are generally eliminated or well controlled by adequate anticonvulsant therapy

Febrile Seizures

INTRODUCTION

- A febrile seizure is a spell that occurs between the ages of 3 months and 5 years that is associated with fever but without evidence of intracranial infection, other neurologic disorders, or a history of afebrile seizures
- It is unclear whether the triggering factor is the degree of fever, the rapidity of its rise, or both
- Occurs in 2–4% of all children

ETIOLOGY, EPIDEMIOLOGY, & RISK FACTORS

- Seizure activity is related to degree of temperature elevation and child's threshold for seizure (based on the developmental state of the brain)
- There is a genetic predisposition; at least 25% of cases have a positive family history in close relatives, and susceptibility has been linked to several genetic loci
- Generally occurs between 3 months and 5 years of age; peak age of onset is 18–22 months
- Typically occurs on the first day of an illness

PATIENT PRESENTATION

- Simple febrile seizure (80%): Generalized tonic-clonic activity lasting less than 15 minutes with associated fever
- Complex febrile seizure (15%): Focal seizure activity lasting beyond 15 minutes
  - Multiple seizures may occur within a 24-hour period
  - Abnormal neurologic status
  - Afebrile seizure in a parent or sibling
- When complex febrile seizures occur, the risk of epilepsy is increased

DIFFERENTIAL DX

- Epileptic seizure provoked by fever
- CNS infection (eg, bacterial meningitis, viral encephalitis)
- Toxins (eg, salicylates, theophylline, Shiga toxin, anticholinergics)
- Electrolyte disturbances (eg, hypoglycemia, hypocalcemia, hypernatremia, hyponatremia)
- Shaking chills

DIAGNOSTIC EVALUATION

- History and physical examination are usually diagnostic; patients are generally in the typical age range, have no prior neurologic disease, and have no focal deficits on physical exam
- Complete blood count may show leukocytosis
- EEG during the event will show seizure activity, but EEG is not helpful if the child is not seizing (it may be normal, slow, or epileptiform following seizures)
- Consider cerebrospinal fluid analysis if meningitis is suspected (eg, children <12 months of age, seizure occurring after the second day of illness)
- Transient hyperglycemia may accompany febrile seizures
- Routine testing of serum electrolytes if of low yield
- Neuroimaging should only be considered if the child has an abnormally large head or abnormal neurologic exam

TREATMENT & MANAGEMENT

- In the acute setting, evaluate and secure the airway, breathing, and circulation and administer supplemental oxygen as necessary
- Antipyretic measures may be helpful at the time of febrile illness but have not been shown to prevent recurrence
- In the acute setting, administer antiepileptics to end prolonged seizures
- Treat underlying infections as necessary
- Reassure the family as to the benign nature of the disease
- Hospital observation is not required for simple febrile seizures
- Anticonvulsants are not usually recommended for prophylaxis; however, in cases of recurrent febrile seizures, three groups of anticonvulsants (barbiturates, benzodiazepines, and valproic acid) have been found effective in preventing the recurrence of febrile seizures

PROGNOSIS & COMPLICATIONS

- Does not result in brain damage, neurologic defects, mental retardation, or learning disorders
- Recurrence risk is 35% over lifetime and 25% during the following 12 months
- One-third of affected children experience a second episode; less than 10% have more than three episodes
- 50% of children younger than 1 year of age experience a recurrence compared with 28% who have initial febrile seizure after 1 year of age
- Affected children are at slightly increased risk for epilepsy; the risk is more significant if complex febrile seizures occur

Breath-Holding Spells

INTRODUCTION

- Breath-holding spells are brief apneic episodes usually provoked by an emotional response (eg, anger, pain)
- Although the name may imply that this is a voluntary act that occurs during inspiration, these are actually involuntary, paroxysmal events that occur during expiration
- The child may turn blue or pale, lose consciousness, become rigid, or have seizure-like shaking
- Spells usually start in the toddler age group and resolve by 5 years of age

ETIOLOGY, EPIDEMIOLOGY, & RISK FACTORS

- Occurs due to a developmental disturbance in central autonomic regulation, leading to loss of consciousness
- May occur as often as several times per day or as infrequently as once per year
- Cyanotic breath-holding spells account for 90% of cases; they are precipitated by emotional stimuli (eg, anger, frustration)
- Pallid breath-holding spells account for the remaining 10% of cases; they are provoked by sudden unexpected stimuli (eg, bump on the head) and occur due to hyperresponsive vagal reflexes that cause transient bradycardia
- Incidence of 4–5% in toddlers
- Typical age of onset is between 6 and 18 months
- May be familial

PATIENT PRESENTATION

- The child cries and then holds breath
- Loss of consciousness
- Often becomes stiff or rigid
- Opisthotonos is common
- Recovers within 1 minute
- Cyanosis occurs in cases of cyanotic breath-holding spells
- Anoxia and cerebral hypoperfusion may result in seizure-like activity (ie, tonic-clonic movements)
- "Temper tantrums" are nonessential contributing factors

DIFFERENTIAL DX

- Syncope (eg, vasovagal, orthostatic hypotension)
- Seizure
- Arrhythmia (eg, prolonged QT syndrome, superventricular tachycardia, atrioventricular block)
- Cardiac anomalies (eg, aortic stenosis, pulmonic stenosis, tetralogy of Fallot)
- Dysautonomia (Riley-Day)
- Arnold-Chiari malformation
- Anterior mediastinal tumor

DIAGNOSTIC EVALUATION

- Clinical description, observation, or video recording is important for diagnosis
- EEG is usually not indicated unless there is prolonged anoxic seizure activity with breath-holding spells or if the clinical description of the spells suggests seizures
- Consider EKG to rule out prolonged QT syndrome or other cardiac causes, particularly if the event is precipitated by exercise or excitement
- Clinical laboratory testing is usually not necessary
- Consider a complete blood count in high-risk cases (iron deficiency lowers the threshold for breath-holding spells)

TREATMENT & MANAGEMENT

- Supportive treatment and parental reassurance
- Maintain supine position during spells to facilitate cerebral blood flow
- Atropine or other anticholinergics may be useful in pallid breath-holding spells, but these are not often used
- Iron supplementation may also be helpful
- Parents should be encouraged to not change disciplinary measures to avoid spells

PROGNOSIS & COMPLICATIONS

- Almost all cases cease by age 7–8
- Patients are predisposed to syncope in late childhood or adolescence; syncopal episodes are generally triggered by emotional stimuli
- Fatalities are rare and are probably due to aspiration

Neurocutaneous Syndromes

INTRODUCTION

- The neurocutaneous syndromes, also known as phakomatoses, consist of a group of disorders that tend to result in hamartoma malformations and neoplastic growths affecting the skin and the nervous system, as well as other organs
- The more common neurocutaneous syndromes include neurofibromatosis (NF), tuberous sclerosis complex (TSC), Sturge-Weber disease (SW), von Hippel-Lindau syndrome (VHL), Osler-Rendu-Weber syndrome, and ataxia-telangiectasia syndrome
- Each syndrome has distinct clinic features and genetic profiles
- Patients have a genetic tendency to form ectodermal tumors (skin, central nervous system, eyeball, retina)

ETIOLOGY, EPIDEMIOLOGY, & RISK FACTORS

Neurofibromatosis Type 1 (von Recklinghausen Disease, NF1)
- Neurofibromas are benign Schwann cell tumors felt as nodules along peripheral nerves
- "NF1 occurs in 1 in 2600–3000 live births and is inherited in an autosomal dominant manner; 50% of individuals with NF1 have an affected parent and 50% have the altered gene resulting from a de novo gene mutation."
- The NF1 gene has been mapped to chromosome 17q11.2
- Neurofibromin, the gene product, is thought to be a tumor suppressor gene; it belongs to a family of GTPase-activating proteins that downregulate a cellular proto-oncogene (p21-ras), an important determinant of cell growth and regulation
- Autosomal dominant transmission or sporadic mutations found in up to 50% of cases
- Neurofibromatosis type 2 (bilateral acoustic neuromas) is far less common in children

Tuberous Sclerosis Complex
- An autosomal dominant disease characterized by the growth of benign hamartomas in multiple organs, including the brain, kidney, skin, and lung
- New mutations account for 65% of cases
- Occurs in 1 in 5000–10,000 live births
- The TSC1 gene maps to chromosome 9q34 and encodes a protein termed hamartin
- The TSC2 gene maps to chromosome 16p13.3 and encodes the tuberin protein

PATIENT PRESENTATION

- Neurofibromatosis type 1: Café-au-lait spots, axillary and inguinal freckles, Lisch nodules on iris, cutaneous and subcutaneous tumors, optic gliomas, bony cysts, pathologic fractures, hypertension, scoliosis, spinal root tumors, learning disabilities
- Neurofibromatosis type 2: Hearing loss, tinnitus, vertigo, facial pain, gait ataxia, headache
- Tuberous sclerosis complex: May present in infancy with infantile spasms; presents in childhood with seizures, ash leaf spots, shagreen patches, retinal hamartomas, renal angiomyolipomas, cardiac rhabdomyomas, cortical tubers, subependymal nodules, and subependymal giant-cell astrocytomas

DIFFERENTIAL DX

- Neurofibromatosis
- Tuberous sclerosis complex
- Albright syndrome
- Posterior fossa tumors
- Metastatic brain cancer
- Other causes of infantile spasms:
  - Cerebral dysgenesis (eg, Aicardi syndrome)
  - Lissencephaly (eg, Miller-Dieker syndrome)
  - Holoprosencephaly
  - Hemimegalencephaly
  - Phenylketonuria
  - Toxoplasmosis
  - Syphilis
  - Cytomegalovirus
  - Metabolic disorders

DIAGNOSTIC EVALUATION

- Diagnosis of neurofibromatosis type 1 requires two or more of the following:
  - Five or more café-au-lait spots (>5 mm in prepubertal children; >15 mm in postpubertal)
  - Two or more neurofibromas or one plexiform neurofibroma
  - Axillary or inguinal freckles (Crow sign)
  - Optic gliomas
  - Two or more Lisch nodules (iris hamartomas)
  - Bone lesions (sphenoid dysplasia, thinning of long bone, pseudoarthrosis)
  - First-degree relative with neurofibromatosis type 1
- Diagnosis of tuberous sclerosis complex typically includes two or more major criteria:
  - Cortical tuber
  - Subependymal nodule
  - Subependymal giant-cell astrocytoma
  - Facial angiofibroma or forehead plaque
  - Ungual or periungual fibroma (nontraumatic)
  - Hypomelanotic macules (three or more)
  - Shagreen patch (connective tissue nevus)
  - Multiple retinal nodular hamartomas
  - Cardiac rhabdomyoma
  - Renal angiomyolipoma
  - Pulmonary lymphangioleiomyomatosis

TREATMENT & MANAGEMENT

- No cure exists; treatment is based on managing the symptoms and associated tumors

Neurofibromatosis Type 1

- Patients require yearly neurologic examination and visual testing to rule out optic nerve glioma and other central nervous system complications; based on the exam findings, patients may require further imaging and treatment
- Surgery may be necessary for accessible tumors
- Orthopedic procedures are indicated for orthopedic deformities
- Ophthalmologic surveillance for optic gliomas

Tuberous Sclerosis Complex

- Follow patients with a brain MRI and renal imaging (ultrasound, CT scan, or MRI) every 1–3 years
- Neurodevelopmental testing at the time of beginning first grade
- Based on the complications, additional follow-up testing may be required
- Treatment and prevention of seizures, as necessary
- Surgical removal of epileptogenic tubers
- Transcatheter embolization of renal angiomyolipomas
- Laser treatment of facial angiofibromas

PROGNOSIS & COMPLICATIONS

- 50% of individuals with neurofibromatosis type 1 will have only cutaneous neurofibromas, café-au-lait spots, or Lisch nodules
- 30–40% of patients will develop one or more serious complications in their lifetime, including malignancy, learning disability, cerebrovascular disease, hypertension, or scoliosis
- Tuberous sclerosis complex patients may have refractory epilepsy and renal complications
  - Epilepsy is the most common medical condition (80–90% of patients)
  - In about one-third of patients, epilepsy starts out as infantile spasms
  - 50% of the patients have autism spectrum disorder
  - Cardiac rhabdomyomas usually recede after the newborn period so they can be managed conservatively

Guillain-Barré Syndrome

INTRODUCTION

- Guillain-Barré syndrome, also known as acute inflammatory demyelinating polyradiculopathy, is the most common cause of acute flaccid paralysis in polio-free regions
- It is an immune-mediated polyneuropathy that causes demyelination primarily of the motor nerves, although sensory nerves may be affected to a lesser degree
- Early recognition and proper monitoring and treatment can be life saving
- Initial examination reveals symmetric weakness (usually of the proximal legs), decreased reflexes, and minimal loss of sensation
- The Miller-Fisher variant presents with ophthalmoparesis, areflexia, and ataxia

ETIOLOGY, EPIDEMIOLOGY, & RISK FACTORS

- Frequently postinfectious, especially following gastrointestinal and respiratory infections
  - *Campylobacter jejuni* is the most common infectious cause
  - Other infectious etiologies include Epstein-Barr virus, cytomegalovirus, measles, mumps, enteroviruses, herpes simplex virus, *Mycoplasma*, *Borrelia burgdorferi*, hepatitis A and B, *Chlamydophila pneumoniae*
- Guillain-Barré syndrome is one of the most common causes of acute weakness in children living in countries with immunization programs
  - Although the disease has been reported after vaccinations, the danger may be overstated
- Incidence is 1 in 100,000 for children aged less than 16
- Approximately 800 pediatric cases occur yearly in the U.S.
- Rarely occurs in children less than 2 years of age
- Males are affected approximately 1.5 times more often than females in all age groups
- Not thought to have racial or economic predispositions
- There is no known genetic factor

PATIENT PRESENTATION

- In most cases, symptoms begin 1–4 weeks after antecedent illness
- Typically begins with fine paresthesias in the toes and fingertips; minimal loss of sensation
- Ascending, typically symmetric, weakness progressing toward the trunk, neck, and bulbar muscles occurs over 1–2 weeks
- Diminished or absent reflexes on exam
- Cranial nerves are affected in 30–40% of cases; bilateral facial weakness is most common
- Back pain and lower limb pain are common
- Bulbar dysfunction and weakness of respiratory muscles may lead to respiratory failure requiring intubation
- Autonomic dysfunction (eg, tachycardia, fluctuating blood pressures, gastrointestinal disturbance) occurs in 50% of cases
- Miller-Fisher variant includes ophthalmoplegia, ataxia, and areflexia

DIFFERENTIAL DX

- Acute myositis
- Enteroviral infections (eg, poliomyelitis)
- Botulism
- Acute intermittent porphyria
- Tick paralysis
- Transverse myelitis
- Periodic paralysis
- Critical illness
- Polyneuropathy or myopathy
- Compressive myelopathy
- Anterior spinal artery syndrome
- Myasthenia gravis
- HIV
- Lyme disease
- Sarcoidosis
- Drug or heavy metal toxicity
- Bilateral strokes
- Hysteria

DIAGNOSTIC EVALUATION

- A clinical diagnosis based on history and physical examination
- Cerebrospinal fluid analysis (after 1 week of symptoms) reveals normal pressures, elevated protein (>45 mg/dL), and no significant rise in WBC count (fewer than 10 cells, typically mononuclear); cultures are typically negative for viruses and bacteria
- Electrophysiologic testing reveals partial motor conduction block, slowed nerve conduction velocities, abnormal temporal dispersion, prolonged distal latencies, slowed nerve conduction velocities due to segmental demyelination, and absent H reflexes or abnormal prolonged F waves due to proximal nerve root involvement
- MRI is used to rule out transverse myelitis; spinal nerve root enhancement may be seen
- Biopsy is rarely necessary

TREATMENT & MANAGEMENT

- Historically, children typically recover completely, but recovery may take up to 6 months; current management is still largely based on supportive therapy, but intravenous immunoglobulin (IVIG) or plasmapheresis is indicated when ambulation or respiratory function is affected
  - Both IVIG and plasmapheresis have been shown to reduce morbidity
- Hospital admission and intensive care may be required due to autonomic instability, arrhythmias, or respiratory failure
- Supportive care includes frequent vital sign checks and pulmonary function testing; negative inspiratory pressures can be followed in older children
- Steroids alone have no proven benefit
- Maintenance of adequate nutrition and prevention of complications is essential
- Physical therapy to facilitate recovery and improve functioning

PROGNOSIS & COMPLICATIONS

- Progression occurs over 1–2 weeks; within 2–4 weeks, most patients begin to show recovery
- 20–25% of affected patients require mechanical ventilation
- Mortality rates are as high as 5%
- The majority of patients have full motor recovery
- Recovery is descending in nature; reflexes are the last to recover
- About 7% of patients relapse

Migraine

INTRODUCTION

- Migraines occur in approximately 7% of all children; some studies suggest that the majority of pediatric headaches are due to migraines
- They are frequently pulsatile or throbbing in nature and are associated with nausea, vomiting, photophobia, and phonophobia
- Children should be asymptomatic between events
- There appears to be a strong genetic component; most children with migraines have a family history of migraines

ETIOLOGY, EPIDEMIOLOGY, & RISK FACTORS

- Migraines are frequently worsened by bright lights, loud noises, diet (eg, chocolate, alcohol), trauma, certain medications (eg, oral contraceptive pills), exercise, fatigue, fasting, and stress; they are often relieved by rest
- Autosomal dominant inheritance
- Adolescent females are at highest risk
- 50% of cases begin prior to age 20
- Chronic conditions (eg, epilepsy, collagen vascular diseases) and previous trauma may predispose to headaches
- The mechanism appears to be a primary neuronal dysfunction resulting in a sequence of intracranial and extracranial changes; the pathogenesis may be related to an imbalance in activity between brainstem nuclei regulating antinociception and vascular control
  - A primary event may occur in the brainstem involving diffuse projections from the locus ceruleus to other parts of the brain
  - Vasodilatation plays an important role in the characteristic severe throbbing head pain
- The previously popular vascular theory of migraines suggested they were caused by dilatation of blood vessels and the aura resulted from vasoconstriction; however, this is no longer considered correct

PATIENT PRESENTATION

- Common migraine: Intense headache (throbbing pain, frontal or temporal, unilateral or bilateral), nausea, and photophobia; may last for a day or longer
- Classic migraine: Symptoms of common migraine preceded by an aura period that lasts a few minutes (most often visual, such as flashing lights); may be associated with temporary neurologic deficits (eg, hemiplegia, aphasia, sensory deficits, vertigo)
- Distinguish from other types of headaches:
  - Tension headache: Diffuse, bilateral pain lasting hours to days; *not* associated with nausea, vomiting, photophobia, or aura
  - Cluster headache: Severe unilateral pain, generally around the eye, temple, or forehead, lasting minutes to hours; usually occurs at night

DIFFERENTIAL DX

- Tension headache
- Cluster headache
- Mass lesion
- Chiari malformation
- Pseudotumor cerebri
- Stroke
- Meningitis
- Aneurysm
- Arteriovenous malformation
- Sinus infection
- Temporomandibular joint syndrome
- Central nervous system vasculitis

DIAGNOSTIC EVALUATION

- Diagnosis is based on history and physical examination; diagnostic tests are useful only to rule out other causes
- Characteristic features of drawings of the headaches experienced by affected children have been shown to helpful in accurately making a diagnosis of migraine
- In patients with severe headache but no history of migraines, persistent headaches, or neurologic findings, more sinister causes of headache should be ruled out:
  - ○ Serum and cerebrospinal fluid studies to rule out infection
  - ○ Head CT scan to rule out subarachnoid hemorrhage or mass (eg, tumor, subdural hematoma)
  - ○ Thyroid-stimulating hormone (TSH) to assess for hyper- or hypothyroidism
  - ○ EEG to assess for seizures
  - ○ If the child has experienced a recent lumbar puncture or spine procedure, consider lumbar MRI to rule out pseudomeningocele

TREATMENT & MANAGEMENT

- Identify triggers (eg, trauma, sunlight, insomnia, hormones, stress, diet, dehydration), and modify reversible factors (eg, diet, sleep disturbances)
- Acute attacks: Place the child in a dark, quiet room and treat with acetaminophen, NSAIDs, sumatriptan and related serotonin agonists, ergotamines, or other analgesics, sedatives, and antiemetics
- For patients who experience more than one migraine per week, prophylactic medications should be considered, including Periactin (an antihistamine), β-blockers and/or calcium-channel blockers, tricyclic antidepressants (eg, amitriptyline), and anticonvulsants (eg, topiramate, levetiracetam, valproic acid, gabapentin)
- Cluster headaches are treated with supplemental oxygen, corticosteroids, and migraine preparations
- Tension headaches are often treated with tricyclic antidepressants

PROGNOSIS & COMPLICATIONS

- Family history is often helpful in determining prognosis
- Recurrent migraines can be associated with psychiatric disorders, such as depression, anxiety, and social withdrawal
- Many children miss multiple days of school
- Pediatric migraines, unlike adult migraines, are often more brief and intense and include vomiting, making medication administration difficult
- Menstrual cycles and hormonal effects may worsen headaches and may require hormonal treatment to regulate cycles
- Children may either outgrow or experience onset of migraines during puberty

Ataxia

INTRODUCTION

- Ataxia is defined as a disturbance in the smooth, accurate coordination of movements; it is most commonly manifested as an unsteady gait
- Ataxia occurs due to dysfunction of the cerebellum or its connections
- It can present as an acute or chronic, progressive illness
- Associated signs and symptoms, such as papilledema, myoclonus, and retinopathy, help determine the underlying etiology

ETIOLOGY, EPIDEMIOLOGY, & RISK FACTORS

- Acute etiologies include tumors, toxic ingestion (eg, phenytoin), brainstem encephalitis, migraine, postinfectious or autoimmune (eg, acute cerebellar ataxia, Guillain-Barré, multiple sclerosis), trauma, vascular disorders (eg, cerebellar hemorrhage, stroke), and conversion reaction
- Chronic etiologies include tumors (eg, ependymoma, medulloblastoma), congenital malformations (eg, Dandy-Walker malformation), and hereditary causes (eg, olivopontocerebellar degeneration, ataxia-telangiectasia, adrenoleukodystrophy, Friedreich ataxia)
- Toxic ingestion is a common cause in ages 1–4
- Acute cerebellar ataxia occurs between 2 and 7 years
- Conversion disorder is common in adolescent females
- Multiple sclerosis is typically a disease of young adults

PATIENT PRESENTATION

- Wide-based, staggering gait
- Unsteady, inaccurate limb movement
- Scanning speech (increased separation of syllables, varied volume)
- Sensory disturbance; loss of proprioception results in slapping of feet during gait
- Positive Romberg test
- Nystagmus with eye movement
- Other signs of brainstem involvement include visual loss, vertigo, tinnitus, alternating hemiplegia, and dysphagia

DIFFERENTIAL DX

- Vertigo
- Hysteria
- Opsoclonus-myoclonus
- Epilepsy
- Chorea

DIAGNOSTIC EVALUATION

- History and physical examination are paramount
  - Assess for recent illness (eg, varicella infection), ingestion of toxins or drugs, trauma, previous episodes of ataxia, headaches, progressive gait disturbance, and family history of migraine or spinocerebellar ataxia
  - Determine the time course (acute onset, episodic, progressive, chronic/nonprogressive)
  - Physical examination should include assessment for skin rashes, telangiectasias, cardiac exam, abdominal masses, ears, and sinuses
  - Neurologic exam should focus on cranial nerves and cerebellar examinations
  - The presence of papilledema is concerning for causes of increased intracranial pressure
  - Extraocular eye movements and nystagmus should be carefully tested
  - Reflex, Babinski, proprioceptive sense, and Romberg tests should be performed
- Initial testing may include toxicology screen; lumbar puncture (only after neuroimaging to rule out increased intracranial pressure) if suspect infection, Guillain-Barré syndrome, or multiple sclerosis; and homovanillic acid and vanillylmandelic acid levels
- Metabolic testing: Serum amino acids, vitamin E, cholesterol + subtypes, lactate, pyruvate, α-fetoprotein, ammonia, lysosomal enzymes, transferrin electrophoresis, electromicroscopy of lymphocytes for inclusion bodies, muscle biopsy for mitochondrial disease
- Further testing includes thoracic and abdominal MRI to rule out neuroblastoma, EEG to assess for seizures, and genetic testing for Friedreich ataxia and spinocerebellar ataxia

TREATMENT & MANAGEMENT

- In most cases, supportive treatment is sufficient
- Exogenous toxins should be removed from the patient's system, if possible
- Neoplasms, abscesses, and hemorrhage require neurosurgical intervention
- Patients with Friedreich ataxia and mitochondrial disease need cardiac evaluation
- Ataxia due to the Miller-Fisher variant of Guillain-Barré syndrome usually has a very good prognosis; intravenous immunoglobulin (IVIG) or plasmapheresis may be used
- Opsoclonus/myoclonus syndrome can be treated with ACTH or IVIG
- Acute demyelinating encephalomyelitis is treated with steroids
- Some genetic and metabolic diseases are treatable:
  - Supplemental vitamin E for ataxia with vitamin E deficiency (AVED)
  - Supplemental biotinidase for biotinidase deficiency
  - Supplemental niacin for Hartnup disease
  - Dietary restriction of phytanic acid for Refsum disease
  - Acetazolamide for episodic ataxia
- CT scan or MRI if suspect a mass lesion or demyelination

PROGNOSIS & COMPLICATIONS

- Tumors often have good prognoses, depending on the type of tumor (refer to the *Brain Tumors* entry)
- Acute cerebellar ataxia may take weeks or months to recover; some have persistent deficits
- Multiple sclerosis generally follows a progressive, relapsing-remitting pattern
- Toxic ingestion usually recovers completely
- Encephalitis outcomes depend on the causative agent
- Postconcussive ataxia usually remits
- Recovery from stroke and cerebellar hemorrhage is variable; outcomes depend on the site of the infarct
- Genetic syndromes may be associated with progressive neurodegeneration

Chorea

INTRODUCTION

- Chorea consists of brief, irregular, nonrhythmic, unsustained, involuntary movements that flow from one part of the body to another; it is often accompanied by athetosis, which are slow, writhing, involuntary movements
- These movement disorders are thought to result from dysfunction of the basal ganglia
- Normal infants make movements resembling chorea; this resolves by 8 months
- Children with attention deficit disorder and hyperactivity may have distal chorea or chorea minima

ETIOLOGY, EPIDEMIOLOGY, & RISK FACTORS

- Cerebral palsy is a common cause in children (one-third of affected patients have choreo-athetosis); occurs due to to sprouting and denervation supersensitivity of receptors in the basal ganglia
- Drugs are a common cause (eg, antiepileptics, psychotropics, phenytoin, Reglan, theo-phyllines, stimulants)
- Systemic etiologies include hyperthyroidism, SLE, pregnancy, and Sydenham chorea
  - 20% of cases of rheumatic fever include chorea (Sydenham chorea); it usually occurs 4 months after group A beta-hemolytic *Streptococcus* infection and is caused by molecular mimicry between streptococcal and central nervous system antigens leading to forma-tion of cross-reactive antibodies that disrupt basal ganglia function
- Genetic etiologies include Huntington disease, Wilson disease, Hallervorden-Spatz syndrome, Fahr syndrome, glutaric aciduria type I, benign familial chorea, ataxia-telangiectasia, mitochondrial encephalopathies, and Lesch-Nyhan syndrome
- Other etiologies include kernicterus; tumors (eg, glioma); postcardiopulmonary bypass surgery ("postpump chorea"), which begins 2 weeks after the procedure with hypotonia, oral-facial dyskinesias, and affective changes; and postinfectious (eg, *Mycoplasma*, herpes simplex virus, Epstein-Barr virus, Echo 25, varicella)

PATIENT PRESENTATION

- Identified by a quick, jerk-like movement that is not rhythmic
- These movements are incorporated into volun-tary movement
- Patients may look restless; they can make unusual sounds
- May be symmetric or asymmetric
- Often involves the face, arms, or legs
- Milking hand grip, spooning, and pendular extremity movements occur due to extremities held in a hypotonic position
- Accompanying behavioral problems (eg, obses-sive-compulsive disease, tics)
- 5% of SLE patients have chorea as a presenting neurologic symptom

DIFFERENTIAL DX

- Seizures
- Tics
- Ballismus
- Athetosis
- Tardive dyskinesia

DIAGNOSTIC EVALUATION

- Diagnosis depends on correct identification of the movement disorder and correlation with other features of the etiologic condition
- History should assess for prior streptococcal infections, rheumatic fever, arthritis, fever, rash, birth history, family history, and home medications
- Physical exam includes ophthalmologic exam for Kayser-Fleischer rings, cardiac exam, joint exam, and skin exam
- Neurologic exam should include eye movements, dysarthria, evaluation of tone, and motor impersistence
- Laboratory testing includes electrolytes, glucose, calcium, magnesium, TSH, parathyroid hormone, liver function tests, complete blood count, blood smear (for acanthocytes), throat culture, anti–streptolysin O titer, lactate, pyruvate, ceruloplasmin, amino acids, lyme titer, antinuclear, anticardiolipin, antiphospholipid, and anti–ds-DNA antibodies, rheumatoid - factor, and lipid profile
- Consider genetic testing for Huntington disease
- Heart evaluation with echocardiography and EKG is mandatory since the association of Sydenham chorea with carditis is found in up to 80% of patients
- Lumbar puncture may be useful in infectious or postinfectious cases and for multiple - sclerosis
- Neuroimaging includes CT scan or MRI

TREATMENT & MANAGEMENT

- Treatment is reserved for patients in whom chorea is so severe that it interferes with - normal function
- Simple measures such as rest and avoidance of stress often alleviate symptoms
- Dopamine blockers (eg, haloperidol, pimozide) can be used to decrease the movement disorder

Treat the Underlying Disorder as Appropriate
- In cases of toxin-induced chorea, removal of the offending agent is usually sufficient
- Sydenham chorea can be treated with valproate, pimozide, benzodiazepines, phenothiazine, or haloperidol; steroids, IVIG, or plasmapheresis have been used as well
  - Treat the infection with high-dose penicillin for 10 days followed by daily prophylaxis for life or at least until age 21
  - Cardiology consultation
  - Address behavior, nutrition, and sleep issues
- Huntington chorea does not have a definitive therapy; seizures may be controlled with medications, and the movement disorder may be improved with haloperidol and reserpine
- Postcardiopulmonary bypass chorea may require sedation to prevent exhaustion
- Systemic lupus erythematosus is treated with high-dose steroids

PROGNOSIS & COMPLICATIONS

- Sydenham chorea improves over weeks to months, although full recovery may not occur, and emotional lability may persist
- Huntington chorea starts in childhood in about 10% of cases; it is relentlessly progressive, with death occurring within 8–12 years; rigidity is more common than chorea in children, who may also have seizures, emotional flattening, cerebellar signs, or impaired eye movements
- Most children recover from postcardiopulmonary bypass surgery within 2 months
- Systemic lupus erythematosus has poor overall outcome
- Emergent withdrawal syndrome: Lingual-facial-buccal dyskinesia appears after neuroleptic drugs are abruptly discontinued or greatly reduced in dosage

Head Trauma

INTRODUCTION

- Trauma is the leading cause of death in children younger than 1 year of age
- Approximately 200,000 children per year are hospitalized secondary to head trauma
- Boys have twice the risk compared with girls
- Nonaccidental trauma (abuse) is a significant contributor
- Use of CT scan for pediatric head trauma increased from 13% in 1995 to 29% in 2000
- Recently, some studies suggest that children who have head CTs may be at increased risk for malignancies later in life; consequently, a number of studies are investigating which subsets of the pediatric "head trauma" population warrant imaging

ETIOLOGY, EPIDEMIOLOGY, & RISK FACTORS

- Falls and child abuse are the most common causes of head trauma in infants
- Falls and motor vehicle accidents (as passenger) are the most common causes in preschool-age children
- Falls, motor vehicle accidents (as passenger), and sports-related trauma are the most common causes among school-age children
- Motor vehicle accidents (as driver or passenger) and sports-related trauma are the most common causes in adolescents
- 5–10% of pediatric head trauma patients are discharged to long-term care facilities
- Overall mortality from pediatric head injury can approach 20% in some studies
- Patients presenting with Glasgow Coma Scale of 3–5 have a 50% chance of permanent neurologic injury
- Overall, children fare better than adults with similar head injuries
- Key anatomic differences render the pediatric patient more susceptible to certain injuries:
  - The head is larger in proportion to body surface area compared with adults
  - The pediatric brain has a higher water content than the adult, which increases the severity of acceleration/deceleration injuries
  - The pediatric brain is more unmyelinated and is thus more susceptible to shear injuries

PATIENT PRESENTATION

- Hemotympanum (bloody discharge from temporal bone fracture)
- Battle sign: Postauricular ecchymosis signifying basilar skull fracture
- Raccoon's eye (bleeding into the infraorbital region from a basilar skull fracture)
- Cerebrospinal fluid otorrhea or rhinorrhea
- Signs and symptoms of increased intracranial pressure:
  - Infants: Full fontanel, separated sutures, papilledema, and expanding head size
  - Altered mental status, seizures
  - Cushing triad (hypertension, bradycardia, decreased and irregular respirations)
  - Abnormal posturing (decerebrate or decorticate)
  - Diplopia and strabismus
  - Nausea, vomiting

DIFFERENTIAL DX

- Nonaccidental trauma
- Underlying coagulopathy
- Migraine
- CNS neoplasm

Altered Mental Status
- *A*lcohol (intoxication or withdrawal)
- *E*ndocrine, electrolytes, encephalopathy (eg, uremia)
- *I*nsulin (hyper- or hypoglycemia)
- *O*xygen deprivation
- *U*remia
- *T*rauma, toxins, temperature (eg, hypo- or hyperthermia)
- *I*nfection (eg, meningitis)
- *P*sychiatric, postictal state,
- *S*ubarachnoid hemorrhage, seizures

DIAGNOSTIC EVALUATION

- Any patient with head trauma **must** be evaluated for associated cervical spine injury
- A full clinical assessment of the child is indicated to assess for other injuries (eg, long bone fractures, abdominal trauma)
- Apply the Pediatric Glasgow Coma Scale (GCS) for children younger than 5:
  ○ GCS of 13–15 indicates minor head injury
  ○ GCS of 8–12 indicates moderate head injury
  ○ GCS less than 8 indicates severe head injury
- Laboratory studies should include CBC, chemistry panel, coagulation studies, fibrinogen, and blood type and cross
- Consider urine toxicology screen and urine pregnancy testing, if appropriate
- Head CT scan will evaluate for increased intracranial pressure, contusions, hematomas (subdural, epidural, or parenchymal), and hemorrhage (subarachnoid is the most common)
  ○ Ultrasound (instead of CT scan) should be considered in neonates or small infants
  ○ MRI has a limited role in the acute evaluation due to cost and availability
- The University of California-Davis devised a clinical prediction rule for blunt head trauma:
  ○ Five clinical predictors are used to assess risk of severe injury: (1) Vomiting after the injury; (2) abnormal mental status; (3) clinical signs of skull fracture; (4) headache; and (5) scalp hematoma in children younger than 2 years
  ○ If none of these predictors is present, there is about 1% chance of a significant injury that will be readily detected by CT scan

TREATMENT & MANAGEMENT

- Assess and manage airway, breathing, and circulation
- Stabilize the neck with a cervical collar and be prepared to control the airway, if necessary
- Early neurosurgical consultation for suspected or diagnosed intracranial injury
- The decision to order a CT scan in a pediatric patient should include an evaluation of the risks of possible sedation, radiation exposure, higher hospital cost, and prolonged stay
- Depressed, basilar, or diastatic (wide separation) skull fractures require neurosurgical consultation and admission to the hospital
- Isolated, nondepressed skull fractures with <3 mm of diastasis do not require admission
- Open skull fractures (penetrating injuries) require antibiotics with coverage of *S. aureus*
- If suspect increased intracranial pressure (ICP), treat immediately with intubation, administration of mannitol, and elevation of the head of the bed to improve venous drainage
  ○ The use of mannitol for elevated ICP has become standard of care; however, a meta-analysis by the Cochrane Foundation failed to find a consistent mortality benefit
- Aggressive treatment of acute seizures is essential to reduce intracranial pressure and risk of hypoxia, which also increases intracranial pressure
  ○ Short-acting benzodiazepines (eg, lorazepam) should be used to abort seizure activity, followed by phenytoin or phenobarbital for seizure prophylaxis
- The use of therapeutic hypothermia in head injuries is theoretical and not evidence based

PROGNOSIS & COMPLICATIONS

- Children younger than 4 have poorer outcomes
- Duration of coma, severity of increased intracranial pressure, and ischemic injury to the brain all adversely affect outcome
- Postconcussive seizures may occur early (within hours to days) after injury
- Late-onset seizure or epilepsy occurs in 5% of cases
- Concussions may cause headaches and behavior and memory disturbance for days to months
- Highest rates of recovery from memory impairment occur during the first year after injury
- Injury patterns in young children strongly related to abuse include subdural hematoma, retinal hemorrhages, and diffuse brain injury

Pseudotumor Cerebri

INTRODUCTION

- Pseudotumor cerebri is characterized by elevated intracranial pressure in the setting of normal cerebral spinal fluid indices and no mass lesions on neuroimaging tests
- Should be considered in the differential diagnosis of chronic headaches
- Also called idiopathic intracranial hypertension

ETIOLOGY, EPIDEMIOLOGY, & RISK FACTORS

- Most prepubertal children have an identifiable cause:
  - Drugs: Steroid withdrawal, oral contraceptive pills, tetracycline, nalidixic acid, vitamin A, thyroid replacement, phenothiazines
  - Systemic disease: Iron deficiency, systemic lupus erythematosus, Guillain-Barré syndrome, leukemia, chronic otitis media or sinusitis with venous thrombosis, polycythemia
  - Metabolic: Hyperthyroidism, obesity, pregnancy, hypoparathyroidism, adrenal insufficiency, menarche, initiation of treatment for hypothyroidism
  - Trauma
- Proposed causes include increased cerebrospinal fluid production, cerebral edema, decreased cerebrospinal fluid absorption, and elevated cerebral venous pressure
- May occur at any age during childhood
- More likely to occur in obese individuals, females, and adolescents
- Annual incidence of 0.9 per 100,000 individuals

PATIENT PRESENTATION

- Headache, which is often pulsatile and may awaken the child from sleep
  - Headache may worsen with maneuvers that increase intracranial pressure, such as coughing or bending over
- Diplopia due to compression of the 6th cranial nerve
- Blackouts of vision lasting seconds may occur in one or both eyes, usually upon standing
- Optic disc edema (usually bilateral but may be asymmetric)
- Nonverbal children may present with irritability
- Nausea and vomiting
- Neck pain
- Retro-ocular pain that worsens with eye movement

DIFFERENTIAL DX

- Tumor
- Meningitis
- Hydrocephalus
- Intracranial hemorrhage
- Intracranial abscess
- Venous sinus thrombosis
- Pseudopapilledema

DIAGNOSTIC EVALUATION

- A diagnosis of exclusion; the evaluation is usually based on the modified Dandy criteria:
  - An awake and alert patient
  - Presence of signs and symptoms of increased intracranial pressure (eg, pupillary dilation, ptosis, increased blood pressure, decreased heart rate, change in respiratory pattern)
  - Absence of localized findings on neurologic examination, except paresis of the abducens nerve (cranial nerve 6)
  - Normal cerebrospinal fluid findings except for increased pressure (>200 mmH$_2$O in nonobese patients and >250 mmH$_2$O in obese patients)
  - Absence of deformity, displacement, or obstruction of the ventricular system on neuroimaging studies
  - No other identifiable cause of increased intracranial pressure
- The diagnosis requires a thorough history to assess for drug exposures (eg, corticosteroids), trauma, and recent weight gain
- Ultrasound of the optic nerve has been proposed as a noninvasive way to diagnose and monitor children with idiopathic intracranial hypertension
- In one study, 70% of patients had an empty sella, presumably caused by the longstanding effects of pulsatile high-pressure cerebrospinal fluid causing downward herniation of an arachnocele through a defect in the diaphragma sella

TREATMENT & MANAGEMENT

- Eliminate the offending agent, if identified (eg, offending medications)
- Diuretic therapy (eg, acetazolamide, furosemide) is used to decrease formation of cerebrospinal fluid
- Weight loss in obese patients
- Steroids may be used, but they tend to cause rebound effects and weight gain
- Serial lumbar punctures with measurement of opening pressures can also be helpful to monitor response to therapy
- Monitor the neuro-ophthalmologic exam, including visual field function
- Surgical intervention (eg, optic nerve sheath fenestration, lumboperitoneal or ventriculoperitoneal shunting) may be necessary in patients who continue to have visual compromise despite aggressive medical therapy

PROGNOSIS & COMPLICATIONS

- Most patients without visual deficits do well without sequelae
- Optic nerve damage is the only serious complication
  - Affected patients begin with increased blind spots, then visual field loss, then loss of visual acuity
- The majority of patients with visual deficits will improve, although some will have worsening courses
- Some patients develop post–lumbar puncture headaches requiring analgesia and bed rest

Brain Tumors

INTRODUCTION

- Brain tumors are the most common solid malignancy in children and the second most common malignancy overall, second only to leukemias
- Overall survival rate is 60–70%; despite major advances in treatment, many types of brain tumors continue to have dismal prognoses
- Chromosomal abnormalities have been identified in many brain tumors

ETIOLOGY, EPIDEMIOLOGY, & RISK FACTORS

- The World Health Organization (WHO) classifies brain tumors into the following:
  - Tumors of neuroepithelial tissue: Neuronal/embryonal cells and neuroglial cells (astrocytes, oligodendrocytes, ependymal cells, choroid plexus)
  - Tumors of peripheral nerves
  - Tumors of the meninges
  - Lymphomas and hematopoietic malignancies of the CNS
  - Tumors of the sellar region
  - Tumors metastatic to the central nervous system
- Tumors can also be classified by histology or topography:
  - Glial cell tumors are most common (70–80% of cases) and include astrocytoma (the most common tumor in children), ependymoma, and glioblastoma multiforme (GBM)
  - Neuroectodermal tumors include medulloblastoma (cerebellar primitive neuroectodermal tumors), craniopharyngioma, and dermoid tumors
- Unlike adults, 70% of pediatric brain tumors are infratentorial (in the posterior fossa)
- Genetic risk factors include neurofibromatosis-1, tuberous sclerosis, basal cell nevus syndrome, and Turcot syndrome

PATIENT PRESENTATION

- Presentation depends on growth rate, location, and tumor type
- Increased ICP results in headache/vomiting, diplopia or impaired vision, papilledema (bulging fontanelle occurs in infants)
  - Can present just as irritability and lethargy
  - Cushing triad (bradycardia, hypertension, and irregular respirations) is an ominous sign of severely increased intracranial pressure
- Focal neurologic deficits or cranial nerve palsy
- Behavior and mental status changes; seizures
- Gait and balance disturbances (eg, ataxia)
- Endocrine abnormalities may occur due to hypothalamic or pituitary tumors
- Head tilting and neck stiffness may result from cerebellar tonsil herniation
- Developmental delay
- Weight gain, weight loss, or failure to thrive

DIFFERENTIAL DX

- Migraine
- Stroke
- Pseudotumor cerebri
- Intracranial hemorrhage
- Neurocutaneous disorders (eg, neurofibromatosis, tuberous sclerosis, Sturge-Weber, ataxia-telangiectasia)
- Acute demyelinating disease
- Brain abscess or focal infection
- Herpes simplex or postinflammatory encephalitis
- Vasculitis
- Vascular malformation (eg, aneurysm, arteriovenous malformation)
- Granulomatous disease

DIAGNOSTIC EVALUATION

- When clinical suspicion arises, neuroimaging studies can identify a mass lesion and the presence of increased intracranial pressure
  - MRI with gadolinium or CT scan with contrast is the best test
  - CT scan can detect 95% of tumors; however, MRI is best to evaluate the posterior fossa
  - MRI also defines the relationship between the tumor and critical neurovascular structures (for surgical reduction)
  - Most cases also require MRI of the spine for staging
  - Magnetic resonance angiogram (MRA) will determine if there is a vascular component to the tumor and will differentiate tumors from vascular malformations
- Cerebrospinal fluid and histopathologic analysis may identify genetic or chemical tumor markers (eg, beta-hCG, alpha-fetoprotein)
- Visual and auditory evoked potentials may help to evaluate tumors that invade the optic or auditory nerves
- Metastatic workup may include bone marrow aspiration or bone scan, depending on tumor pathology
- Surgical biopsy is usually necessary for diagnosis, except in certain rare cases (eg, brainstem glioma)

TREATMENT & MANAGEMENT

- Surgical resection is the most important initial therapy; it provides tissue samples for histologic diagnosis and relieves elevated intracranial pressure
  - Gross total resection should be attempted whenever safe, but biopsy and/or debulking may be the only feasible approach(es)
  - Can also allow for other supportive measures (eg, placement of a ventriculoperitoneal shunt)
- Brain tumors are generally responsive to radiation
  - Radiation is often used following resection because many tumors cannot be completely removed by surgery
  - However, radiation should be avoided or postponed as long as possible (at minimum, until after age 3 years since nerve myelination is not yet complete)
- Chemotherapy is usually a second-line agent, in part because the effects are limited by the blood-brain barrier (BBB); it is primarily used for recurrent disease but is also useful in germ cell tumors and embryonal tumors
  - May also be used to avoid or postpone radiation therapy in young children
- Steroids may be used to decrease inflammation and mass effect of tumor

PROGNOSIS & COMPLICATIONS

- Survival depends on age at diagnosis and tumor type and location; unlike other tumors, the anatomic location of brain tumors is often more important than the grade or stage
- In general, children younger than 2 have much lower survival rates than other age groups
- Due to BBB and lack of lymphatics in CNS, brain tumors do not regularly metastasize
- Primitive neuroectodermal tumors (eg, medulloblastoma) tend to seed the subarachnoid space and may metastasize to other CNS locations, bone, and bone marrow
- Cerebellar astrocytomas have the best prognosis
- Late effects of radiation include intellectual deficits, learning disabilities, hypopituitarism, myelopathy, spine deformity, and second malignancy
- Novel therapies and delivery systems may offer future improvements in survival

Infectious Disease

Acute Otitis Media

INTRODUCTION

- Otitis media is a common condition seen in both outpatient and emergency settings; it is the most common cause of pediatric patient visits (40% of all pediatrician visits)
- Defined as inflammation and effusion of the middle ear
- Results in characteristic changes of the tympanic membrane on physical examination
- The classic presentation is a young child with a recent upper respiratory infection and sudden onset of fever, crying, and ear pain

ETIOLOGY, EPIDEMIOLOGY, & RISK FACTORS

- Most cases occur between 6 and 18 months of age
- Very common: Most young children experience 1–1.5 episodes per year, and recurrences are common
- May be of bacterial or viral origin
  - Bacterial etiologies include *Streptococcus pneumoniae*, *Moraxella catarrhalis*, and *Haemophilus influenzae* (nontypable strain)
  - Viral causes include any respiratory virus (eg, RSV, influenza)
  - Neonatal disease may be caused by the above organisms, as well as *E. coli*, *Klebsiella*, *Enterobacter*, group B streptococci, and *Staphylococcus aureus*
- Risk factors include daycare environments, bottle feeding, passive smoke exposure, recent or concurrent respiratory viral illness or environmental allergies, male gender, family history of recurrent otitis media in childhood, early age of first infection, craniofacial anomalies (eg, cleft palate), or any immunodeficiency (eg, antibody deficiency or ciliary dyskinesia)

PATIENT PRESENTATION

- Ear pain occurs in 70–80% of cases
- Crying or irritability
- Coryza
- Fever
- Sleep disturbance
- Otorrhea
- Tympanic membranes may have a characteristic appearance
  - Red or yellow, bulging, and thickened
  - Aberrant light reflex
  - Decreased mobility with pneumatic otoscopy
  - Perforation with drainage
- Younger children tend to have fewer and less specific symptoms

DIFFERENTIAL DX

- Acute otitis externa
- Chronic otitis media with effusion
- Chronic suppurative otitis media
- Viral upper respiratory tract infection
- Redness of the tympanic membrane from crying
- Mastoiditis

DIAGNOSTIC EVALUATION

- History and physical examination are usually sufficient for diagnosis
- Tympanogram (a graphic depiction of the mobility of the tympanic membrane) shows decreased compliance
- Tympanocentesis is only necessary to confirm the pathogen in neonates, if severe pain is present, or if failure of therapy occurs
- Risk factors for antibiotic-resistant *S. pneumoniae* include age younger than 36 months, daycare environment or numerous siblings, and antibiotic use during the previous 2 months

TREATMENT & MANAGEMENT

- If there are no risk factors for antibiotic-resistant *S. pneumoniae*, treat with amoxicillin
  - Begin with amoxicillin 40–50 mg/kg/day for 10 days
  - If this fails to cure the infection, increase the dose of amoxicillin to 80–90 mg/kg/day
  - If this still fails to cure the infection, switch to amoxicillin-clavulanate or cefuroxime
- If the patient has risk factors for antibiotic-resistant *S. pneumoniae*, begin therapy with high-dose of amoxicillin (80 mg/kg/day), with or without clavulanate
- In cases of recurrent infections, consider surgical placement of tympanostomy tubes and possible adenoidectomy

PROGNOSIS & COMPLICATIONS

- Prognosis is good; spontaneous resolution without sequelae is common
- If treated with antibiotics, rapid decrease of symptoms usually occurs
- Complications may include perforation of tympanic membrane, mastoiditis, meningitis, conductive hearing loss, lateral sinus thrombophlebitis, and facial nerve paralysis

Streptococcal Pharyngitis

INTRODUCTION

- Also known as "strep throat," this condition is one of the most important causes of acute pharyngitis
- Streptococcal pharyngitis is important not only because of the immediate morbidity but also due to its relationship to other serious conditions, such as rheumatic fever and poststreptococcal glomerulonephritis
- It can be rapidly diagnosed in any clinical setting by a simple test, and antibiotics can be prescribed to prevent rheumatic fever and other sequelae

ETIOLOGY, EPIDEMIOLOGY, & RISK FACTORS

- The infection is caused by *Streptococcus pyogenes* (group A β-hemolytic *Streptococcus*)
  - It is the cause of acute pharyngitis in 15–20% of children
  - Occurs in all ages but predominantly in children 5–12 years old
  - Colonization by *S. pyogenes* is present in as many as 15% of healthy children
  - Transmitted person-to-person via respiratory droplets
- Scarlet fever is an erythematous rash that may occur in the setting of streptococcal pharyngitis
- Acute streptococcal pharyngitis may occur in isolation, as part of scarlet fever, or associated with a peritonsillar abscess
- Although upper respiratory and cutaneous infections with *S. pyogenes* are common in the pediatric population, infection may also cause serious invasive disease, such as toxic shock syndrome or necrotizing fasciitis
- *S. pyogenes* is also a common cause of bacterial superinfection following acute varicella infection

PATIENT PRESENTATION

- Incubation period of 2–5 days
- Variable clinical spectrum ranging from subclinical infection with few symptoms (especially in younger children) to toxic-appearing manifestations
- Fever, headache, malaise, abdominal pain, dysphagia, and vomiting are common
- Exam may show erythematous pharynx, exudative tonsillitis, palatal petechiae, uvular edema, strawberry tongue, circumoral pallor, scarlatiniform rash, or swollen, tender, anterior cervical lymphadenopathy
- A papular, "sandpaper-like," diffuse rash begins in the neck and chest area, extending especially to the flexor creases; desquamation may occur over the trunk, hands, and feet after the first week of illness

DIFFERENTIAL DX

- Other causes of pharyngitis:
  - Adenovirus
  - Enterovirus
  - Parainfluenza
  - Rhinovirus
  - Epstein-Barr virus
  - Diphtheria
  - *Arcanobacterium haemolyticum*
  - Kawasaki syndrome
  - Drug eruption
  - Toxigenic *Staphylococcus aureus* infection
  - Measles
  - Roseola

DIAGNOSTIC EVALUATION

- Throat culture is the gold standard for diagnosis; it is 90–95% sensitive when performed correctly
  - A rapid strep test via throat swab is cheaper and quicker but less sensitive (sensitivity of 70–90%; specificity of 95–100%); thus, a positive test warrants therapy, but a negative test should be confirmed with a standard throat culture before streptococcal pharyngitis is ruled out
  - Specimens should be obtained from both tonsillar surfaces and the posterior pharyngeal wall
  - Detects the group A streptococcal carbohydrate antigen
- *S. pyogenes* is less likely as the cause of pharyngitis if hoarseness, cough, conjunctivitis, diarrhea, or rhinorrhea is present

TREATMENT & MANAGEMENT

- Antimicrobial therapy will prevent the development of sequelae, especially rheumatic fever, and may decrease the duration of acute illness
- Treatment should be started within 9 days after the onset of acute illness to prevent rheumatic fever
- Penicillin for 10 days remains the treatment of choice
  - Penicillin-resistant *S. pyogenes* has not been seen in clinical practice; clinical failures of penicillin therapy may be due to poor compliance
  - Penicillin derivatives (eg, cephalosporins) may be more palatable for young children
  - Clindamycin or macrolides are used in penicillin-allergic patients; however, resistance to macrolides exists
- Treatment of asymptomatic carriers and contacts is controversial and should be considered on a case-by-case basis

PROGNOSIS & COMPLICATIONS

- Sequelae may include parapharyngeal or peritonsillar abscess, retropharyngeal abscess, acute glomerulonephritis, and acute rheumatic fever
- Appropriate treatment of pharyngitis will prevent the development of rheumatic fever but not acute glomerulonephritis
- Isolation precautions: Children should be kept from contact with other children until 24 hours after the initiation of therapy

Sinusitis

INTRODUCTION

- Sinusitis has been becoming more common in the pediatric population
- It is diagnosed primarily by the duration of symptoms, which differentiates it from viral upper respiratory tract infections that do not require antibiotic therapy
- Sinusitis can be acute, chronic, or recurrent
- Often associated with allergic rhinitis

ETIOLOGY, EPIDEMIOLOGY, & RISK FACTORS

- Defined as inflammation of one or more of the normally sterile paranasal sinuses
  - The inflamed mucosa of the sinuses (eg, allergies, viruses, chemical irritation) leads to obstruction and infection
  - Bacterial etiologies include *Streptococcus pneumoniae*, *Haemophilus influenzae*, *Moraxella catarrhalis*, *Streptococcus* groups A or B, and *Staphylococcus aureus*
  - Any respiratory virus may cause sinusitis
- Approximately 35 million cases occur annually in the U.S.

PATIENT PRESENTATION

Acute Sinusitis
- Upper respiratory infection-like symptoms persisting beyond 7–10 days
- Purulent rhinitis
- Frontal or maxillary pain
- Postnasal drip with coughing, especially at night
- Fever
- Periorbital edema
- Epistaxis

Chronic Sinusitis
- Complaints are more nonspecific
- Fever (usually low grade)
- Nasal discharge
- Halitosis

DIFFERENTIAL DX

- Allergic rhinitis
- Upper respiratory tract infection
- Unilateral choanal atresia
- Hypertrophy of adenoids
- Primary ciliary dyskinesia
- Cystic fibrosis
- Foreign body in nasal cavity

DIAGNOSTIC EVALUATION

- A clinical diagnosis is made by inspection of the anterior nasal cavity and middle meatus with an otoscope
  - Characteristic findings include the presence of pus in a cavity, obstruction of nasal passages, and hypertrophy and congestion of the nasal mucosa
- Sinus X-ray or CT scan is used only in children older than 6 and only to confirm clinical suspicions
  - May show opacification of a sinus cavity, mucosal thickening (>4 mm), and air-fluid levels in the sinus cavity
  - Three X-ray views (AP, lateral, and occipitomeatal) are needed to see all paranasal sinuses
- Bacterial cultures are obtained in cases of chronic or recurrent sinusitis or if the patient is immunocompromised with possible unusual pathogens

TREATMENT & MANAGEMENT

- Amoxicillin (with or without clavulanic acid) is usually first-line therapy
- Macrolides or second-generation cephalosporins are frequently used as well
- Viral infections should be treated only with symptomatic care
- Symptomatic treatment of allergic rhinitis with decongestants may help
- Intranasal steroids can be a useful adjunct, especially in chronic cases

PROGNOSIS & COMPLICATIONS

- Complications include periorbital or orbital cellulitis, mastoiditis, osteomyelitis of local bone (osteitis), intracranial infections (brain abscess, cavernous sinus thrombosis, or meningitis), pyocele, or mucocele
- Prompt appropriate treatment of acute sinusitis results in improvement of symptoms within 48 hours

Laryngotracheobronchitis (Croup)

INTRODUCTION

- Laryngotracheobronchitis, or croup, is characterized by a "barky" cough, stridor, and hoarseness
- Usually affects infants and toddlers under 3 years of age
- The primary causative organism is parainfluenza virus, which causes laryngitis in adolescents and adults
- Children can be observed at home but may require an emergency department visit for inhaled epinephrine or steroid treatment

ETIOLOGY, EPIDEMIOLOGY, & RISK FACTORS

- Inflammation of the subglottic tissues and/or tracheal mucosa results in luminal narrowing secondary to airway edema
- Generally a benign, self-limited disease; however, 20–30% of children require hospitalization, and 1–3% require intubation
- Most commonly of viral origin: Parainfluenza type 1 is most common cause (60% of cases); other viruses include parainfluenza 2 and 3, respiratory syncytial virus (RSV), adenovirus, and influenza
- Most common between 6 months and 3 years of age
  - Greatest incidence occurs during the second year of life; rare after age 6
- Person-to-person transmission via respiratory droplets or fomite exposure; the virus then spreads from the nasopharynx to the larynx and trachea
- Seasonal peak in late fall and early winter
- Boys are affected more often than girls (ratio, 2:1)

PATIENT PRESENTATION

- Prodromal symptoms include coryza, nasal congestion, sore throat, and cough, and progresses to fever
- Characteristic "bark-like" cough, hoarseness, and inspiratory stridor (stridor is notably worse at night)
- Patients with mild disease may have a normal lung exam (with or without an expiratory wheeze)
- Mild to moderate disease presents with stridor following agitation or at rest, without signs of respiratory distress
- Severe disease results in respiratory distress, including stridor at rest, nasal flaring, retractions, poor air exchange, and mental status changes
- Typical duration of illness is 3–7 days, with peak of symptoms at 3–5 days
- No signs of toxicity (as opposed to epiglottitis)

DIFFERENTIAL DX

- Foreign body obstruction
- Epiglottitis
- Bacterial tracheitis
- Retropharyngeal abscess
- Diphtheria
- Vascular ring or sling
- Peritonsillar abscess
- Laryngomalacia or tracheomalacia
- Aspiration
- Inhalation injury (thermal or chemical)

DIAGNOSTIC EVALUATION

- Typically a clinical diagnosis
- X-rays may be used but are usually not necessary for diagnosis
  - Steeple sign: Narrowing of laryngeal air column (due to mucosal edema) for 5–10 mm below the vocal cords on frontal neck films
  - Ballooning: Overdistension of the hypopharynx during inspiration on lateral neck films
- Complete blood count may show leukocytosis with elevated lymphocytes

TREATMENT & MANAGEMENT

- Nebulized epinephrine may be used in moderate to severe cases of viral croup to decrease laryngeal mucosa edema; nebulized budesonide may also used to decrease laryngeal mucosa edema
- Intramuscular corticosteroids (dexamethasone) have been shown to improve symptoms and decrease the need for hospitalization and intubation
- Endotracheal intubation is required in patients with severe airway obstruction (ie, increasing stridor, retractions, cyanosis, signs of exhaustion, altered mental status) and/or patients who fail to respond to the above treatments
- Heliox (mixture of helium and oxygen) may decrease the need for intubation

PROGNOSIS & COMPLICATIONS

- Mild croup does not require hospitalization
- The decision to hospitalize should be made after 3–4 hours of observation (usually in the emergency department)
- Severe croup requires systemic corticosteroids and more frequent use of nebulized epinephrine, and may require admission to an intensive care unit; heliox (if available) may prevent the need for intubation
- Complications include bacterial tracheitis due to *Staphylococcus aureus*, *Haemophilus influenzae*, *Streptococcus pneumoniae*, or *Moraxella catarrhalis*; the acute onset of respiratory compromise that mimics epiglottitis should be considered bacterial tracheitis until proven otherwise

Epiglottitis

INTRODUCTION

- Epiglottitis is now rare since the advent of *Haemophilus influenzae type B* (HiB) vaccine
- However, it is a true emergency that can result in severe airway compromise and high morbidity and mortality

ETIOLOGY, EPIDEMIOLOGY, & RISK FACTORS

- Bacterial etiologies include *Haemophilus influenzae* type B (accounts for 90% of pediatric cases), *Streptococcus pneumoniae*, *Moraxella catarrhalis*, *Haemophilus parainfluenzae*, and *Pseudomonas* species
- Viral etiologies include herpes simplex virus, parainfluenza viruses, varicella-zoster virus, and Epstein-Barr virus
- The incidence of epiglottitis has decreased significantly since the introduction of the HiB vaccine
- Males are affected more than females
- Typically occurs during ages 2–7 but may occur at any age, even during adulthood

PATIENT PRESENTATION

- Abrupt onset of high fever (>40°C) with rapid development of sore throat, hoarse voice, dysphagia, and respiratory distress (marked stridor with subcostal and supraclavicular retractions)
- Toxic appearance with irritability and anxiety
- Cherry-red, swollen epiglottis
- Patients tend to assume a characteristic tripod position in order to optimize the airway: They sit erect with chin hyperextended, mouth wide open, and body leaning forward
- Cyanosis may occur
- Drooling occurs in up to 80% of affected children

DIFFERENTIAL DX

- Bacterial tracheitis
- Croup
- Retropharyngeal abscess
- Foreign body aspiration
- Diphtheria
- Mononucleosis
- Thermal or chemical airway burn
- Trauma to airway
- Laryngomalacia
- Severe pharyngitis

DIAGNOSTIC EVALUATION

- Primarily a clinical diagnosis; it is often suspected at first glance of the sick patient
- Most of the evaluation (laboratory studies, films, and even the examination) should be done only after a safe airway is ensured; many patients warrant direct transport to the operating room for immediate airway stabilization and examination under anesthesia
- Laboratory testing includes complete blood count (may show leukocytosis) and blood culture
- Epiglottic culture should be collected, if possible
- Lateral neck X-ray shows a swollen epiglottis ("thumb print sign"), thickened aryepiglottic folds, and dilation of the hypopharynx
- Chest X-ray may reveal concurrent pneumonia

TREATMENT & MANAGEMENT

- Treatment is first surgical, then medical
  - Evaluating and securing the airway are critical in patients with suspected epiglottitis
  - Endotracheal intubation should be done by an airway expert; if endotracheal intubation cannot be performed and the patient is in extremis, tracheostomy is indicated
- Treat with second- or third-generation cephalosporins (eg, cefuroxime, ceftriaxone, or cefotaxime) for 7–10 days
- There is no proven efficacy of corticosteroids

PROGNOSIS & COMPLICATIONS

- Sequelae may include sepsis, shock, pneumothorax, tracheal stenosis, cerebral anoxic injury, and/or death
- Mortality may be as high as 10%; however, if the airway is secured immediately, mortality is closer to 1%
- Cyanosis is associated with a poor prognosis

Orbital and Periorbital Cellulitis

INTRODUCTION

- Although both are infections around the eyes, it is important to differentiate between the two:
  - Periorbital cellulitis is inflammation of the eyelids and surrounding eye structures
  - Orbital cellulitis is inflammation of the same structures with associated proptosis, movement limitations, and impairment of vision
- Typically, the two are differentiated by assessing for the proptosis and impaired extraocular movement restriction associated with orbital cellulitis
- Orbital cellulitis is much more severe and may be associated with CNS infection

ETIOLOGY, EPIDEMIOLOGY, & RISK FACTORS

- May be caused by: Direct extension of infection from adjacent structures (eg, sinusitis, local dermatitis), direct infection from a penetrating or blunt wound, or seeding of eye structures during bacteremia
- Direct extension from adjacent structures is the most common method of transmission (especially sinusitis)
- If due to sinusitis, the causative organisms include *Streptococcus pneumoniae*, *Haemophilus influenzae*, *Staphylococcus aureus*, and group A *Streptococcus*
- Viruses (primarily adenovirus) are common causes of periorbital cellulitis
- The mean age of presentation with orbital cellulitis is 7 years
- Orbital cellulitis is more common is winter, when sinusitis is common

PATIENT PRESENTATION

Orbital Cellulitis
- Eyelid swelling and erythema
- Impairment of extraocular movement
- Proptosis (protrusion of the eye)
- Chemosis (edema of the conjunctiva)
- Decline in visual acuity
- Eye pain
- High fever with toxic appearance

Periorbital Cellulitis
- Eyelid swelling and inflammation
- No restriction of eye movement or vision
- No proptosis
- Chemosis is rare
- Generally afebrile and nontoxic

DIFFERENTIAL DX

- Allergic eye involvement
- Orbital fracture
- Primary or metastatic tumor of eye
- Severe conjunctivitis
- Retained foreign body in eye
- Eyelid abscess
- Exophthalmos secondary to thyroid dysfunction

DIAGNOSTIC EVALUATION

- History should assess the type and degree of eye symptoms, associated ear/nose/throat symptoms, and systemic symptoms
- Physical exam should thoroughly evaluate the eyes:
  - Assess visual acuity before other eye examination
  - Assessment of extraocular movement is essential, although it may be difficult if significant eyelid edema is present
  - Examine the conjunctiva for chemosis or conjunctivitis
  - Examine the eyelids, globe, and conjunctiva for signs of trauma or a foreign body
- Laboratory testing includes complete blood count with differential
- Blood culture is indicated if there is a high neutrophil count, bandemia, or suspicion of orbital cellulitis
- CT scan of the orbit and sinuses is indicated if the patient has proptosis or restriction of extraocular movement; it is also useful to evaluate for adjacent sinusitis or abscess formation
- Culture of associated abscess via surgical drainage may be necessary

TREATMENT & MANAGEMENT

- ENT and/or ophthalmic consultation is mandatory in any case of suspected orbital cellulitis
- Systemic antibiotics are usually targeted against likely sinusitis organisms: First-line agents include ampicillin-sulbactam, clindamycin, cefuroxime, and ceftriaxone
- Once improvement occurs and the child is afebrile, switch to oral antibiotics (amoxicillin-clavulanate or cefuroxime) and complete a full 10- to 14-day course of therapy
- Surgical abscess drainage and culture may be necessary
- Noticeable improvement should occur within 48–72 hours after antimicrobial therapy is initiated
- Antihistamine and steroid use is controversial
- If orbital trauma led to cellulitis, consider tetanus prophylaxis

PROGNOSIS & COMPLICATIONS

- Involvement of the optic nerve may result in blindness (1% of cases)
- Extension of orbital infection into the brain may lead to meningitis (2%), cavernous sinus thrombosis (1%), or brain abscess (1%)

Meningitis

INTRODUCTION

- Meningitis is an important pediatric disease that may be fatal if the diagnosis is missed
- Young children may not be able to communicate symptoms and the symptoms may be less specific, so a high index of suspicion is required
- Evaluation is part of a "rule out sepsis" protocol in febrile children less than 2 months of age

ETIOLOGY, EPIDEMIOLOGY, & RISK FACTORS

- 70% of cases occur in children younger than 2 years
- Bacterial meningitis is especially common in winter
  - Group B *Streptococcus*, *Listeria monocytogenes*, and *E. coli* are the most common bacterial etiologies during the neonatal period
  - *Streptococcus pneumoniae*, *Neisseria meningitidis*, and *Haemophilus influenzae* type B (HiB) are the most frequent bacteria beyond the neonatal period
  - HiB vaccine has dramatically decreased the incidence of *H. influenzae* meningitis
  - *Neisseria meningitides* incidence peaks at 6–12 months and teens
  - Risk factors for bacterial meningitis include respiratory infections, ventriculoperitoneal shunt, mastoiditis, head trauma, immunodeficiency, and hemoglobinopathies
- Viral meningitis is more common in spring and summer; common viral etiologies include enteroviruses, mumps, herpes simplex virus, and arboviruses (eg, West Nile virus, California/LaCrosse virus)
- Immunocompromised patients are at risk for *Pseudomonas*, *Serratia*, and *Proteus*
- Fungal, mycobacterial, and aseptic (drug-induced) meningitis also occur

PATIENT PRESENTATION

- Flu-like illness
- Headache
- Vomiting
- Neck stiffness
- Photophobia
- Arthralgias, myalgias
- Poor feeding, anorexia
- Opisthotonos
- Fever, hypothermia
- Shock
- Seizures
- Altered consciousness (lethargy, irritability)
- Purpuric rash in cases of *Neisseria* meningitis
- Kernig sign: With patient in supine position with hip and knee flexed to 90 degrees, further extension of the knee causes neck pain
- Brudzinski sign: Flexing the neck of a supine patient results in reflexive hip and knee flexion

DIFFERENTIAL DX

- Migraine
- Brain abscess
- Brain tumor
- Leukemia
- Heavy metal poisoning
- Systemic lupus erythematosus
- Kawasaki disease
- Gastroenteritis
- Drugs
- Hemolytic-uremic syndrome
- Subdural hematoma
- Subarachnoid hemorrhage
- Sinusitis
- Mollaret syndrome
- Head trauma

DIAGNOSTIC EVALUATION

- History and physical examination with a strong index of suspicion are paramount
  - History should include the type and severity of symptoms, duration of symptoms, sick contacts (including childcare and group housing), and history of altered mental status
  - Physical examination should pay attention to photophobia, Kernig and Brudzinski signs, and a meticulous skin examination
- Laboratory studies include complete blood count, electrolytes (ensuing SIADH may cause severe hyponatremia), and blood cultures
- Lumbar puncture with cerebrospinal fluid analysis is often diagnostic
  - Assess opening pressure, cell count, differential, glucose, protein (compare with systemic values), bacterial culture, and PCR for viruses
  - Avoid lumbar puncture if signs of elevated intracranial pressure, prolonged or focal seizures, focal neurologic signs, increased purpuric rash, Glasgow Coma Scale less than 13, or pupillary asymmetry or dilatation are present
  - If suspect increased intracranial pressure, a head CT scan should be performed prior to lumbar puncture
- Cerebral imaging and EEG should be done in cases of atypical seizures

TREATMENT & MANAGEMENT

- Immediate and aggressive supportive therapy for shock, seizures, and disseminated intravascular coagulation may be necessary
- Begin empiric treatment immediately with a third-generation cephalosporin plus vancomycin in children; neonates should receive ampicillin (to cover *Listeria*) plus either a third-generation cephalosporin or aminoglycoside
- The etiologic agent and clinical course dictate duration of treatment; adjust antibiotics once culture results and sensitivities are available
- In cases of *N. meningitidis* meningitis, administer prophylaxis for all household and nursery school contacts
- In cases of HiB, administer prophylaxis for all household contacts, even if previously immunized
- Meningococcal vaccine for college students and in endemic areas
- Steroids are standard of care for tuberculous meningitis and may prevent hearing loss

PROGNOSIS & COMPLICATIONS

- Long-term sequelae (30% of cases) include mental or motor retardation, learning disabilities, obstructive hydrocephalus, sensorineural hearing loss, cortical blindness, hemiparesis, ataxia, seizures, complications of intravascular coagulopathy, and Waterhouse-Friderichsen syndrome
- *Citrobacter* and *Salmonella* have higher mortality rates due to possible brain abscess formation
- Perform hearing screening after diagnosis and during follow-up
- Consider neuropsychiatric and neurodevelopmental testing

Osteomyelitis

INTRODUCTION

- Inflammation of bone, most often caused by bacterial infections
- 50% of cases occur during the first 5 years of life
- Missing this diagnosis can result in considerable morbidity, even an amputation
- If considering osteomyelitis in the differential diagnosis, consult orthopedics and do all appropriate imaging if in doubt

ETIOLOGY, EPIDEMIOLOGY, & RISK FACTORS

- Long bones (especially the femur and tibia) are most frequently involved
- Males are affected more commonly than females
- One-third of patients have a history of minor trauma involving the affected region prior to the onset of osteomyelitis
- The majority of cases occur secondary to hematogenous spread; may also occur secondary to surgery, trauma, or contiguous infection of soft tissue
- The most common bacterial etiologies include *Staphylococcus aureus* and group A streptococci
- Less frequent bacterial causes include *Streptococcus pneumoniae*, coagulase-negative *Staphylococcus, Bacillus*, and enteric Gram-negative anaerobes
- *M. tuberculosis* and fungal infections may also cause disease

PATIENT PRESENTATION

- Intermittent or constant bone pain at the site of infection
- Reluctance to move the affected limb or region (most common in young children)
- Focal swelling, tenderness, warmth, and erythema
- High fever may be present; osteomyelitis should be in the differential diagnosis of fever of unknown origin
- Nonspecific symptoms (eg, anorexia, malaise, vomiting) are common

DIFFERENTIAL DX

- Fracture
- Juvenile arthritis
- Cellulitis
- Rheumatic fever
- Pyogenic arthritis
- Lyme disease
- Postinfectious arthritis
- Leukemia
- Child abuse
- Animal bites
- Cat scratch disease
- Serum sickness
- Polyarteritis nodosa
- Bone malignancy

DIAGNOSTIC EVALUATION

- History and physical examination
- Laboratory studies include complete blood count with differential and blood culture
- Joint fluid culture, if present
- Culture of the affected bone via needle aspirate or surgical biopsy may be necessary
- X-rays of bone are indicated, but a negative X-ray does not rule out disease because bone changes may take 10–14 days to become visible
- MRI and radionuclide bone scan are more sensitive for bone lesions; however, bone scan does not specifically identify osteomyelitis
- Nonspecific indicators of possible osteomyelitis include elevated erythrocyte sedimentation rate (ESR), elevated C-reactive protein, and elevated white blood cell count
- PPD should be placed to rule out tuberculosis

TREATMENT & MANAGEMENT

- Administer empiric IV antibiotics according to age:
  - In children younger than 3 months, administer nafcillin plus gentamicin or cefotaxime
  - In children older than 3 months, administer cefazolin, clindamycin, nafcillin, or oxacillin
- Once the specific organism is identified, treat with appropriate antibiotics for 4–8 weeks
- If signs and symptoms do not improve within 72 hours of appropriate therapy, consider repeat bone aspiration

PROGNOSIS & COMPLICATIONS

- If treated appropriately, prognosis is good
- Close follow-up is necessary with weekly ESR and CBC to monitor response to treatment and possible development of antibiotic-related neutropenia
- Chronic osteomyelitis may result in necrotic bone, requiring surgical debridement
- Clinical response, etiologic agent, and normalization of ESR will decide duration of therapy
- 5–10% recurrence rate despite adequate therapy

Infectious Mononucleosis

INTRODUCTION

- Commonly known as "mono," this disease is a self-limited viral infection
- The most likely significant factor is splenic enlargement and friability, which necessitates avoiding contact sports
- The most harmless associated finding is a rash, which can appear in patients who are inadvertently treated with penicillin

ETIOLOGY, EPIDEMIOLOGY, & RISK FACTORS

- Epstein-Barr virus (EBV) is the most common cause and accounts for 90% of cases; cytomegalovirus (CMV) accounts for the remainder of cases
- The primary source of infection is oropharyngeal secretions, which are transmitted through close personal contact, such as kissing, sharing toys, and so forth; rarely, the disease may be transmitted via blood transfusion
- The virus infects B lymphocytes in the lymphoid tissue of the pharynx and then disseminates throughout the lymphoid system
- EBV is ubiquitous in nature
  - There is no seasonal pattern
  - Incubation period of 4–6 weeks
  - By age 5, 50% of children in the U.S. are infected by EBV; asymptomatic carriage with lifelong intermittent excretion is common
  - Other EBV-linked syndromes include Burkitt lymphoma and nasopharyngeal carcinoma
- Infectious mononucleosis is exceedingly common on college campuses

PATIENT PRESENTATION

- Severity of illness depends on age
  - Infection during childhood generally only results in subclinical disease or nonspecific signs and symptoms
  - Older children, adolescents, and adults have a more significant clinical picture
- The syndrome begins with a flulike illness (malaise, fatigue, and headache) for 3–5 days
- Fever (up to 105°F)
- Exudative pharyngitis and severe sore throat
- Generalized, tender lymphadenopathy
- Hepatosplenomegaly
- Rash, especially if treated with ampicillin or penicillin

DIFFERENTIAL DX

- Streptococcal pharyngitis and other viral pharyngitis syndromes
- Hepatitis
- Bacterial meningitis
- Cat scratch disease
- Leukemia
- Postinfectious myocarditis
- Herpes simplex virus
- Human herpesvirus 6
- HIV
- Toxoplasmosis
- Rubella

DIAGNOSTIC EVALUATION

- History and physical examination are often classic for the disease
- Evaluation for mononucleosis should be done in strep-negative patients with impressive pharyngitis or lymph nodes
- The classic diagnostic triad is lymphocytosis (80–90% of WBCs), greater than 10% atypical lymphocytes on peripheral smear, and serologic testing positive for EBV
- The Monospot test is quick and cheap but has low sensitivity, and false-positive results may occur in patients with lymphoma or hepatitis; more useful after the first week of illness
- Serologies:
  - IgM and IgG are elevated early in disease
  - Early antigen (EA) disappears after 6 months
  - EBNA (EBV nuclear antigen) appears several months after infection
- Liver function tests may be mildly elevated
- Mild thrombocytopenia

TREATMENT & MANAGEMENT

- Supportive therapy, hydration, and bed rest
- Pain control for pharyngitis and lymphadenopathy
- Corticosteroids may be administered in severe cases, particularly to reduce swelling in cases of airway compromise
- Steroids should be considered in patients who are unable to tolerate oral intake, who are unable to manage their secretions, or who become dyspneic
- Antivirals (acyclovir) have no proven clinical benefit for the general population
- Antibiotics should only be given in patients who have concomitant streptococcal disease; consider a macrolide (eg, azithromycin) to avoid the characteristic rash
- Avoid contact sports for at least 1 month after diagnosis
- Patients with splenomegaly should be periodically reexamined to assess spleen size
- Surgical treatment is necessary in cases of splenic rupture

PROGNOSIS & COMPLICATIONS

- Self-limited disease in most patients
- Most patients will have infectious mononucleosis only once
- May result in hepatitis, aseptic meningitis, encephalitis, Guillain-Barré syndrome, or lymphoma
- Rarely, splenic rupture, orchitis, myocarditis, or pneumonia may occur

Varicella

INTRODUCTION

- Varicella is still seen sporadically in the U.S. despite a widespread vaccination program
- It is primarily a clinical diagnosis based on its polymorphic appearance; historically, it was often confused with smallpox
- Complications include secondary bacterial infection and varicella pneumonia

ETIOLOGY, EPIDEMIOLOGY, & RISK FACTORS

- Varicella-zoster virus is transmitted via respiratory droplets or direct contact
- The virus begins to replicate in the upper respiratory epithelium and spreads to regional lymph nodes, followed by primary low-grade viremia that leads to visceral spread; a secondary viremia develops within 1 week, which disseminates the infection to the skin and causes the characteristic rash
- The infectious period begins 2 days before skin lesions appear and ends when the lesions crust, usually 5 days later
- An episode of varicella confers immunity; second episodes are exceedingly rare
- Maximum incidence of varicella is in children aged 1–6 years
- Maximum transmission occurs during late winter and spring
- Highly contagious; secondary attack rate is 80–90% for contacts

PATIENT PRESENTATION

- The characteristic rash usually begins on the head and spreads to the trunk and extremities
- Varicella's hallmark is the simultaneous presence of rash in different stages
- Each lesion starts as a red macule and passes through stages of papule, vesicle ("pearl" or "dewdrop on a rose petal"), and pustule, and then crusts
- An otherwise healthy child usually has 250–500 lesions, but may have as few as 10 or as many as 1500
- New lesions continue to erupt for 3–5 days
- Lesions usually crust within 1 week and heal completely by 2 weeks
- Other accompanying manifestations include headache, malaise, anorexia, cough and coryza, sore throat, and low-grade fever

DIFFERENTIAL DX

- Contact dermatitis
- Drug reaction
- Enterovirus
- Insect bites
- Impetigo
- Smallpox
- Urticaria
- Herpes simplex virus

DIAGNOSTIC EVALUATION

- A clinical diagnosis based on the characteristic appearance of the rash
- Tzanck smear of scrapings from the base of vesicles will show multinucleated giant cells
- Postvaccine varicella exanthema is less classic and more difficult to diagnose
- Serologic tests can be done to assess prior exposure to varicella but have little diagnostic value during acute infection

TREATMENT & MANAGEMENT

- Symptomatic relief of fever and itching
- Avoid aspirin in children as it is associated with Reye syndrome
- Antivirals (acyclovir) are used in some cases (eg, progressive or severe varicella, life-threatening complications including encephalitis or pneumonia, neonatal infection, adolescent or adult infection, cancer patients, immunocompromised patients)
- Universal vaccination with live virus has significantly reduced morbidity and mortality; it confers protection to 75–100% of those immunized
  ○ Children with immunodeficiencies (eg, HIV, cancer, steroids, or other immunosuppressive regimens) should not receive the varicella vaccine or any other live vaccine product
- Nonimmune, pregnant women should not have contact with patients with varicella because of the risk of congenital varicella, which can result in intrauterine fetal death, intrauterine growth retardation, microcephaly, cortical atrophy, microophthalmos, chorioretinitis, hypoplastic limbs, and skin abnormalities

PROGNOSIS & COMPLICATIONS

- The infection is contagious from 2 days before skin lesions appear until the 6th day of rash or until the lesions crust
- Nearly 1 in 50 cases of varicella may be associated with complications (eg, varicella pneumonia, encephalitis)
- Secondary bacterial infection may occur with invasive group A *Streptococcus*, a serious infection that may evolve rapidly into necrotizing fasciitis or toxic shock syndrome

Rocky Mountain Spotted Fever

INTRODUCTION

- The most common rickettsial infection in the U.S.
- "Rocky Mountain" is a misnomer; there is actually a higher documented prevalence in the Eastern U.S.
- Rocky Mountain spotted fever (RMSF) should be considered in any person with fever and a history of tick bite or exposure
- The infection can be lethal but is very curable with early diagnosis and appropriate therapy

ETIOLOGY, EPIDEMIOLOGY, & RISK FACTORS

- A tickborne infection caused by *Rickettsia rickettsii*
  - At least 6 hours of tick attachment is necessary for transmission
  - Incubation period is 2–8 days following the tick bite
  - After inoculation, the organism propagates intracellularly and then spreads throughout the body via the lymphatics or bloodstream
  - The infection has tropism for endothelial cells; subsequent endothelial cell injury leads to immune-mediated vasculitis, hemorrhage, edema, thrombosis, and multiorgan dysfunction
  - A history of a tick bite is present in only two-thirds of cases
- RMSF is the second most commonly reported tickborne disease in the U.S.
- Most cases (90%) occur between April and September, when ticks have maximal activity and people participate in outdoor activities
- Infection is most prevalent in the Southeast and South Central states; it is more common in suburban and rural locations but may also occur in urban areas
- Children are at greater risk than adults; highest incidence during ages 5–9 years

PATIENT PRESENTATION

- Symptoms usually appear within 2 days to 2 weeks of tick bite
- The early phase of disease has only nonspecific symptoms, including fever, malaise, myalgias, arthralgias, severe headache, nausea, vomiting, abdominal pain, and cough
- Rash occurs in 80–90% of cases; begins peripherally (wrists/palms and ankles/soles) and proceeds centrally
- Patients often appear toxic
- Headache is the most common neurologic manifestation; altered mental status or level of consciousness may occur
- Hepatomegaly and splenomegaly are present in one-third of patients

DIFFERENTIAL DX

- Nonspecific viral illness
- Meningococcemia
- Infectious mononucleosis
- Infectious hepatitis
- Ehrlichiosis
- Leptospirosis
- Secondary syphilis
- Typhoid fever
- Hypersensitivity to drugs
- Atypical measles
- Rickettsial pox
- Disseminated gonococcus

DIAGNOSTIC EVALUATION

- There is no reliable test during the early phase of disease; during this time, clinical recognition of the disease is most important
- Detection of antirickettsial IgG antibody is diagnostic
- Enzyme immunoassays (EIA) and IgM antibody immunoassays are newer tests for diagnosis
- Biopsy of a skin lesion can be diagnostic if *Rickettsia* organisms are seen by immunofluorescence methods
- Nonspecific laboratory findings include abnormal leukocyte levels (may be increased, decreased, or normal; usually left-shifted), mild anemia and thrombocytopenia (severe in 10%), hyponatremia, increased ALT, decreased albumin, increased BUN, and increased antidiuretic hormone and aldosterone
- Cerebrospinal fluid analysis is generally normal

TREATMENT & MANAGEMENT

- Never delay treatment pending a confirmatory laboratory diagnosis; if suspect RMSF, begin treatment immediately
- IV fluids and supplemental oxygen
- Correct electrolytes and coagulopathies
- Doxycycline is the antibiotic of choice, even in children younger than 8 years (staining of teeth by tetracyclines is acceptable in light of the potential severity of RMSF)
- Antibiotics should be continued for a minimum of 5–7 days and until the patient is afebrile for at least 1 day

PROGNOSIS & COMPLICATIONS

- Treatment within 3 days after onset of symptoms is associated with significantly lower mortality; therefore, a high index of suspicion is important
- Mortality ranges from 2% in children to 9% in elderly persons
- Complications may include CNS involvement, pulmonary involvement, liver impairment, renal failure, splenomegaly, myocarditis, and severe thrombocytopenia
- Children with glucose-6-phsophate dehydrogenase deficiency are at increased risk for severe disease
- Most patients who recover from the acute disease are cured of the infection

Lyme Disease

INTRODUCTION

- A tickborne disease characterized by a pathognomonic, annular rash
- May not be readily diagnosed because the patient may not recall tick bite or present for treatment
- Patients who undergo prompt diagnosis and treatment have an excellent prognosis
- Late diagnosis or delayed treatment may lead to neurologic and cardiac complications

ETIOLOGY, EPIDEMIOLOGY, & RISK FACTORS

- Caused by the spirochete *Borrelia burgdorferi*
- Humans are infected when bitten by an infected deer tick
- Generally, the tick must stay attached for 24 hours for transmission to occur
- Occurrence of disease correlates with distribution and frequency of tick infections
- Primarily occurs in three geographic regions in the United States: Northeast (Maryland to Massachusetts), upper Midwest (Wisconsin and Minnesota), and the West Coast
- Endemic in Canada, Europe, Russia, China, and Japan
- Most cases occur between April and October, when ticks have maximal activity and people are outdoors

PATIENT PRESENTATION

- Early localized disease (typically 7–14 days after tick bite) is associated with the characteristic rash and mild constitutional symptoms
  - Erythema migrans: Red macula or papule at the site of the bite, expanding over days to weeks to form a large, annular, erythematous lesion >5 cm
  - Mild neck stiffness, myalgia, arthralgia, fever, and malaise
- Early disseminated disease (3–5 w after tick bite) may include neurologic and cardiac involvement
  - Multiple erythema migrans
  - Cranial nerve VII palsy (Bell palsy), meningitis, conjunctivitis, headache, fatigue, and carditis
  - Arthralgia, myalgia
- Late manifestations (months to years later) include recurrent arthritis (knee), subacute encephalopathy, and polyneuropathy

DIFFERENTIAL DX

- Cellulitis
- Myocarditis/endocarditis
- Flulike illness
- Viral/bacterial meningitis
- Erythema multiforme
- Juvenile arthritis
- Idiopathic Bell palsy
- Henoch-Schönlein purpura
- CNS tumor
- Rheumatic fever
- Serum sickness
- Septic arthritis
- Postinfectious meningoencephalitis
- Contact dermatitis
- Mononucleosis
- Chronic fatigue syndrome

DIAGNOSTIC EVALUATION

- History and physical examination may reveal a history of tick attachment, travel to endemic areas, or the presence of erythema migrans
- Laboratory studies include blood testing and serologies
  - Complete blood count may show leukocytosis
  - Erythrocyte sedimentation rate is usually elevated
  - *Borrelia*-specific IgM peaks 3–6 weeks after onset of symptoms; *Borrelia*-specific IgG then develops and persists indefinitely
  - *Borrelia* will not grow in cultures
- The perimeter of cutaneous lesions may be biopsied

TREATMENT & MANAGEMENT

- Treat early, localized disease with oral doxycycline (if > age 8) or oral amoxicillin for 14–21 days
  - Tetracycline administration in young children results in permanent staining of teeth
- Treat early, disseminated disease and late disease based on presentation:
  - Multiple erythema migrans, isolated facial palsy, and/or arthritis: Same oral antibiotics as above, but treat for 28 days
  - Persistent or recurrent arthritis, carditis, meningitis, and/or encephalitis: IV or intramuscular ceftriaxone or IV penicillin for 14–21 days
- Prophylactic antibiotics after deer tick exposure are not recommended, but patients should be educated about signs and symptoms of Lyme disease

PROGNOSIS & COMPLICATIONS

- Excellent prognosis with proper treatment
- If untreated, symptoms persist for several weeks or months and late disease manifestations evolve
- Even if treated successfully, the patient may experience fatigue, arthralgia, and myalgia for weeks to months after therapy
- Antibodies induced by the infection are not protective against further exposures
- Prevent tick bites by wearing protective clothing and careful inspection of skin and hair for ticks
- Jarisch-Herxheimer reaction (fever, chills, malaise) may occur upon initiation of therapy due to bacteriolysis and release of cellular products; NSAIDs may be beneficial

Vulvovaginitis

INTRODUCTION

- Vulvovaginitis is the most common gynecologic problem in premenarchal girls
- Defined as vulvar or vaginal inflammation, but also may be used to describe vulvar pain or itching without obvious signs of inflammation
- Due to infections or various physical or chemical irritants
- Common in young, prepubertal children, as well as pubertal or postpubertal, sexually active women
- Infectious causes are further subdivided into those that are usually not sexually transmitted and those that are sexually transmitted; sexually transmitted vulvovaginitis usually occurs in sexually active adolescents with different organisms than vulvovaginitis in younger children

ETIOLOGY, EPIDEMIOLOGY, & RISK FACTORS

- Noninfectious etiologies are more common in children and include local chemical or allergic irritation, improper or inconsistent hygiene, and poor aeration or tight-fitting clothing
- The most common nonsexual infectious causes are often respiratory or enteric pathogens that are transmitted via self-inoculation, including *Streptococcus pyogenes*, *Haemophilus influenzae*, *Staphylococcus aureus*, *Gardnerella vaginalis*, anaerobes, *Mycoplasma hominis*, *E. coli*, *Salmonella*, *Shigella*, and pinworm infestation; viral pathogens include varicella and adenovirus
- Children with underlying chronic dermatologic disorders are at higher risk for noninfectious vulvovaginitis due to sensitivity to irritants
- Less frequent causes include trauma, contact dermatitis, herpes simplex virus, secondary bacterial infection due to retained foreign bodies, medications, and (rarely) systemic illness (eg, toxic shock syndrome, Crohn disease)
- Sexual abuse may be a cause
- In adolescents, the primary etiologies include *Candida* infection, trichomoniasis, or bacterial vaginosis

PATIENT PRESENTATION

- Diffuse vulvovaginal pain, burning, and itching
  - Itching can predominate if pinworms are the cause
- Dysuria
- The vulvovaginal region appears irritated (erythema, excoriation)
- Seropurulent vaginal discharge may be present; in infectious cases, the discharge may be more purulent and malodorous
  - In *Candida* infections, a thick, white, adherent vaginal discharge occurs
  - In bacterial vaginosis, a gray-white, foul-smelling vaginal discharge occurs
  - In trichomoniasis, a profuse, frothy, green-yellow discharge occurs
- In group A streptococci vulvovaginitis, a well-demarcated, scarlet-colored dermatitis of vulvar or perianal tissues may be present

DIFFERENTIAL DX

- Anatomic abnormality
- Foreign bodies
- Sexual abuse
- Hygiene
- Allergic reaction
- Lichen sclerosus
- Physiologic leukorrhea
- Paget disease
- Atopic dermatitis
- Psoriasis
- Lichen simplex chronicus
- Neoplasm
- Vulvodynia

DIAGNOSTIC EVALUATION

- History and physical examination should assess for recent infections, exposure to irritants, hygienic practices, and possible sexual contact
- A microbiologic investigation is indicated if vaginal discharge with moderate to severe inflammation is present upon examination
- Diagnostic tests include examining vaginal secretions with wet prep, smear for Gram stain, and culture
- Other exclusion methods may be used if sexual abuse is suspected (eg, pinworm test or chlamydia/gonorrhea probe)
- Isolation or suspicion of a sexually transmitted organism in young, prepubertal children should prompt evaluation for abuse
- Urinalysis and urine culture
- In sexually active adolescents, assess for cervicitis with a pelvic exam and prepare a wet prep for pH and KOH test
  - Bacterial vaginosis: clue cells on wet prep with pH >4.5
  - Trichomoniasis: motile trichomonads with pH >4.5
  - Candida: budding yeast or pseudohyphae on wet prep with pH of 4–4.5
- Pregnancy testing
- If foreign body is suspected, ultrasound may be indicated

TREATMENT & MANAGEMENT

- Treat with antibiotics directed toward the specific pathogenic organisms; an adequate response can generally be achieved with a course of oral penicillin, cephalosporins, or erythromycin
  - *Candida* infections can be treated with oral fluconazole
  - Bacterial vaginosis and trichomoniasis can be treated with metronidazole; sexual partners of those with trichomoniasis should be treated
- Most episodes do not have a specific cause; in such cases, treatment should focus on improved hygiene and sitz baths
  - Sitz bath: Patients should be instructed to sit in warm water for 10–15 minutes once or twice a day; the vulva *should not* be scrubbed
- Clothes should be washed in a mild detergent with no rinse or dryer additives
- Loose-fitting clothes with cotton underwear can be helpful
- Small amounts of ointment (eg, Vaseline) can be used to protect the vulvar skin
- Avoid bubble baths or soaps/shampoo in bathtub

PROGNOSIS & COMPLICATIONS

- Few complications occur in the pediatric population
- For children with uncomplicated vulvovaginitis, if there is failure to improve with hygienic practices listed above, consider further evaluation for sexual abuse
- If severe and untreated, vulvovaginitis may progress to upper genital tract infections, such as pelvic inflammatory disease; prepubertal girls are at less risk of ascending infection

Pelvic Inflammatory Disease

INTRODUCTION

- Pelvic inflammatory disease (PID) encompasses a spectrum of inflammatory disorders of the upper genital tract, including endometritis, salpingitis, pelvic peritonitis, and tubo-ovarian abscess
- Occurs due to ascending infection from microorganisms in the vagina and cervix and is a complication of sexually transmitted diseases; it is inherently a polymicrobial infection
- Lower tract infection may or may not be symptomatic before PID develops
- PID can be associated with serious morbidity if treatment is delayed or inadequate; thus, it is important to have a low threshold to initiate empiric treatment as presenting signs and symptoms of PID are very commonly mild or subtle

ETIOLOGY, EPIDEMIOLOGY, & RISK FACTORS

- Causative organisms include *Chlamydia trachomatis, Neisseria gonorrhoeae*, and endogenous vaginal microflora (eg, *M. Hominis, Gardnerella vaginalis, H. influenzae*, enteric Gram-negative organisms, *Peptococcus, Streptococcus agalactiae, Bacteroides fragilis*, and cytomegalovirus
- Adolescents are at highest risk due to their high rates of sexually transmitted infections
- Risk factors include young age at first intercourse, multiple sexual partners, intrauterine device insertion, douching, lower socioeconomic status (due to delay or obstacles to health care access), inconsistent use of barrier method of contraception, history of previous episodes of PID, and bacterial vaginosis
- Affects 11% of women of reproductive age; 1 million cases per year in the U.S.
- Usually develops around the time of menses because there is greater access to the upper genital tract
- No pathogen is isolated in many cases, and patients are treated empirically
- Usually begins with cervicitis, and then progresses to endometritis, salpingitis, oophoritis, and ultimately tubo-ovarian abscess

PATIENT PRESENTATION

- There is a wide spectrum of symptoms and presentation
- Lower abdominal pain is the most common presenting complaint
  - Usually bilateral, dull, aching, and constant
  - Pain is accentuated by motion, exercise, or coitus
- Abnormal vaginal discharge is present in 75% of cases
- Unanticipated vaginal bleeding or increased menstrual bleeding
- Dysmenorrhea
- Dyspareunia
- Dysuria
- Fever, nausea, vomiting, anorexia, and malaise are less common and may present late in the course of disease

DIFFERENTIAL DX

Gynecologic Diagnoses
- Endometriosis
- Ectopic pregnancy
- Complications of ovarian cyst
- Adnexal or ovarian torsion
- Adnexal tumors
- Rupture of adnexal mass

Gastrointestinal Diagnoses
- Appendicitis
- Inflammatory bowel disease
- Constipation
- Gastroenteritis

Others
- Pelvic thrombophlebitis
- Functional abdominal pain
- Cystitis or pyelonephritis
- Renal colic

DIAGNOSTIC EVALUATION

- The minimum criterion for diagnosis is uterine *or* adnexal *or* cervical motion tenderness
- Additional criteria (supports the diagnosis but not absolutely required for diagnosis) includes fever >101°F, abnormal cervical or vaginal mucopurulent discharge, increased WBC count on vaginal secretions, increased ESR or CRP levels, and laboratory documentation of *Chlamydia* or *N. gonorrhoeae* infection
- History and physical examination typically reveal a tender lower abdomen, adnexa, and/or cervix; adnexal mass or enlargement on exam suggests abscess
- Laboratory testing includes complete blood count (leukocytosis is common), cervical or pelvic cultures for *Chlamydia* and *N. gonorrhoeae*, pregnancy testing (urine or serum β-hCG), urinalysis, and culture
- Consider testing for other sexually transmitted diseases (eg, HIV, syphilis)
- Pelvic ultrasound may be indicated to assess for pelvic abscess or inflammatory complex
- Definitive diagnosis is made by laparoscopy, endometrial biopsy, or ultrasound or MRI showing thickened, fluid-filled tubes or free fluid in the pelvis; however, these are not routinely performed

TREATMENT & MANAGEMENT

- There are multiple antibiotic regimens for parenteral or oral therapy; common choices include a second- or third-generation cephalosporin (eg, cefoxitin, cefotetan, ceftriaxone) to cover Gram-negative bacteria, or doxycycline plus gentamicin or ofloxacin or levofloxacin
- Clindamycin or metronidazole may be used for anaerobic coverage, especially if bacterial vaginosis is suspected
- Indications for hospitalization when the diagnosis is in doubt and surgical emergency cannot be excluded: pelvic abscess appears on ultrasound, pregnancy, failure to respond to or tolerate outpatient management, severe illness, the presence of nausea or vomiting (failure to tolerate oral medications), HIV with low CD4 count, and patients taking immunosuppressive medications
- Hospitalized patients who are improving on parenteral therapy may transition to oral antibiotics after 24 hours of parenteral therapy
- Sexual partners should be evaluated and treated if sexual activity occurred 60 days prior to onset of symptoms
- Patients must complete 14 days of antibiotic therapy; do not stop treatment earlier even if cultures are negative
- A direct correlation exists between the incidence of STDs and PID; be sure to ask women about high-risk sexual behavior and counsel about safe sex practices

PROGNOSIS & COMPLICATIONS

- Must have follow-up within 48–72 hours of initiating treatment to ensure improvement
- 20% of patients require hospitalization
- A delay in diagnosis or treatment may result in long-term sequelae, including infertility due to fallopian tube stricture or dysfunction
- Women with a history of PID have a 10-fold increased risk for ectopic pregnancy
- Chronic pelvic pain may result
- Fitz-Hugh-Curtis syndrome (perihepatitis) may occur
- Because of these long-term complications, initiation of treatment should not be delayed, even if culture results are not known or are negative

Human Papillomavirus

INTRODUCTION

- Anogenital human papillomavirus (HPV) is the most common viral sexually transmitted infection in the U.S. (5.5 million cases per year)
- HPV is the most common cause of abnormal Pap smear in women, and certain serotypes can lead to squamous cell carcinoma of the cervix, anus, vulva, vagina, penis, and oropharynx
- HPV also causes anogenital, cutaneous, and mucosal warts
- HPV DNA can be found in the oral cavity and nasopharynx in infants born to HPV-infected mothers
- There is no cure for HPV infection, but the infection may clear on its own, especially in mild cases; recurrences of lesions can occur as well

ETIOLOGY, EPIDEMIOLOGY, & RISK FACTORS

- HPV is a DNA virus with >70 serotypes; about 40 are spread through sexual contact
- Incubation is usually 3–4 weeks but can be many years
- In adolescents and adults, transmission primarily occurs via sexual contact
- In children, transmission can be vertical or via autoinoculation or heteroinoculation (self-inoculation from somewhere else in the body)
- Transmission of anogenital warts in children younger than 2 years usually occurs via auto- or heteroinoculation, but sexual abuse should be considered
- Genital HPV is associated with serotypes 6, 11, 16, 18, 31, and 45
- Serotypes 16, 18, 31, and 45 are associated with squamous cell carcinoma of the cervix and anus, and some cases of vulva, penis, vagina, and oropharynx cancer
- Malignant changes of genital warts result in 90% of cervical cancer cases
- Laryngeal papillomas are acquired via aspiration of infected secretions during passage through the birth canal; HPV acquired at birth may not cause manifestations for several years
- Nongenital warts are usually caused by different serotypes than anogenital papillomas; transmission occurs by close contact
- 80% of females in the U.S. acquire HPV during the reproductive years
- Cutaneous warts are highly prevalent in school-aged children (up to 50%)

PATIENT PRESENTATION

- Epithelial tumors (warts) of skin and mucous membranes
- Cutaneous warts (nongenital)
- Mucosal warts (anogenital, nasal, oral, and/or conjunctival)
- Respiratory papillomatosis, resulting in stridor
- The growths may be sessile or pedunculated and range in size from several millimeters to many centimeters
- Warts are usually asymptomatic but can have itching, discomfort, tenderness, and bleeding
- Postcoital bleeding may occur

DIFFERENTIAL DX

- Molluscum contagiosum
- Skin malignancy
- Skin polyp
- Skin tags
- Pyoderma gangrenosum
- Severe atopic dermatitis
- Dyshidrotic eczema
- Nevi
- Scabies infestation
- Severe eczema
- Seborrheic keratoses
- Enlarged sebaceous glands or cysts

DIAGNOSTIC EVALUATION

- The mainstay of diagnosis is recognizing the characteristic clinical appearance
- Clinical diagnosis is usually sufficient for cutaneous warts
- Biopsy is diagnostic for all types of warts and may also be curative if the complete lesion is removed
- Sexually active females with genital warts require a Pap smear; diagnosis of cervical HPV infection may be enhanced by the use of colposcopy with application of 3–5% acetic acid on the lesions
  - Many women are asymptomatic despite HPV infection and possible cervical precancerous changes; therefore, regular Pap smears are necessary in all sexually active women
- PCR testing for detecting high-risk types of HPV DNA in cervical cells collected via Pap smear is useful in identifying women who are at high risk for developing precancerous changes
- Cultures are not available for diagnosis
- Sexual abuse should be suspected when anogenital warts occur in prepubertal child
- Anyone with anal warts requires anoscopy to assess for internal lesions
- Consider other sexually transmitted infections in those diagnosed with HPV
- HIV testing is often warranted

TREATMENT & MANAGEMENT

- Most nongenital warts regress spontaneously; however, they may persist or relapse for months to years
- Treatment reduces symptoms but cannot eliminate virus
- Chemical or physical destruction of infected epithelia (eg, via salicylic acid products or cryotherapy)
- For laryngeal warts, repeat surgery may be necessary to keep airway patent
- Cryotherapy or electrocautery for oral warts
- Anogenital warts often spontaneously regress; otherwise, they may be destroyed or removed via podophyllin resin, cryotherapy, trichloroacetic acid, imiquimod, electrocautery, laser surgery, or surgical excision
- Young children usually followed by pediatric dermatologist or gynecologist
- Vaccine (Gardisil) is now available
  - The vaccine protects against four serotypes: 16 and 18, which cause 70% of cervical cancer cases, and 6 and 11, which cause 90% of genital warts
  - Nonpregnant females aged 9–26 are eligible for vaccination
  - Should be administered prior to the onset of sexual activity, typically at a well child visit at ages 11–12
  - The vaccine is administered in three doses (at 0, 2, and 6 months)

PROGNOSIS & COMPLICATIONS

- Recurrences are common and occur by reactivation of HPV, rather than reinfection
- HPV infection (particularly mucosal lesions) may be associated with epithelial dysplasia; unlike mucosal lesions, skin warts almost never undergo malignant changes
- Extension or dissemination of laryngeal papilloma to trachea, bronchi, or lung parenchyma is a rare complication but is associated with high morbidity and mortality
- HPV is the causal agent of at least 90% of cases of cervical cancer
- Regular cytologic screening for cervical cancer is recommended in patients with anogenital lesions
- Vaccine is newly available
- Red flags on history or physical exam should prompt consideration of sexual abuse

Toxic Shock Syndrome

INTRODUCTION

- Toxic shock syndrome (TSS) is an acute, multisystem, febrile illness caused by toxin-producing strains of staphylococci and streptococci
- TSS represents a severe manifestation of disease caused by either organism
- It can be rapidly progressive resulting in serious morbidity and mortality if not recognized and treated promptly and aggressively
- Classically associated with menstruating women and tampon use, but can also occur in nonmenstrual-related conditions in children, men, and women
- May mimic other common diseases; it is important to include TSS in the differential diagnosis of any patient with unexplained fever, rash, and toxic appearance

ETIOLOGY, EPIDEMIOLOGY, & RISK FACTORS

- TSS develops in a nonimmune host via growth of a toxin-producing organism from an infected site; toxins act as superantigens that activate the immune system and release cytokines
- Staphylococcal TSS traditionally affects menstruating women secondary to tampon use
  - Toxic shock syndrome toxin-1 (TSST-1) is implicated in 75% of cases, followed by enterotoxin B and C
  - Menstrual-related TSS has decreased since the elimination of hyperabsorbable tampons; now, up to 45% of cases are nonmenstrual
  - Incidence of 1–5 per 100,000 menstruating women
- Streptococcal TSS is caused by *Streptococcus pyogenes* exotoxins A or B
  - Affects both genders and all ages
  - Transmission is likely via person-to-person contact
  - Incidence is 5–10 cases per 100,000 population
  - In children, varicella infection increases the risk of developing strep TSS
- Nonmenstrual cases include those caused by wound infections, postsurgical infections, abscess, cellulitis, tracheitis, pneumonia, and necrotizing fasciitis

PATIENT PRESENTATION

- A multisystem disease with sudden onset
- Patient appears sick or "toxic"
- Fever, chills
- Hypotension
- Myalgias
- Headache
- Dizziness
- Vomiting
- Diarrhea
- Erythroderma rash ("sunburned-appearing" skin)
- Conjunctival injection
- Nonfocal neurologic signs, such as confusion, somnolence, and irritability

DIFFERENTIAL DX

- Kawasaki disease
- Adenovirus or other acute viral syndrome
- Systemic lupus erythematosus
- Drug eruption
- Measles
- Rocky Mountain spotted fever
- Meningococcemia
- Acute rheumatic fever
- Ehrlichiosis
- Leptospirosis

DIAGNOSTIC EVALUATION

- Criteria for staphylococcal TSS includes:
  - Temperature greater than 38.9°C
  - Systolic blood pressure less than 90 mmHg (or lower than 5th percentile in children) or the presence of orthostatic hypotension
  - Rash with desquamation (usually on the palms and soles)
  - Involvement of three or more of the following organ systems: gastrointestinal, musculoskeletal, renal, hepatic, CNS, blood, or mucous membranes
- Criteria for streptococcal TSS include:
  - Isolation of group A streptococci
  - Hypotension
  - Two or more of the following: coagulopathy (DIC), adult respiratory distress syndrome, soft tissue necrosis, rash with desquamation, or involvement of the liver or kidneys
- Bacteremia and positive blood cultures are more likely in cases of streptococcal TSS; additionally patients with streptococcal TSS more commonly have pain, tenderness, and elevated CPK levels
- Lab abnormalities for both types of TSS include thrombocytopenia, anemia, hypoalbuminemia, hypocalcemia, elevated liver enzymes, and elevated BUN/creatinine
- 90% of adults have detectable antibodies to TSST-1, with a lower frequency in pediatric population; however, affected patients with TSS have low titers of TSST-1 antibodies

TREATMENT & MANAGEMENT

- Hemodynamic stabilization with large volumes of IV fluids is often necessary due to capillary leakage, fluid losses (eg, vomiting, diarrhea), and vasodilatation; vasopressor support may be necessary if fluid resuscitation is not sufficient
- Correct electrolyte abnormalities and coagulopathies as necessary
- Debride infected surgical wounds; drain and irrigate abscesses; remove postsurgical foreign bodies; remove tampons in menstrual cases
- Obtain cultures from possible sites of infection
- Administer antibiotics targeted against staphylococci and streptococci (eg, nafcillin, oxacillin, first-generation cephalosporin)
- Clindamycin may inhibit toxin production
- A 10- to 14-day course of antibiotics is usually required
- IVIG may be indicated in severe cases (one dose of 1–2 g/kg)

PROGNOSIS & COMPLICATIONS

- Mortality from staphylococcal TSS is approximately 4%
- Mortality from streptococcal TSS is approximately 30%
- Female patients with staphylococcal infection should be warned against the use of tampons
- Capillary leak with third spacing of fluids and subsequent severe hypotension, hypoperfusion, and ultimately organ failure (shock) may occur
- Other complications include renal failure, heart failure, and respiratory distress syndrome (due to shock)

Pediatric (Perinatal) HIV

INTRODUCTION

- HIV is the seventh leading cause of death in children
- HIV infection is a chronic RNA viral infection; documented presence of viral infection confirms the diagnosis whether symptomatic or asymptomatic
- AIDS occurs when HIV infection compromises the immune system and opportunistic infections develop; organisms that cause opportunistic infections in AIDS patients normally do not harm those with normal immune systems
- Can occur in all pediatric age groups, including neonates, children, and adolescents
- Recent advances have reduced perinatal transmission to infants

ETIOLOGY, EPIDEMIOLOGY, & RISK FACTORS

- Transmission occurs via sexual contact, percutaneous or mucous membrane exposure, vertical spread (30% of cases occur in utero, 70% occur during labor and delivery), or breastfeeding
- Perinatal transmission from mother to child during pregnancy accounts for 90% of all pediatric AIDS cases in the U.S.; the remaining 10% of cases occur due to contaminated blood products, sexual abuse, or unknown causes
- Factors that increase the risk of perinatal transmission include high maternal viral load, low maternal CD4+ count, maternal drug abuse, HIV virulence, birth weight less than 2500 g, and rupture of membranes >4 hours
- Perinatal transmission is reduced when antenatal, intrapartum, and infant prophylaxis is administered (zidovudine, AZT)
- There is 0.3% seroprevalence of HIV among pregnant women in the U.S.
- Greater incidence in racial and ethnic minorities
- Median age of onset is 12–18 months

PATIENT PRESENTATION

Historical Factors Suggesting HIV
- *Pneumocystis carinii* pneumonia (PCP) is the most common presentation
- Lymphoid interstitial pneumonitis
- Recurrent bacterial infections (eg, otitis media, sinusitis, meningitis)
- Candida esophagitis or oral candidiasis
- Disseminated CMV, HSV, or varicella
- Tuberculosis or *Mycobacterium avium* complex

Physical Findings Suggesting HIV
- Generalized lymphadenopathy
- Persistent or recurring adenopathy
- Hepatosplenomegaly
- Failure to thrive
- Parotid enlargement
- Developmental delay
- Papular rash (HIV dermatitis)
- Recurrent diarrhea

DIFFERENTIAL DX
- Lymphadenitis
- Malabsorption syndrome
- Failure to thrive (other causes)
- Epstein-Barr virus infection
- Cytomegalovirus infection
- Hypogammaglobulinemia
- Severe combined immune deficiency
- Common variable immune deficiency

DIAGNOSTIC EVALUATION

- Infants younger than 18 months require two separate positive HIV DNA PCR tests for evidence of the virus; serologic tests before 18 months reflect the mother's serologic status
- Children older than 18 months require two separate positive enzyme immunoassays (EIA), Western blot assays, or viral detection tests (if EIA or Western blot are used before 18 months of age, the results may reflect the mother's serologic status)
- Complete blood count with differential may reveal anemia, thrombocytopenia, neutropenia, or atypical lymphocytes
- Liver enzymes may be elevated
- CD4+ lymphocyte count should be obtained at baseline and followed; declining counts are a marker of disease progression
- Quantitative immunoglobulins should be measured at baseline since a diagnosis of hypogammaglobulinemia would invalidate the result of a negative antibody test
  - Quantitative immunoglobulins have no prognostic significance
  - Usually elevated in children with HIV, but may be low or normal
- HIV studies include HIV viral load, HIV p24 antigen assays (less sensitive), and HIV culture
- Other diagnostic elements are based on presentation (eg, patients with respiratory distress may require bronchoscopy for cultures, patients with persistent lymphadenopathy may require fine-needle biopsy)

TREATMENT & MANAGEMENT

- Antiretroviral therapy should be given to all HIV-infected children younger than 12 months of age or those with more than 100,000 viral load, or as soon as infection is diagnosed
- For older children and adolescents, timing of therapy is based on CD4+ count, clinical status, and viral load
- Combination therapy is the rule; typically, two to three drugs are started, including a nucleoside reverse transcriptase inhibitor and/or a nonnucleoside reverse transcriptase inhibitor and a protease inhibitor
- The goal of treatment is to decrease viral load
- Compliance is crucial; partial compliance is worse than noncompliance
- Breastfeeding should be avoided
- All pregnant women should be counseled about HIV and offered testing because of the reduction in perinatal transmission with AZT therapy
- Prophylaxis should be given to prevent opportunistic infections
- Other immune-based therapy includes IVIG in children with repeated bacterial infections such as pneumonia, otitis media, invasive bacterial infection, or sinusitis
- All normal childhood vaccines should be given, including influenza vaccination; however, live vaccines should only be given if the CD4+ count is normal

PROGNOSIS & COMPLICATIONS

- Mean survival is 10 years; this is likely to increase with improved antiretroviral agents
- Disease may be rapidly progressive (10–15% die by age 4), chronic progressive, or follow an adult-like pattern
- Diagnosis of HIV in children is often the sentinel event to diagnosis in the mother
- Vertical transmission is significantly lowered by AZT prophylaxis in the mother and parenteral zidovudine administration during labor and delivery
- Oral zidovudine should be administered to the infant within 12 hours after birth and continued until 6 weeks of age while HIV status is being determined
- Caesarean section delivery diminishes risk

Hepatitis A

INTRODUCTION

- Hepatitis A is an acute, self-limited disease with a favorable outcome in most cases
- It is part of a heterogeneous group of hepatitis viruses that cause similar acute clinical illnesses
- Acute hepatitis is the primary manifestation
- Hepatitis A does *not* cause chronic infection
- There is a variable clinical presentation in children ranging from asymptomatic to fulminant hepatitis (although the latter is rare)
- Younger children usually have milder or asymptomatic infections compared with older children, adolescents, and adults; the highest rates of infection occur in children aged 5–14

ETIOLOGY, EPIDEMIOLOGY, & RISK FACTORS

- A nonenveloped, single-stranded RNA picornavirus
- Occurs worldwide but is endemic in certain areas, including South and Central America and certain parts of Africa
- Spreads via person-to-person contact
  - Fecal-oral transmission via contamination of materials or food; can have foodborne or waterborne outbreaks
  - Blood and perinatal transmission are rare
  - Transmission occurs during the preicteric phase
  - Increased risk of infection in contacts of infected persons, daycare centers, homosexuals, those traveling internationally, IV drug users, and those with known chronic liver disease
- Incubation period of 15–50 days
- Nationwide epidemics occur every 10 years; half of those infected during epidemics will not have an identifiable source of infection
- Higher rates occur in areas of low socioeconomic status and poor sanitation, although infection is independent of sex or race

PATIENT PRESENTATION

- Presentation is variable with preicteric phases followed by icteric phase:
  - Asymptomatic (no liver enzyme abnormalities)
  - Subclinical (asymptomatic, mild liver enzyme abnormalities)
  - Anicteric (symptomatic, but without jaundice)
  - Icteric (symptomatic, with jaundice)
  - Fulminant liver failure (mental confusion, emotional instability, bleeding, coma)
- Young children are generally less symptomatic
- Early symptoms (preicteric) last up to 5 days: fever, nausea, vomiting, malaise, anorexia, headache, diarrhea, abdominal pain
- Late symptoms (icteric) last a few days to 1 month: Dark urine, icterus, right upper quadrant tenderness, hepatomegaly, splenomegaly
- Extrahepatic complaints (eg, arthralgias, cutaneous vasculitis, and pruritus) are rare

DIFFERENTIAL DX

- Autoimmune hepatitis
- Other hepatitis viruses
- Adenovirus
- Enterovirus
- Epstein-Barr virus infection
- Drug-induced hepatitis
- Cytomegalovirus infection
- Hemolytic disease (eg, early stages of hemolytic uremic syndrome)
- Gallstones
- Wilson disease

DIAGNOSTIC EVALUATION

- History and physical examination
- Liver function tests
  - ALT and AST values of 200–5000
  - ALT is elevated much higher than AST (whereas ALT is more specific to the liver, AST is often elevated with injury to skeletal muscle)
  - Elevation of ALT occurs 2–3 weeks after the incubation period
  - Total bilirubin may become abnormal when ALT peaks and lasts 1 day to 1 month
  - There is no distinct pattern of enzyme abnormalities that distinguishes hepatitis A infection from other etiologies of hepatitis
- Prothrombin time (PT) to assess the extent of liver injury
- Serologic testing:
  - Anti-HAV appears after the onset of jaundice
  - Anti-HAV IgM is present at the onset of illness and disappears within 4–6 months
  - Anti-HAV IgG develops shortly after the appearance of IgM and persists indefinitely
- Fecal shedding of the hepatitis A virus can occur up to 1 week after the onset of jaundice

TREATMENT & MANAGEMENT

- Primarily supportive treatment
- Avoid hepatotoxic drugs (eg, acetaminophen)
- Antiviral medications are not indicated
- Pre-exposure prophylaxis via vaccination or immunoglobulins:
  - Administer hepatitis A vaccine to all children from 12–23 months of age, as well as to persons in the following circumstances (if not already vaccinated): foreign travel to endemic areas, communities with consistently elevated infection rates, chronic liver diseases, clotting factor disorders, homosexual and bisexual men, IV drug users, and persons at risk of occupational exposure
  - Administer immunoglobulin to children younger than 12 months
- Postexposure prophylaxis for household, close, and sexual contacts of confirmed cases, newborn infants of recently infected mothers, and daycare center contacts
  - Immunoglobulin is recommended as prophylaxis if within 2 weeks of exposure
  - Vaccine can be given to unimmunized postexposure contacts; however, it must be given along with immunoglobulin
- Patients with hepatitis A infection who work as food handlers or in daycare centers should not attend work for 1 week after illness

PROGNOSIS & COMPLICATIONS

- Disease is typically self-limited with complete recovery (even in prolonged cases)
- Fulminant hepatitis is rare
- Symptoms usually last less than 2 months
- No chronic carrier state exists
- Mortality of 0.1–0.2%
- Relapsing hepatitis occurs in 10% of patients
- Prevention involves good hygiene (hand washing), ensuring a safe water supply, and preexposure immunization and postexposure prophylaxis, when indicated

Hepatitis B

INTRODUCTION

- Hepatitis B virus (HBV) is a hepatitis virus that may cause primary acute hepatitis and chronic hepatitis; it is a common cause of neonatal hepatitis via highly efficient perinatal transmission
- Those who do not clear the virus after an acute infection can go on to develop two chronic states: persistent infection characterized by chronic liver disease with abnormal liver enzymes and liver histology, or an asymptomatic carrier state with normal liver enzymes
- Onset is usually insidious; can also be asymptomatic or have an extrahepatic prodromal period prior to the onset of jaundice

ETIOLOGY, EPIDEMIOLOGY, & RISK FACTORS

- A double-stranded DNA hepadnavirus
- Has a worldwide distribution with over 2 billion infected individuals; endemic in Southeast Asia and Southern Africa
- Transmitted via blood, body fluids, and blood products (eg, transfusions, needle sharing, hemodialysis, mucous membrane exposure to blood or bodily fluid via sexual activity, occupational exposure, maternal-fetal transmission); less frequently, transmission can occur via oral-oral contact or any intimate physical contact
- The greatest risk of childhood transmission is in children born in highly endemic areas
- Vertical transmission occurs in 2.4% of infants born to chronic carriers despite vaccination at birth, suggesting that intrauterine infection occurs in some cases
- Persons with chronic disease are the primary reservoirs of infection
- Chronic infection occurs in 95% of infants with perinatal infection (without prophylaxis), 30% of children 1–5 years old, and 2–6% of older children
- One-third of infected patients have no identifiable risk factors
- Males are affected more commonly than females, and blacks are affected more commonly than whites
- Incubation period of 45–160 days

PATIENT PRESENTATION

- May be asymptomatic (most common presentation in young children); symptoms rare in the perinatal period
- Presenting symptoms include anorexia, nausea, malaise, low-grade fever, jaundice, clay-colored stools, dark urine, and abdominal pain
- Extrahepatic manifestations occur as an immune complex vasculitis affecting the skin (eg, Gianotti-Crosti syndrome, urticaria), joints (arthralgias, arthritis), small arterioles (vasculitis), and renal glomeruli (glomerulonephritis)
- May rarely present with fulminant hepatic failure (persistent jaundice, encephalopathy, coagulopathy)

DIFFERENTIAL DX

- Other viral hepatitis infections
- Cytomegalovirus infection
- Drug-induced hepatitis
- Enterovirus infection
- Herpes simplex
- Epstein-Barr infection
- Autoimmune hepatitis
- Alcoholic cirrhosis

DIAGNOSTIC EVALUATION

- The pattern of liver enzyme elevations is indistinguishable from other types of acute hepatic infections
- Diagnosis is based on serologies, presence/absence of hepatitis B virus antigens, and hepatitis B DNA PCR
- Hepatitis B e antigen (HBeAg) indicates active replication (in acute and chronic infection) and high infectivity; becomes elevated before the onset of symptoms
- HBsAg is present in acute infection; it appears in the latter part of the incubation period; infected individuals who are unable to clear HBsAg become chronic carriers or develop chronic infection
- HBsAg and HBV DNA are positive in acute and chronic infections; in asymptomatic chronic carriers, HBsAg is positive, HBeAg is negative, and HBV DNA negative
- Anti-HBc IgM is the first antibody to be detectable; it becomes elevated upon onset of acute symptoms and may also be positive in those with chronic active hepatitis; it is negative in those who are carriers or who have cirrhosis
- Anti-HBs appears late (2 weeks to 2 months after HBsAg becomes undetectable)
- Anti-HBs IgG and Anti-HBc IgG are formed when the acute disease is over and persist indefinitely; they usually appear 3–4 months after clearance of HBsAg
- The presence of anti-HBe indicates decreased infectivity and low risk of transmitting virus
- Anti-HBs IgG is also seen in those who have immunity from vaccination
- HBsAg, HBeAg, and HBV DNA are positive in chronic persistent disease

TREATMENT & MANAGEMENT

- Hepatitis B vaccine is an important part of pre- and postexposure prophylaxis
  - The three dose vaccine series is given to all infants as part of routine immunization series
  - Confers 95% seroprotection rate after vaccination
- Treat chronic symptomatic infection with recombinant interferon-α-2b; lamivudine may also be effective
- Infants born to hepatitis B–positive mothers should be treated with hepatitis B vaccine within 12 hours of birth; hepatitis B immunoglobulin (HBIG) should be given concurrently at a different site
  - If maternal status is unknown, the vaccine should be given within 12 hours of birth while maternal hepatitis status is determined; HBIG can be given within 7 days if maternal status is found to be positive or cannot be determined by 7 days
  - In infants weighing less than 2 kg and for whom maternal status is unknown, the vaccine should still be given within 12 hours of birth; however, HBIG should also be given within 12 hours if maternal status cannot be determined by 12 hours of life
- Breastfeeding can be continued by hepatitis B–positive mothers
- HBIG should be given in those with accidental percutaneous or mucosal exposure
- Children with HBV infection should be monitored for complications
- Adolescents should be counseled on safe sex practices and risks of unprotected sex

PROGNOSIS & COMPLICATIONS

- Chronically infected children are at increased risk of chronic liver disease (cirrhosis, chronic active hepatitis, chronic persistent hepatitis) and liver cancer during adulthood
- Age and immunocompetence affect the course of infection
- Patients infected at birth have a lifetime risk of hepatocellular carcinoma of 50% among males and 20% among females
- Alcohol consumption is an independent risk factor for progression to cirrhosis; known carriers are advised not to drink alcohol and minimize hepatotoxic medications
- More severe hepatic injury occurs upon concurrent infection with hepatitis D
- Fulminant hepatitis occurs in 1–2% of cases; risk is increased by hepatitis D coinfection
- Mortality of 0.5–2% in uncomplicated cases

Hepatitis C

INTRODUCTION

- Hepatitis C virus (HCV) is the most common cause of chronic viral hepatitis in the U.S.
- Prevalence is highest in adults 30–49 years old, but it affects all ages and tends to be underdiagnosed in children
- Prior to universal screening of blood products, hepatitis C used to be a major cause of "non-A, non-B hepatitis"
- 60–80% of infections result in chronic disease (in 20–40% of cases, the virus is cleared by the host's immune system)
- Fulminant hepatitis occurs in 1–2% of infections

ETIOLOGY, EPIDEMIOLOGY, & RISK FACTORS

- A single-stranded RNA flavivirus with worldwide distribution
- Incubation period of 15–180 days (mean, 50 days)
- Since universal screening of blood products began, the risk of hepatitis C transmission from a single blood transfusion has substantially decreased; vertical transmission has become the most common mode of pediatric infection
  - 5% of infants born to anti-HCV–positive mothers will acquire hepatitis C
  - Perinatal transmission rate is higher in mothers with concomitant HIV infection (14% of infants will acquire hepatitis C infection)
  - Increased risk of perinatal transmission occurs with prolonged rupture of membranes and use of internal fetal monitoring devices
  - Caesarian section delivery decreases risk of transmission
- Transmission also occurs through direct percutaneous exposure to blood of hepatitis C–infected persons (eg, IV drug abuse, hemodialysis, tattooing, high-risk sexual behavior)
- Chronic infection results from difficulty by the host's immune system to eliminate the virus due to the virus' rapid mutation rate
- For most infected children, there is no identifiable exposure

PATIENT PRESENTATION

- Acute disease is usually milder than in cases of acute hepatitis A or B:
  - Low-grade fever, malaise, nausea, anorexia, fatigue, right upper quadrant pain
  - Jaundice
  - Pale stools and tea-colored urine
- Chronic disease is usually asymptomatic in children:
  - Chronic fluctuations in liver enzymes occur in 50% of cases
  - Signs of chronic liver disease may include hepatomegaly, ascites, splenomegaly, and spider angioma
  - Extrahepatic manifestations may include serum sickness, pancreatitis, rash, glomerulonephritis, aplastic anemia, mixed cryoglobulinemia, and arthralgias

DIFFERENTIAL DX

- Hepatitis B
- Other viral hepatitis (eg, cytomegalovirus, Epstein-Barr virus, enterovirus)
- Reye syndrome
- Drug-induced hepatitis
- Shock liver
- Alcoholic hepatitis
- Autoimmune hepatitis

DIAGNOSTIC EVALUATION

- Because patients are often asymptomatic during both acute and chronic infection, diagnosis often depends on risk factors and subsequent screening
- ALT is usually <600 (1.5–10 times normal); ALT usually becomes elevated 6–8 weeks after infection
  - Chronic infections may have normal ALT
- Anti-HCV IgG antibody and HCV RNA assays are available for diagnosis
- Enzyme immunoassay of HCV IgG is used as initial screening test; it may be detected within 6–8 weeks after infection
- Recombinant immunoblot assay (RIBA) of HCV IgG is used to confirm results
- HCV RNA can be detected by PCR within 1–2 weeks after exposure and several weeks before the onset of clinical hepatitis
  - Qualitative PCR testing is used to detect the presence of infection; it is used to diagnose early infection of infants (in whom antibody testing reflects maternal antibodies), as well as to confirm acute infections, distinguish resolved from persistent infection, and follow treatment
  - Quantitative PCR (viral load testing) is useful in deciding when to treat and to follow treatment efficacy
- False positives and negatives are possible
- All infants born to infected mothers should be screened

TREATMENT & MANAGEMENT

- Few data are available for management or treatment in children
- Early treatment offers the best hope for elimination of the virus
- Interferon therapy has been used effectively in adults; however, relapses occur, and there may be significant side effects
- Combined treatment with recombinant interferon and ribavirin has been used in adults with some success; however, pediatric experience with this therapy is limited, and it is not approved for children; additionally, ribavirin can be teratogenic
- Liver biopsy is the most accurate method of evaluating the extent of disease and is recommended prior to starting antiviral therapy
- Liver transplantation may be indicated for end-stage liver failure
- Continued follow-up is important to follow liver function tests and screen for hepatocellular carcinoma
- Avoid further insults to the liver: Patients should abstain from alcohol and hepatotoxic medications (eg, acetaminophen) and should receive vaccinations for hepatitis A and B
- Multiple serotypes exist; thus, no vaccine has been effective
- Breastfeeding can be continued by HCV-positive mothers
- Infected adolescents should be counseled on transmission to sexual partners

PROGNOSIS & COMPLICATIONS

- Chronic hepatitis C in childhood is a mild disease but does not often spontaneously remit; treatment during childhood is important because the disease tends to become more severe in adulthood
- Cirrhosis and hepatocellular carcinoma are serious complications
- Most patients are asymptomatic for 20–25 years before developing cirrhosis; few become acutely symptomatic
- Patients with underlying liver disease (eg, other hepatitis viruses, alcoholic liver disease, hemochromatosis) have a poorer prognosis and will become symptomatic quicker
- 50% of chronic hepatitis patients will develop cirrhosis
- Coinfection with HIV results in a more rapid progression to hepatocellular carcinoma

Hemolytic-Uremic Syndrome

INTRODUCTION

- Hemolytic-uremic syndrome (HUS) is defined as a combination of hemolytic anemia, thrombocytopenia, and acute renal failure
- It is the most common cause of acute renal failure in children
- It occurs in previously healthy children and typically starts with watery diarrhea (gastroenteritis) that evolves over several days to weeks into hemorrhagic colitis, hemolysis, thrombocytopenia, and acute renal failure with oliguria or anuria
- Two types exist: The most common form (D+ HUS) is preceded by gastroenteritis, as described above; the atypical form (D− HUS) is not preceded by diarrhea and is more sporadic and less common in children (this entry primarily discusses D+ HUS)

ETIOLOGY, EPIDEMIOLOGY, & RISK FACTORS

- Most common in children younger than 4
- Toxigenic *E. coli* (O157:H7) infection precedes HUS in more than 70% of cases; other causes include shiga toxins produced by *Shigella*
  - 10–15% of patients infected with toxigenic *E. coli* develop HUS; risk is increased in patients receiving antibiotics
  - Infected meat (eg, undercooked hamburger) is the most common source of *E. coli*–associated HUS; other sources include unpasteurized milk, contaminated apple juice or water, and alfalfa sprouts
- Verotoxin produced from the toxigenic strain of *E. coli* attaches to endothelial cells and results in vascular injury; this vascular injury leads to mechanically damaged red blood cells and platelets that are subsequently consumed by the spleen, leading to local coagulopathy, microthrombi, microangiopathic hemolysis, and ultimately end-organ damage
- In cases of D− HUS, etiologies include *S. pneumoniae*, drugs, pregnancy, and OCP use
- The kidney is usually most severely affected, but any organ may be involved, especially the CNS (more common in adults)

PATIENT PRESENTATION

- Initial presentation of infection ranges from mild watery or bloody diarrhea to severe hemorrhagic colitis
- HUS develops 3–7 days later in 10–15% of infected patients
- Fever
- Abdominal pain
- Evidence of dehydration on physical exam
- Pallor, fatigue, weakness
- Irritability, lethargy
- Renal disease may be mild or severe, resulting in variable incidence of hematuria, proteinuria, acute renal failure (oliguria, anuria), hypertension, or edema
- Petechiae due to thrombocytopenia; frank bleeding is rare
- CNS symptoms in 20–30%; seizures most common
- Pancreatic insufficiency (due to microthrombi)

DIFFERENTIAL DX

- Gastroenteritis
- Appendicitis
- Inflammatory bowel disease
- Food poisoning
- Gastrointestinal bleeding
- Sepsis with disseminated intravascular coagulation (DIC)
- *Clostridium difficile* colitis
- Drugs
- Pregnancy
- Thrombotic thrombocytopenic purpura
- Malignant hypertension
- Intussusception

DIAGNOSTIC EVALUATION

- Triad of microangiopathic hemolytic anemia, thrombocytopenia, and renal insufficiency
- Unexplained acute renal failure, with or without neurologic findings, should prompt an evaluation with CBC and peripheral blood smear
- Stool culture remains the gold standard for diagnosis; however, isolation of *E. coli* from the stool may not be possible by the time HUS has developed because the highest likelihood of isolating the organism occurs during the initial 6 days of illness
- Complete blood count reveals normocytic anemia (median hemoglobin, 8 g/dL) and thrombocytopenia
- Reticulocyte count is elevated
- Peripheral smear classically shows schistocytes and microangiopathic hemolysis
- Direct Coombs test should be negative
- Other coagulation tests (PT, PTT) are usually normal; may see increase in fibrin degradation products
- Decreased haptoglobin, increased LDH
- Abnormal renal function studies (elevated BUN/creatinine)
- Renal biopsy is rarely indicated unless there is prolonged renal failure longer than 2 weeks
- Urinalysis reveals hematuria or proteinuria; may see casts on microscopic urinalysis
- Liver function tests may reveal unconjugated hyperbilirubinemia

TREATMENT & MANAGEMENT

- Medical management with supportive care and nutrition
- Control renal failure by monitoring fluids and electrolytes carefully
- Control hypertension to prevent encephalopathy
- Dialysis is indicated if fluid status and electrolyte abnormalities cannot be controlled or corrected medically (ie, when hyperkalemia, uremia, or volume overload states affect cardiopulmonary function)
- Antidiarrheal agents should *not* be used because they may prolong the clinical and bacteriologic course of disease; one study reported that HUS is more likely to develop in patients with *E. coli* infection who received antimotility agents
- Avoid antibiotic treatment; available data indicate antimicrobials offer no substantial benefit and may be detrimental
- If symptomatic with anemia, consider red blood cell transfusion
- Platelet transfusion is rarely necessary but may be indicated prior to surgical procedures (eg, insertion of central lines or dialysis catheter)

PROGNOSIS & COMPLICATIONS

- Overall prognosis good, with the majority of patients recovering renal function
- Up to 50% of children will require acute dialysis
- Chronic renal failure develops in as many as 10% of patients
- 5–10% mortality during the acute phase, generally secondary to CNS events
- Long-term follow-up is required due to the risk for renal insufficiency, proteinuria, and hypertension
- Prognosis is worse with proteinuria lasting beyond 1 year
- Can develop long-term complications of proteinuria, hypertension, and late end-stage renal disease years later, even if full recovery occurs initially
- Recurrences are rare except in the atypical D− form

Tuberculosis

INTRODUCTION

- Tuberculosis (TB) is one of the most common worldwide causes of infection-related death
- TB is caused by infection with *Mycobacterium tuberculosis*, an acid-fast bacillus
- It is an important cause of morbidity and mortality in children, especially in the very young
- The diagnosis may be difficult because children often present with extrapulmonary manifestations rather than the classic constellation of pulmonary symptoms
- Children usually initially develop latent infection; however, active disease is not uncommon in children between age 5 and adolescence
- HIV is the strongest risk factor for development of TB

ETIOLOGY, EPIDEMIOLOGY, & RISK FACTORS

- In children, TB occurs primarily in minorities, immigrants, and those living in inner cities and in poverty
- Risk factors for development of TB include HIV infection, immigration from areas of high incidence, poor access to medical care, and living in homeless shelters, prisons, or overcrowded areas
- In HIV patients, the annual risk of developing TB is 7–10%
- In infected, immunocompetent patients, the *lifetime* risk of developing disease is less than 10%; that is, the majority of infected persons never develop active disease
- Transmitted from person-to-person via respiratory droplets
- Highly contagious and difficult to diagnose (it may resemble many other diseases)
- Approximately 15 million people in the U.S. are PPD-positive
- The World Health Organization has declared TB a global public health emergency
- The source of childhood infections is usually from a high-risk adult, rather than from child-to-child transmission
- Positive cultures often are not obtained in children

PATIENT PRESENTATION

- Known as "the great mimicker" because the presentation often appears similar to many other diseases
- Pulmonary manifestations (eg, cough, fever, weight loss, night sweats) are more common in adults
- Extrapulmonary manifestations are more common in children:
  - TB cervical adenitis is the most common presentation outside the chest and lungs
  - Failure to thrive
  - Fever of unknown origin
  - Meningitis
  - Osteomyelitis

DIFFERENTIAL DX

Pulmonary Disease
- Nontuberculous pneumonia
- Nocardiosis
- Bronchiectasis
- Legionellosis
- Coccidioidomycosis
- Histoplasmosis

Nonpulmonary Manifestations
- Failure to thrive
- Nontuberculous meningitis
- Nontuberculous osteomyelitis
- Fever of unknown origin

DIAGNOSTIC EVALUATION

- The most specific diagnostic test is the Mantoux skin test with 5 units of PPD injected intra-dermally into the forearm
- PPD reaction occurs after 24–48 hours; the test should be read within 48–72 hours after placement
  - Less than 5 mm induration is a negative test
  - Greater than 15 mm induration is a positive test for individuals with no personal or environmental risk factors
  - 5–15 mm induration should be interpreted according to the patient's risk factors (eg, immigrant, HIV, cancer chemotherapy, incarceration)
- If the PPD is positive, obtain a chest X-ray
  - Findings consistent with TB include infiltrates (usually the upper lobes), pneumonia, pleural effusion, and hilar adenopathy
  - If chest X-ray is positive, obtain a sputum sample for acid-fast bacilli stain and culture (children younger than 12 cannot produce enough force to reliably produce sputum; a gastric aspirate should be collected in these children)
- The most definitive test for diagnosis is a mycobacterial culture; however, it is not easy to isolate the organism
- TB *exposure*: PPD and chest X-ray are negative
- TB *infection*: PPD is positive, but chest X-ray is negative
- TB *disease*: PPD and chest X-ray are positive

TREATMENT & MANAGEMENT

- Treat TB infection with isoniazid (INH) prophylaxis for 9 months
  - Administer supplemental vitamin B_{12} to adolescents and adults to prevent INH-induced neuropathy
- Treat TB disease with isoniazid, rifampin, and pyrazinamide daily for 2 months, followed by isoniazid and rifampin for an additional 4 months
  - Adjust therapy according to drug susceptibility of isolates from sputum or gastric aspirates
  - If an adult source case is known with susceptibility, this can direct therapy; if the source is not known or the child is critically ill or in an area with known drug resistance, then it is important to obtain cultures from child
  - The usual duration of treatment is 6 months or until repeat specimens are negative
  - Direct-observed medication administration by a health care worker is indicated to ensure compliance
  - If miliary disease, meningitis, or bone/joint disease is present, the patient should receive 12 months of treatment
  - Streptomycin or ethambutol may be added to therapy for drug resistance
- Vaccination with the bacille Calmette-Guérin (BCG) vaccine does not prevent infection, but it may reduce the incidence of serious disease

PROGNOSIS & COMPLICATIONS

- Treatment is complicated by the need for multiple drugs over a prolonged time, which reduces compliance rates and allows development of resistance against many of the traditional first-line drugs; the existence of multidrug-resistant tuberculosis further adds to this public health problem
- Strict infection control measures are necessary (eg, isolation of hospitalized patients and use of ultrafiltration masks)
- Up to 3 million deaths occur annually worldwide

Fever without Source

INTRODUCTION

- Fever without source is used to describe cases of acute fever (lasting <1 week) without an obvious source
- Esp. important in children <36 months as this is when most severe, focal infections occur
- It is difficult but important to distinguish between serious bacterial infections and self-limited viral infections
- The majority of children have self-limited viral infections that resolve without sequelae; however, meningitis and "occult bacteremia" must be ruled out
- 10–20% of primary care visits are due to fever; however, 20% of childhood fevers have no apparent cause

ETIOLOGY, EPIDEMIOLOGY, & RISK FACTORS

- The definition of fever, causative pathogens, and risk factors are different for differing age groups (<1 month of age, 1–3 months of age, and 3–36 months of age)
- Fever in neonates (<1 month of age) is defined as temperatures higher than 38°C; organisms to consider are late perinatal pathogens (eg, group B *Streptococcus*, *E. coli*, *Listeria monocytogenes*, and herpes simplex virus)
  - If fever occurs in this age group, have higher suspicion for serious bacterial infections, which may occur without localizing signs
- In infants 1–3 months of age, *S. pneumoniae* emerges as a likely cause, and the perinatal pathogens occur less frequently; these infants are at high risk for occult bacteremia
- Fever in children 3–36 months is most commonly caused by *Streptococcus pneumoniae*, group B streptococci, *Neisseria meningitidis*, *Haemophilus influenzae* type B, *E. coli*, and *S. aureus*; the introduction of vaccinations for *S. pneumoniae* (Prevnar) and *H. influenzae* type B have substantially reduced the incidence of serious infections in this age group
- Socioeconomic status, race, and gender do not affect risk of occult bacteremia
- Common sources of fever include sepsis, meningitis, pneumonia, urinary tract infection, septic arthritis, omphalitis, gastroenteritis, pneumonia, otitis media, and skin and soft tissue infections

PATIENT PRESENTATION

- Fever
- Lethargy/decreased activity
- Toxic appearance
- Irritability
- Decreased crying and/or eye contact
- High-pitched cry (suspect meningitis)
- Social withdrawal
- Pallor
- Vomiting or diarrhea
- Poor feeding
- Abnormal vital signs
- Weight loss
- Rash
- Increased work of breathing, and/or nasal flaring, retractions, and grunting

DIFFERENTIAL DX

- Bacteremia
- Respiratory tract infection
- Meningitis
- Urinary tract infection
- Bronchitis
- Viral infection
- Osteomyelitis
- Gastroenteritis
- Endocarditis
- Rheumatic fever
- Malaria
- Tuberculosis
- Postvaccination fever

DIAGNOSTIC EVALUATION

- Careful history and physical examination, including ill contacts and immunization history
- Repeated daily clinical exams
- In neonates, perform a complete evaluation for sepsis, including complete blood count, blood culture, urinalysis and urine culture (obtained by bladder catheterization), and lumbar puncture with cerebrospinal fluid culture with Gram stain
  - Chest X-ray, stool culture, and stool guaiac should be considered based on clinical symptoms and history
- In infants, perform a complete evaluation for sepsis (as above) if suspect a serious bacterial evaluation; however, infants who are well appearing and with normal blood work, urinalysis, and cerebrospinal fluid analysis are less likely to have a serious bacterial infection
- In infants 3–36 months of age, the risk of serious bacterial infection is increased if fever is greater than 39°C: Urinalysis should be done in girls, uncircumcised boys up to 12 months of age, and circumcised boys up to 6 months of age; obtain blood culture and lumbar puncture if indicated by presentation and history (should be obtained in anyone who is ill-appearing; has high fever, high white blood cell count, or bandemia on CBC; or is irritable/difficult to console)
- Infants who receive three doses of vaccinations for *S. pneumoniae* (Prevnar) and *H. influenzae* (HiB) are at much lower risk

TREATMENT & MANAGEMENT

- Begin empiric antibiotic therapy immediately for toxic or ill-appearing children
- Infants under 1 month of age should be hospitalized and treated empirically after the evaluation (including lumbar puncture) is complete; treat with ampicillin plus either a third-generation cephalosporin or gentamicin
- Infants 1–3 months can be followed up within 24 hours by the primary care provider if they have normal blood work, urinalysis, and cerebrospinal fluid studies
- In nontoxic children older than 1 month of age, daily clinical follow-up is sufficient until cultures return or new symptoms present
- Follow-up is critical; thus, social issues should be evaluated (eg, reliability of the parents to assess their child, access to phone and hospital, ease of communication if culture is positive)
- Parents should be informed about signs that may suggest worsening illness (eg, lethargy, irritability, poor feeding, decreased socialization/interaction)
- Children with urinary tract infections may require hospitalization if unable to take fluids and antibiotics orally, if follow-up is not assured, if ill or have toxic appearance, or if very young with pyelonephritis

PROGNOSIS & COMPLICATIONS

- The Rochester criteria are a set of clinical and laboratory parameters that help to identify febrile infants 1–3 months old who are at low risk of having a serious bacterial infection
  - Reassuring criteria include nonseptic appearance, benign birth history, no source for fever, WBC count of 5000–15,000/mm^3, absolute band count less than 1500/mm^3, normal cerebrospinal fluid analysis, benign urinalysis, or less than 5 WBCs/field in stool specimen (if diarrhea is present)
  - If the child *does not* fulfill Rochester criteria, consider starting empiric antibiotics
- Most fevers without source are benign viral infections
- Serious bacterial infection may lead to death, especially in young children

Fever of Unknown Origin

INTRODUCTION

- Defined as a prolonged fever (longer than 21 days as an outpatient or 1 week as an inpatient) without an apparent cause
- Initial history, physical examination, and diagnostic workup are usually normal; thus, it can be quite challenging from diagnostic standpoint
- Most fevers of unknown origin (FUO) are atypical presentations of common diseases; however, the differential diagnosis is broad and includes both infectious and noninfectious causes
- An explanation for the fever is eventually found in 90% of cases

ETIOLOGY, EPIDEMIOLOGY, & RISK FACTORS

- The most common etiologies are bacterial and viral infections
  - Infections account for about one-third of cases (respiratory tract infections account for half; others include urinary tract infections, CNS infections, septicemia, focal soft tissue infections, and osteomyelitis)
- The most common noninfectious etiologies include rheumatologic (eg, juvenile rheumatoid arthritis, SLE, Behçet disease, vasculitis), autoimmune, and neoplastic disorders
  - FUO is a common presentation for systemic juvenile rheumatoid arthritis and collagen vascular diseases
  - Other noninfectious etiologies include inflammatory bowel disease, drug fever, Munchausen by proxy, central thermoregulation disorder or other CNS lesions (eg, tumors), serum sickness, Kawasaki disease, Henoch-Schönlein purpura, juvenile dermatomyositis, sarcoidosis, pancreatitis, and familial Mediterranean fever
- Unexplained intermittent fever lasting longer than 6 months suggests an autoimmune disorder

PATIENT PRESENTATION

- Fever
  - By definition, lasts more than 21 days as out-patient or longer than 7 days as inpatient
  - Higher than 38.3°C on several occasions
  - Unknown etiology after baseline workup
  - Usually do not see temperatures above 41°C; however, higher fevers (40–41°C) suggest meningitis or other bacterial infections
  - Prolonged fever with meningitis suggests chronic meningitis or partially treated meningitis
- Additional presentation depends on the underlying etiology

DIFFERENTIAL DX

- Infections to consider include:
  - Endocarditis
  - Urinary tract infection
  - Sinusitis or mastoiditis
  - Osteomyelitis
  - Tuberculosis
  - Malaria
  - Chronic bacterial meningitis
  - RMSF
  - Cat scratch disease
  - Visceral abscess
  - Dental infection
  - EBV, CMV, or HSV
  - Syphilis
  - Tularemia, brucellosis
  - Hepatitis; Lyme disease
  - HIV with opportunistic infection

DIAGNOSTIC EVALUATION

- A thorough history is most critical to narrow the differential diagnosis; attention should be paid to animal exposures, recent travel, dietary history, medication history, and genetic background (eg, familial Mediterranean fever)
- Complete physical examination with attention to lymph nodes, oropharynx, skin (for rashes), muscle and joint exam, rectal exam, and eye exam
- The sequence of the evaluation depends on the level of acuity and degree of suspicion for specific diagnoses based on the history and exam; consider the following:
  - CBC with peripheral smear, ESR, CRP, liver/renal function, albumin, globulin, urinalysis
  - Sinus and chest X-rays
  - Blood cultures, urine culture, stool culture with Hemoccult, and CSF culture
  - PPD skin testing
  - Serologies (eg, CMV, EBV, *Brucella, Bartonella*, and others)
  - Bone scan to rule out osteomyelitis
  - Echocardiogram to rule out endocarditis
  - HIV testing
  - Upper GI series with small bowel follow-through (for inflammatory bowel disease)
  - Bone marrow aspiration and biopsy (for malignancy)
  - CT scan or MRI for neoplasms
  - Bronchoscopy
  - Exploratory laparoscopy

TREATMENT & MANAGEMENT

- Empiric antibiotic therapy should be reserved for critically ill patients because this can make some diagnoses more difficult
- Supportive therapy with prolonged observation
- If the patient is stable, evaluation can be done as an outpatient
- The decision to hospitalize depends on the degree of illness and ability to obtain studies; occasionally, patients may need to be hospitalized to carefully document the fever
- It is important to document that fever is actually occurring; up to 20% of patients who report FUO actually have no fever (either because of incorrect method of temperature taking or invention/fabrication of fever)
- Administer appropriate antibiotics once the nidus of infection and specific organism is found
- While evaluating the child, avoid antipyretics in order to observe the true fever curve; antipyretics may be given for comfort after evaluation and documentation of fever
- A diagnostic trial with NSAIDs may be warranted if suspect Still disease

PROGNOSIS & COMPLICATIONS

- Daily inquiries regarding new complaints and complete physical examination must be carried out until reaching a diagnosis
- Some patients never have a final diagnosis
- A large percentage of cases of FUO resolve without diagnosis or treatment and do not recur
- Overall prognosis and complications depend on the primary diagnosis

Acute Myelogenous Leukemia

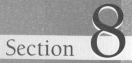

INTRODUCTION

Acute myelogenous leukemia (AML) represents 20% of acute leukemias in children (the remainder are acute lymphocytic leukemia)

Chronic leukemia and myelodysplastic syndromes (MDS) are uncommon in children, but MDS usually predisposes to AML

Acute leukemia is a clonal disorder defined by at least 20% blasts in the bone marrow; blasts represent abnormal cells resulting from malignant transformation of a self-renewing progenitor cell in the bone marrow that undergoes decreased self-destruction (apoptosis) and aberrant differentiation

ETIOLOGY, EPIDEMIOLOGY, & RISK FACTORS

- AML is the malignant transformation and expansion of nonlymphoid precursors in the bone marrow
- Acquired chromosomal abnormalities have been found in 80% of cases
- May occur due to chromosome abnormalities (Down syndrome, trisomy 13), chromatin fragility (Fanconi anemia, Bloom syndrome, ataxia-telangiectasia), chemicals (benzene, smoking, pesticides, petroleum products, and possibly prenatal alcohol or marijuana exposure), X-ray treatment, or drugs (alkylating agents, epidophyllotoxins)
- Also associated with other inherited predisposing conditions: twinning, Kostmann syndrome, Shwachman-Diamond syndrome, neurofibromatosis type 1, Diamond-Blackfan anemia, Klinefelter syndrome, Li-Fraumeni syndrome (germline p53 mutations)
- Also associated with noninherited risk factors, including aplastic anemia, myelodysplastic syndrome, paroxysmal nocturnal hemoglobinuria (PNH)
- Increased incidence with age (peak incidence in adults older than 60)
- Patients with Down syndrome are more than 10 times more likely to develop leukemia, most commonly AML
- A small percentage (5%) of patients have true bilineage leukemia (separate populations of both AML and ALL lineages)
- DIC may occur in cases of M3 AML

PATIENT PRESENTATION

- Symptoms reflect cell line depression (anemia, thrombocytopenia, leukopenia)
  - Anemia-related: Fatigue, pallor, palpitations, dyspnea
  - Thrombocytopenia-related: Poor hemostasis (epistaxis, bleeding, bruising)
  - Leukopenia-related: Infections, fever
- Lymphadenopathy (20% of patients)
- Hepatosplenomegaly (50% of patients)
- Gingival hypertrophy
- Skin infiltration with leukemic cells (leukemia cutis or chloroma)
  Bone pain (20% of patients)
  Nonspecific symptoms include fatigue (the presenting symptom in 50% of cases), fever, weakness, and anorexia or weight loss
  Neurologic deficits (leptomeningeal disease, brain chloroma, leukostasis with high WBCs)

DIFFERENTIAL DX

- Acute lymphocytic leukemia
- Aplastic anemia
- Rheumatoid arthritis
- Systemic lupus erythematosus
- Infectious mononucleosis or other severe viral illness
- Osteomyelitis
- Pertussis
- Idiopathic thrombocytopenic purpura

Acute Lymphocytic Leukemia

INTRODUCTION

- The most common malignancy in children
- Acute lymphocytic leukemia (ALL) and acute myelogenous leukemia (AML) together cause nearly 30% of pediatric malignancies
- Modern treatments decrease late effects of therapy while maintaining excellent cure rates
- Current therapy is stratified by risk and response to treatment; new important variables are emerging to help determine who needs more aggressive therapy and who needs less
- Standard prognostic variables include age and white blood cell count at diagnosis
- Prognosis is based on early response to therapy, cytogenetic analysis, and assessment of minimal residual disease at various time points during treatment

ETIOLOGY, EPIDEMIOLOGY, & RISK FACTORS

- A malignant proliferation of immature lymphoblasts
- Spontaneous mutations are thought to be the major cause of these proliferations
- Mutations may occur due to host factors or environmental factors
  - Host factors include chromosome abnormalities (eg, Down syndrome, trisomy 13); chromatin fragility (eg, Fanconi anemia, Bloom syndrome, ataxia-telangiectasia
  - Environmental factors include chemicals (eg, benzene, tobacco use), ionizing radiation, and drugs (eg, alkylating agents, epidophyllotoxins)
- ALL accounts for 80% of leukemias
  - 80% of ALL cases are of B-cell origin, 20% are of T-cell origin
- Most common in children; peak incidence is 3–4 years of age
- Slightly more common in males and whites
- T-cell leukemia is more common in boys

PATIENT PRESENTATION

- Symptoms reflect cell line depression (anemia, thrombocytopenia, leukopenia)
  - Anemia-related: Fatigue, pallor, palpitations
  - Thrombocytopenia-related: Poor hemostasis (epistaxis, petechiae/purpura, bleeding, bruising)
  - Leukopenia-related: Infections, fever
- Lymphadenopathy
- Hepatosplenomegaly
- Gingival hypertrophy/skin infiltration with leukemic cells (chloroma)
- Bone pain
- Nonspecific symptoms include fatigue or lethargy (the presenting symptom in 50% of cases), fever, weakness, and anorexia or weight loss
- Bulky disease is more likely in T-cell leukemia (mediastinal masses can present with respiratory distress)

DIFFERENTIAL DX

Nonmalignant Processes
- Aplastic anemia
- Osteomyelitis
- Systemic lupus erythematosus
- Infectious mononucleosis
- Pertussis/parapertussis
- Idiopathic thrombocytopenic purpura
- Rheumatoid arthritis

Malignancies
- Acute myelogenous leukemia
- Lymphoma
- Neuroblastoma
- Retinoblastoma
- Rhabdomyosarcoma

DIAGNOSTIC EVALUATION

- CBC reveals abnormal white blood cell count (one-third of cases have elevated WBCs; one-third of cases have low WBCs; one-third are normal), decreased absolute neutrophil count, anemia, and thrombocytopenia
- Bone marrow aspirate is usually diagnostic and reveals bone marrow filled with lymphoblasts
- Workup of a patient with suspected ALL should include:
  - CBC with differential
  - LDH and uric acid (often increased due to rapid cell turnover)
  - Electrolytes, BUN, and creatinine
  - Calcium and phosphorous
  - Chest X-ray (to evaluate for mediastinal mass)
  - Bone marrow aspiration with analysis for morphology, cytogenetics, immunohistochemistry, and flow cytometric analysis
- Lumbar puncture is indicated once the diagnosis is confirmed because ALL can spread intrathecally to the CNS
- Viral titers (varicella immune status, cytomegalovirus, Epstein-Barr virus)
- Coagulation studies (PT/INR)
- Type and cross (for probable transfusion)

TREATMENT & MANAGEMENT

- Chemotherapy is the mainstay of therapy
- Therapy is risk- and response-based
  - Induction chemotherapy to reduce the tumor burden to less than 10^9 cells
  - Consolidation therapy to eradicate residual leukemia
  - Delayed intensification to avoid development of resistance by tumor cells
  - Maintenance therapy to maintain complete remission
  - Intrathecal chemotherapy to prevent relapse in the CNS
  - Patients with high-risk disease receive more intensive therapy
  - Therapy lasts 2 or more years in females and 3 or more years in males (usually as outpatient therapy)
- Bone marrow transplantation is reserved for those patients who relapse or have certain cytogenetic abnormalities

PROGNOSIS & COMPLICATIONS

- Untreated disease is uniformly fatal
- Cure rate is 75–95% (lower in T-cell leukemias), but prognosis remains poor for i
- Remission after 28 days occurs in >95% of cases; most important poor prognosti high WBC count at diagnosis, slow early response to therapy, and age >10 year
- Decreased survival is associated with the presence of the Philadelphia chrom
- Bone marrow is the most common site of relapse; may also relapse in the CN!
- During treatment, patients are at risk for tumor lysis syndrome, which is caus of metabolic products secondary to lysis of blast cells and is characterized b uricemia, hyperkalemia, and hyperphosphatemia; other complications inclu thrombosis, pancreatitis, avascular necrosis, and neurologic complications

DIAGNOSTIC EVALUATION

- It is difficult to distinguish AML from ALL based on presenting signs and symptoms alone
- Like ALL, CBC typically reveals anemia; thrombocytopenia; high, low, or normal WBC
- Auer rods seen on peripheral smear are pathognomonic for AML
- Bone marrow aspirate is diagnostic: More than 20% of cells are nonlymphoid blasts; flow cytometry and immunohistochemical stains clarify the type; cytogenetics is also important
- Blood typing and HLA typing for possible treatment
- Lumbar puncture to determine if there is CNS involvement
- The FAB (French-American-British) classification divides AML into subtypes (M0–M7) based on morphologic and histochemical information:
  M0: Undifferentiated
  M1: Acute myeloblastic without differentiation
  M2: Acute myeloblastic with differentiation
  M3: Acute promyelocytic (APL), hypergranular variant (associated with DIC)
  M3v: Acute promyelocytic, hypogranular variant
  M4: Acute myelomonocytic
  M4eo: Acute myelomonocytic with eosinophilia
  M5a: Acute monocytic
  M5b: Acute monocytic with differentiation
  M6: Acute erythroleukemia
  M7: Acute megakaryoblastic

TREATMENT & MANAGEMENT

- Induction chemotherapy is more intense than in ALL; mortality is high in induction chemotherapy due to severe, prolonged myelosuppression
- Successful supportive care involves prevention and aggressive inpatient management
- Intrathecal chemotherapy to prevent relapse in the CNS
- Patients with a full sibling match should undergo allogeneic bone marrow transplant after they achieve remission
- Patients without sibling match undergo approximately 6 months of combination chemotherapy (vs. 2–3 years for ALL), mostly inpatient
- Intensive timing and dosing of chemotherapy has improved survival rates, equaling those of transplantation
- Allogeneic bone marrow transplant is always recommended for relapses
- Acute promyelocytic leukemia is treated separately with molecular targets (all-*trans* retinoic acid) for PML-RAR gene

PROGNOSIS & COMPLICATIONS

- Untreated disease is uniformly fatal
- Infection is major cause of death during the first 10 wk of intensive chemotherapy; patients are immunosuppressed and have breakdown of anatomic barriers due to oral and GI mucositis
- DIC may occur in M3 AML
- 80% of patients achieve an initial remission
- Disease-free survival at 5 years is 35–60%
- Young age and high WBC count suggest poor treatment outcome
- Certain cytogenetics predict a better prognosis: t(8;21), inversion 16, t(15;17)
- Long-term morbidity and mortality occur due to cardiac, CNS, and hepatic toxicity of chemotherapy and complications of chronic graft-versus-host disease for transplant recipients

Hodgkin Lymphoma

INTRODUCTION

- Hodgkin disease is a malignancy of lymphoid tissue characterized by the presence of Reed-Sternberg (RS) cells or variant
- The treatment for Hodgkin disease was the paradigm for the development of combination chemotherapy protocols and showcases the success of randomized controlled clinical trials in the history of cancer treatment
- Hodgkin disease is responsible for about 8% of childhood cancers but accounts for more than 15% of cancers in patients 15–19 years of age
- Overall, lymphomas are the third most common childhood cancer
- 99% of cases arise in the lymph nodes

ETIOLOGY, EPIDEMIOLOGY, & RISK FACTORS

- Classified into four types: nodular sclerosis, mixed cellularity, lymphocyte predominant, and lymphocyte deplete
  - Nodular sclerosis is most common in adolescents and females
  - Mixed cellularity accounts for 30% of cases and is more common in children under 10
  - Lymphocyte predominant is uncommon but has the best prognosis
  - Lymphocyte deplete is least common (mostly occurs in HIV patients), has the poorest prognosis, and often involves bone or bone marrow
- Hodgkin disease behaves in a characteristic way, by contiguous spread from lymph node to lymph node with a central distribution of affected nodes (eg, mediastinum, neck)
- A role of Epstein-Barr virus (EBV) is suspected (50% of Reed-Sternberg cells are positive for EBV gene expression)
- There is a bimodal distribution of incidence (mid-20s and older than 50); the disease is rare in children under 5 years
- 3 distinct categories: Childhood (<15 years; mostly mixed cellularity, more common in males, tends to occur in low socioeconomic status groups); young adult (15–34 years; mostly nodular sclerosis, tends to occur in higher socioeconomic groups); and older adult (55–74)
- Risk in the sibling of a monozygotic twin increases by nearly 100-fold

PATIENT PRESENTATION

- The majority of patients are asymptomatic
- More than 90% of cases present with firm, painless lymphadenopathy (typically cervical or supraclavicular, but may be axillary or inguinal)
- 50% of patients have mediastinal disease at the time of presentation (cough, dyspnea, dysphagia)
- 20–30% of patients present with systemic symptoms ("B" symptoms), including unexplained fevers (>38.5°C), drenching night sweats, and weight loss (more than 10% of body weight)
- Rarely, patients present with intractable pruritus or alcohol-induced pain in nodal areas

DIFFERENTIAL DX

- Non-Hodgkin lymphoma
- Lymphadenitis
- HIV
- Infectious mononucleosis
- Tuberculosis
- Atypical mycobacteria
- Toxoplasmosis
- Cat scratch disease
- ALPS (autoimmune lymphoproliferative syndrome)

DIAGNOSTIC EVALUATION

- Diagnosis is made by lymph node biopsy demonstrating RS or RS-variant cells
- Flow cytometry shows CD15+ and CD30+ on RS cells
- Workup should include complete blood count, erythrocyte sedimentation rate (ESR), C-reactive protein (CRP), liver function tests, BUN, creatinine, and chest x-ray
- May have associated autoimmune disorders (eg, hemolytic anemia, idiopathic thrombocytopenic purpura) at diagnosis or after treatment
- Bone marrow biopsy; CT scan of the chest, abdomen, and pelvis; gallium scan, and PET scan may be performed for clinical staging
- Surgical staging and/or splenectomy are no longer used for staging
- Cerebrospinal fluid evaluation is not required but should be done if CNS involvement is suspected
- Bone scan is indicated if bony involvement is suspected
- Ann Arbor staging:
  - I: Disease limited to a single lymph node region or organ
  - II: Two or more lymph node regions on the same side of the diaphragm
  - III: Lymph node regions on both sides of the diaphragm
  - IV: Disseminated disease with extralymphatic organ involvement
  - Stages are referred to as A or B depending on presence of systemic ("B") symptoms

TREATMENT & MANAGEMENT

- Low-stage/low-risk (stage I-IIA): 2–4 cycles of multiagent chemotherapy, with or without low-dose radiation therapy to the involved fields
- Intermediate-risk (stages I-IIB or bulky disease, IIIA, or IVA): 4–6 cycles of chemotherapy with involved-field radiation therapy (IFRT)
- High-risk (stages IIIB and IVB): 4–8 cycles of chemotherapy with IFRT
- Combination chemotherapy using MOPP (mechlorethamine, vincristine, procarbazine, and prednisone) alternating with ABVD (doxorubicin, bleomycin, vinblastine, and dacarbazine) is the standard treatment; newer treatment regimens are also used to reduce radiation therapy, alkylating agents, and anthracyclines to minimize late effects in survivors
- Intensive chemotherapy or autologous bone marrow transplant for refractory or recurrent disease

PROGNOSIS & COMPLICATIONS

- Hodgkin disease is curable in 90–95% of children and adolescents
- Elevations in ESR, ferritin, and copper may be indicators of active disease
- Long-term sequelae of treatment include endocrinopathies (especially thyroid dysfunction and growth retardation), infertility, cardiomyopathy or pericarditis, pulmonary fibrosis, osteoporosis, and second malignant neoplasms (especially breast cancer)

Non-Hodgkin Lymphoma

INTRODUCTION

- Non-Hodgkin lymphoma (NHL) is a malignancy of lymphoid cells residing in lymphoid tissues (in contrast to leukemia, where the malignant lymphoid cells reside in bone marrow)
- Non-Hodgkin lymphoma and Hodgkin lymphoma account for 15% of childhood cancer in children 0–19 years of age (non-Hodgkin lymphoma is 7%)
- Overall, lymphoma is the third most common cancer in children
- Non-Hodgkin lymphoma is more common than Hodgkin in children under age 15 years
- 90% of non-Hodgkin lymphomas are of B-cell origin
- One of the most common second malignant neoplasms
- There is no evidence that viral exposure in the U.S. is linked to NHL

ETIOLOGY, EPIDEMIOLOGY, & RISK FACTORS

- Pediatric lymphoma types are different and more aggressive than adult NHL:
  - Burkitt lymphoma (40% of pediatric NHL): A mature B-cell tumor associated with t(8;14) translocation (c-myc); it grows very rapidly (highest tumor turnover of any type) and is most commonly associated with abdominal disease at presentation, followed by head and neck
  - Lymphoblastic lymphoma (30% of pediatric NHL): Primarily a T-cell (85–90%) tumor that is often diagnosed at stages III or IV and often presents with a mediastinal mass (B-cell lymphoblastic tumors usually present at stages I or II but represent only 10–15% of cases)
  - Diffuse large B-cell (10% of pediatric NHL): A mature B-cell tumor with many variants; may have Reed-Sternberg cells and may be difficult to distinguish from Hodgkin disease
  - Anaplastic large cell (10% of pediatric NHL): t(2;5) chromosome translocation is diagnostic; commonly has "B" symptoms and skin involvement
- Common primary sites of presentation includes the lymph nodes, mediastinum, ileocecal area, tonsils, adenoids, and Peyer's patches
- Nonrandom chromosomal translocations are found in both T-cell and B-cell lymphomas
- May be associated with Down syndrome
- Boys affected 2–3× more than girls; no true peak incidence, but incidence has increased in recent years; underlying immunodeficiency yields a 10- to 100-fold increased risk

PATIENT PRESENTATION

- The majority of cases are asymptomatic
- Signs and symptoms depend on location of the primary tumor
- Painless, rapidly progressive lymphadenopathy is a common presentation
- Tends to be peripheral (axillary, epitrochlear, abdominal) with noncontiguous spread (in contrast with Hodgkin disease)
- Mediastinal tumors (usually T-cell in origin) may cause symptoms of localized compression (eg, airway compromise, pleural effusion, superior vena cava syndrome)
- Abdominal tumors (usually B-cell in origin) may cause obstruction or intussusception and may mimic appendicitis

DIFFERENTIAL DX

- Leukemia (most difficult to distinguish from NHL)
- Hodgkin disease
- Lymphadenitis
- Tuberculosis
- Infectious mononucleosis
- HIV
- Atypical mycobacterium
- Toxoplasmosis
- Cat scratch disease
- Other causes of bowel obstruction (eg, intussusception, appendicitis)

DIAGNOSTIC EVALUATION

- Biopsy is necessary for diagnosis
  - The biopsy tissue is analyzed for morphology, immunohistochemical stains, flow cytometry, cytogenetics, and molecular markers
- Patient evaluation and staging include complete physical exam, complete blood count, liver function tests, renal function tests, LDH, chest X-ray, CT scans of the head and chest/abdomen/pelvis, bone scan, gallium scan $\pm$ PET scan, and lumbar puncture
- Bone marrow aspirate to rule out leukemia
- Ann Arbor staging system is not as useful in pediatrics as for adults but is still used (it tends to upstage too many pediatric patients)
- Can also use the Murphy staging system:
  - I: Single nodal site or extranodal tumor, except abdominal or mediastinal primary
  - II: Single extranodal tumor with regional nodes; 2 or more extranodal tumors without nodal involvement or 2 or more nodal regions on the same side of the diaphragm; OR grossly resected primary gastrointestinal tumor $\pm$ nodes
  - III: 2 or more extranodal tumors or nodal areas on opposite sides of diaphragm; primary thoracic disease; gastrointestinal disease not grossly resected; OR paraspinal and epidural disease
  - IV: Central nervous system and/or marrow involvement

TREATMENT & MANAGEMENT

- All patients, regardless of stage or histology, undergo aggressive combination chemotherapy
  - Lymphoblastic lymphoma is treated like acute lymphoblastic leukemia
  - All other non-Hodgkin lymphomas given shorter pulsed cycles of multiagent chemotherapy
  - Chemotherapeutic agents include prednisone, vincristine, cyclophosphamide, doxorubicin, 6-mercaptopurine, and methotrexate
- CNS prophylaxis with intrathecal chemotherapy is necessary in all pediatric patients
- Surgery can be used to remove localized lymphoma in the bowel

PROGNOSIS & COMPLICATIONS

- Non-Hodgkin lymphoma is highly aggressive in children; most tumors grow rapidly
- The most common oncologic emergencies associated with NHL are superior mediastinal syndrome (cough, dyspnea, dysphagia, wheezing, hoarseness, facial edema, chest pain) and tumor lysis syndrome (refer to the leukemia entries for more information)
- The most reliable prognostic factor is the stage of disease at diagnosis
- CNS involvement is associated with an unfavorable prognosis
- For localized disease, the 5-year disease-free survival rate is 85%
- For advanced disease, the long-term survival rate is 65–75%
- Relapsed or refractory disease is very difficult to treat and may require bone marrow transplantation

Neuroblastoma

INTRODUCTION

- Neuroblastoma arises from the primitive neural crest cells in the sympathetic nervous system
- Outcome is highly variable, ranging from spontaneous regression (stage 4S disease) to extremely aggressive disease
- The staging system is highly complex and involves risk group stratification
- Patients are stratified into low-, intermediate-, and high-risk groups based on the International Neuroblastoma Staging System (INSS), which includes age, n-myc amplification status, Shimada classification (histology), and DNA ploidy

ETIOLOGY, EPIDEMIOLOGY, & RISK FACTORS

- The most common extracranial solid tumor and the second most common solid tumor in children; accounts for 8–10% of all childhood cancers
- The most common site of origin is the adrenal gland
- 40% of cases arise from the adrenal glands, 25% from paraspinal ganglions, 15% from the thorax, 5% from the pelvis, and 4% from the neck
- 75% of patients are under 4 years of age at the time of diagnosis; 95% of cases present by age 10
- More common in whites and males
- At diagnosis, more than 40% of patients are classified as high risk, nearly 20% are classified as intermediate risk, and nearly 40% are classified as low risk

PATIENT PRESENTATION

- Most patients have signs and symptoms of metastases at the time of presentation
  - Pallor, weakness
  - Bone pain (limp, refusal to walk)
  - Systemic symptoms (fever, weight loss, irritability, hypertension, diarrhea)
  - Periorbital ecchymoses (raccoon eyes)
  - Skin lesions ("blueberry muffin")
- Asymptomatic mass in abdomen, thorax, pelvis, or neck
- Hepatomegaly
- Paraspinal neuroblastoma can cause spinal cord compression (back pain, weakness, paralysis, and bladder or bowel dysfunction)
- Paraneoplastic manifestations may occur: Horner syndrome, opsoclonus-myoclonus, or intractable diarrhea (caused by tumor secretion of vasoactive intestinal peptide)

DIFFERENTIAL DX

- Hydronephrosis
- Polycystic kidney disease
- Splenomegaly
- Wilms tumor
- Lymphoma
- Leukemia
- Rhabdomyosarcoma
- Ovarian tumors
- TORCH infection (especially in infants)

DIAGNOSTIC EVALUATION

- Diagnosis is made by pathologic examination of tumor tissue or presence of tumor cells in the bone marrow AND detection of elevated urinary catecholamines
- 90% of neuroblastomas excrete catecholamines; their metabolites (vanillylmandelic acid and homovanillic acid) may be detected in the urine
- Workup includes tumor tissue examination for morphology and histology (Shimada classification), DNA index, and n-myc oncogene expression
- Workup should also include complete blood count, skeletal survey, chest X-ray, bone scan, CT scan or MRI of the abdomen and/or primary tumor site, CT scan of the chest if chest X-ray is positive, bilateral bone marrow aspirate and biopsy, and ferritin level
- MIBG scan: A nuclear scan that tests for the presence of neuroectodermal tissue
- Bone scan
- INSS staging:
  - 1: Localized tumor, gross total removal, negative lymph nodes
  - 2A: Localized tumor, incomplete resection, negative nodes
  - 2B: Localized tumor $\pm$ gross total resection, positive ipsilateral nodes
  - 3: Unresectable unilateral tumor crossing midline OR localized unilateral tumor with contralateral positive nodes
  - 4: Disseminated disease
  - 4S: Localized primary tumor with dissemination to skin, liver, and/or marrow

TREATMENT & MANAGEMENT

- Therapy is risk-based
- Neuroblastoma is highly sensitive to doxorubicin, cyclophosphamide, cisplatin, and etoposide
- Low-risk: May be amenable to resection alone (symptomatic patients receive 2–4 cycles of combination chemotherapy)
- Intermediate-risk: Surgery plus chemotherapy (radiation may also be included)
- High-risk: Above modalities plus autologous stem-cell transplantation and postconsolidation therapy with biologic response modifiers (usually retinoic acid)
- Infants with stage 4S are treated with supportive care, unless they are severely compromised, because involution of tumor often occurs spontaneously, and there is better than 80% survival rate with supportive care alone
  - In situ neuroblastoma is found in 1 of 250 autopsies among infants under 3 months, which is 400 times greater incidence than that of clinical disease, demonstrating the high rate of spontaneous resolution in this age group

PROGNOSIS & COMPLICATIONS

- Neuroblastoma is most aggressive in older children
- Disease tends to be more benign in infants and may occasionally spontaneously regress
- Elevated ferritin, DNA index equal to 1, and n-myc oncogene amplification in tumor cells are associated with a poor prognosis
- 5-year survival rates for low- and intermediate-risk disease are excellent
- High-risk disease is still a challenge and carries a poor prognosis
- The late effects of treatment are significant and include hearing impairment or hearing loss; musculoskeletal, neurologic, endocrine, dental, pulmonary, cardiac, and renal complications; and second malignant neoplasms
- Health-related quality of life is lower in survivors with high-risk neuroblastoma

Osteosarcoma and Ewing Sarcoma

INTRODUCTION

- Bone tumors are the sixth most common pediatric cancer
- Osteosarcoma is a malignant tumor of bone-producing osteoblasts
- Ewing sarcoma is a primitive neuroectodermal tumor; the cell of origin remains unknown, but the tumor is thought to arise from primitive mesenchyme
- Ewing sarcoma actually represents a family of tumors including Ewing sarcoma of bone, extraosseous Ewing sarcoma, and peripheral neuroectodermal tumor (PNET) of bone or soft tissue

ETIOLOGY, EPIDEMIOLOGY, & RISK FACTORS

- Together, osteosarcoma and Ewing sarcoma make up 4% of childhood cancers
  - Osteosarcoma is responsible for 400 new cases annually of cancers in children and adolescents under the age of 20
  - Ewing sarcoma is responsible for 200 annual cancer cases in children and adolescents under 20
- Osteosarcoma peaks between the ages of 15 and 19 during the adolescent growth spurt
- Ewing sarcoma peaks between the ages of 11 and 15
- Both tumors are more common in males and in whites
- Osteosarcoma is known to be associated with various conditions, including ionizing radiation (occurs about 10 years after exposure, often as a second malignant neoplasm), hereditary retinoblastoma, Li-Fraumeni (germline p53 mutation) familial cancer syndrome, and Rothmund-Thomson syndrome (an autosomal recessive disorder associated with small stature, skeletal abnormalities, and rash)

PATIENT PRESENTATION

- Both tumors present with pain and swelling around the involved bone, frequently beginning after a sports-related injury
- Gait disturbances and pathologic fractures may also occur
- Systemic symptoms (eg, weight loss, fever) are more common in Ewing sarcoma
- Osteosarcoma most commonly occurs at the knee (60–80% of cases involve the distal femur or proximal tibia or fibula); 10–15% of cases involve the proximal humerus
  - The tumor is usually located in the epiphysis or metaphysis
  - Ewing sarcoma most commonly occurs in the midproximal femur, pelvic bone, tibia, and humerus
  - The tumor is usually located in the diaphysis

DIFFERENTIAL DX

- Osteomyelitis
- Eosinophilic granuloma
- Benign bone tumors
- Metastases secondary to neuroblastoma (in younger children)
- Rhabdomyosarcoma
- Lymphoma
- Chondrosarcoma (the third type of malignant bone tumor)

DIAGNOSTIC EVALUATION

- Plain X-rays are often diagnostic
  - Osteosarcoma: Destruction of bone with formation of new periosteal bone
  - Ewing sarcoma: Lytic bone lesion with periosteal reaction and/or a soft tissue mass
- MRI reveals the extent of tumor involvement for surgical planning
- Biopsy must be performed to send tumor samples for pathology, cytogenetics, and molecular studies
  - 85–95% of Ewing sarcoma cases have Ewing sarcoma fusion protein marker EWS (22q12)
- Chest CT scan, bone scan, and bone marrow aspirate are performed to look for lung, bone, and marrow metastases (marrow only in Ewing sarcoma)
- Labs include complete blood count, electrolytes, renal function, uric acid, liver function tests, LDH, and alkaline phosphatase
- PET scans are under investigation for the staging workup of both tumors
- 20–25% of patients with malignant bone tumors have metastases at presentation
  - Osteosarcoma: Skip lesions occur several centimeters from the primary tumor; lung and bone metastases are also common
  - Ewing sarcoma: Lung, bone, and bone marrow metastases

TREATMENT & MANAGEMENT

- Surgical intervention alone is not enough for these tumors because micrometastases are usually present at diagnosis
- Preoperative chemotherapy is the initial intervention, followed by local control
  - Osteosarcoma: Chemotherapy plus resection of the tumor-containing bone
  - Chemotherapy for osteosarcoma usually consists of doxorubicin, cisplatin, high-dose methotrexate, ifosfamide, ± etoposide
  - Ewing sarcoma: Chemotherapy, resection, and/or radiation
  - Active chemotherapy for Ewing sarcoma includes vincristine, cyclophosphamide, doxorubicin, dactinomycin, ifosfamide, etoposide, topotecan, and irinotecan
- Limb salvage surgery with cadaver allografts or prostheses is typically performed, although amputation is necessary if clean margins cannot be obtained
- Surgical intervention is then followed by postoperative chemotherapy
- In addition to chemotherapy and surgical resection, Ewing sarcoma is responsive to radiation
  - Second malignant neoplasms are more common in Ewing sarcoma, especially when radiation is used

PROGNOSIS & COMPLICATIONS

- Resectability is a good prognostic factor
- Prognosis of axial skeletal tumors is unfavorable in osteosarcoma due to difficulty of complete resection; prognosis of Ewing sarcoma in the distal bones and ribs is more favorable; tumors in the pelvis have unfavorable prognosis
- Markers of poor prognosis are metastases at diagnosis and large tumor size
- 5-year disease-free survival is 20–70%, depending on stage at diagnosis
- Tumor response to presurgical chemotherapy is a predictor of outcome in osteosarcoma (ideally, want to see >90% necrosis in resected specimen after induction chemotherapy)
- Late effects of chemotherapy are common, including cardiotoxicity from anthracyclines (doxorubicin), ototoxicity from cisplatin, and functional issues related to limb salvage

Wilms Tumor

INTRODUCTION

- Wilms tumor is the most common primary malignant renal tumor of childhood
- It generally has a favorable outcome
- Treatment has improved substantially in recent years due to investigation and treatment of the tumor through consortium protocols within the National Wilms Tumor Study Group and collaborating international colleagues
- The primary site of metastasis is to the lungs

ETIOLOGY, EPIDEMIOLOGY, & RISK FACTORS

- The fourth most common pediatric cancer and the most common primary renal tumor in children; accounts for 6% of all childhood cancers
- Although usually sporadic, there are some hereditary forms (autosomal dominant)
- A small deletion in chromosome 11p13 has been detected in tumor cells
- Wilms tumor and neuroblastoma are the most common causes of abdominal masses in children under age 5
- Usually occurs in children younger than 5, with peak incidence between 3 and 4 years of age
- Bilateral tumors occur in 5–10% of cases and are associated with congenital anomalies
  - Median age of presentation of bilateral tumors is 31 months (vs. 44 months for unilateral tumors)
- May be associated with WAGR syndrome (Wilms tumor, aniridia, genitourinary anomalies, mental retardation; associated with deletion of short arm of chromosome 11), Denys-Drash syndrome (constitutional mutation of the WT1 gene), or Beckwith-Wiedemann syndrome (hemihypertrophy, macroglossia, visceromegaly, hypoglycemia, omphalocele; associated with chromosome 11p15)
- Rarely, Wilms tumors can be familial (1.5%) with autosomal dominant inheritance

PATIENT PRESENTATION

- Often asymptomatic
- 85% of cases present with an abdominal or flank mass noticed by the caretaker
- Abdominal pain (20–30%)
- Hypertension (25%)
- Gross or microscopic hematuria due to tumor extension into the renal pelvis occurs (20–30%)
- Anemia may occur due to bleeding into the tumor
- Fever
- Left varicocele may be present due to obstruction of left spermatic vein
- Constitutional symptoms (eg, weight loss, anorexia, fever, malaise, constipation)
- Nearly 6% of patients have associated genitourinary anomalies (eg, hypoplastic kidney, ectopic kidney, horseshoe kidney, duplication of collecting system, cryptorchidism)
- Aniridia (absence or defect of the iris)

DIFFERENTIAL DX

- Congenital hydronephrosis
- Multicystic or dysplastic kidneys
- WAGR syndrome
- Beckwith-Wiedemann
- Perlman syndrome
- Sotos syndrome
- Neuroblastoma
- Rhabdomyosarcoma
- Leiomyosarcoma
- Renal cell sarcoma
- Fibrosarcoma
- Adrenal hemorrhage
- Renal vein thrombosis
- Non-Hodgkin lymphoma
- Clear cell sarcoma
- Rhabdoid tumor

DIAGNOSTIC EVALUATION

- History (especially for family and congenital defects) and complete physical exam (especially to evaluate for blood pressure, hemihypertrophy, and aniridia)
- Abdominal ultrasound with Doppler and CT scan of the abdomen to evaluate for an abdominal mass
- Labs include complete blood count, urinalysis, electrolytes, BUN, creatinine, uric acid, liver function tests, albumin, alkaline phosphatase, and coagulation studies (PT/PTT)
- Evaluate for metastases with chest X-ray and CT scan of the chest
  - For clear cell sarcoma of kidney, assess with skeletal survey and bone scan
  - For clear cell sarcoma or rhabdoid tumor, assess with MRI of the brain
- Surgery remains the primary method of diagnosis, staging, and treatment
- Tumor pathology is important for prognosis:
  - Favorable histology (>90% of tumors) is associated with tubules, blastema, and stroma present
  - Unfavorable histology is anaplastic; can be focal or diffuse
- Tumor cytogenetics is also prognostic; loss of heterozygosity (LOH) of chromosomes 1p and 16q negatively impact the prognosis

TREATMENT & MANAGEMENT

- Staging:
  - Stage I: Tumor confined to the kidney
  - Stage II: Tumor confined to the renal fossa
  - Stage III: Gross residual disease, including nodes
  - Stage IV: Disseminated tumor
  - Stage V: Bilateral tumors
- Surgical resection (radical nephrectomy) is indicated in all patients, including abdominal exploration and surgical staging
  - Complete resection is possible for stage I or II tumors
  - Stages I and II: Resection plus chemotherapy (vincristine and dactinomycin)
  - Stages III and IV: As above, plus radiation therapy and doxorubicin
  - Stage V: Treatment is further complicated by the need to preserve some functioning renal tissue

PROGNOSIS & COMPLICATIONS

- Prognosis depends on histology and stage; the most important indicators of poor prognosis are advanced stage and histologic anaplasia at diagnosis
  - Favorable histology: 80–97% 5-year survival
  - Unfavorable histology: Anaplastic (80% survival for focal; 25–80% for diffuse, depending on stage)
- Newer protocols to stratify patients are based on stage, histology, age, tumor weight, 1p and 16q status, and response rate of lung metastasis
  - This approach may lessen therapy for patients with low-risk disease who have been overtreated on earlier protocols, thus minimizing late effects, while improving outcomes for higher risk patients

Aplastic Anemia

- Aplastic anemia results in severe pancytopenia due to bone marrow hypoplasia
- The mechanism for decreased hematopoiesis remains poorly understood but probably represents a combination of direct cytotoxicity to stem cells along with an activated T-cell immune response
- Two of three cytopenias must be present for diagnosis:
  - Absolute neutrophil count (ANC) <500
  - Platelet count <20,000
  - Reticulocyte count <40×10^9/L, or <1%
  - Bone marrow cellularity <25%

ETIOLOGY, EPIDEMIOLOGY, & RISK FACTORS

- Characterized by peripheral pancytopenia secondary to hypoplasia of the bone marrow
- The mechanism for this decreased hematopoiesis remains poorly understood
- Approximately 1000 new cases are diagnosed in the U.S. each year
- While the disease does occur in children, it is most common in young adults (age 15–30) and elderly patients (age >60)
- Most common form in children is Fanconi anemia
- May be congenital or acquired
  - Most cases are idiopathic (no cause is found in half of acquired cases)
  - Etiologies of acquired cases include radiation-induced, drugs and chemicals (either direct cytotoxic effect or idiosyncratic reaction; eg, chloramphenicol, sulfonamides, antiepileptic medications, anti-inflammatory medications), viral (eg, Epstein-Barr virus, cytomegalovirus, hepatitis, HIV), immune disorders (eg, eosinophilic fasciitis, hypogammaglobulinemia), thymoma, paroxysmal nocturnal hemoglobinuria, myelodysplasia
  - Inherited etiologies include Fanconi anemia, Diamond-Blackfan anemia, Shwachman-Diamond syndrome, dyskeratosis congenita, congenital amegakaryocytic thrombocytopenia, and familial aplastic anemia

PATIENT PRESENTATION

- Petechiae
- Ecchymoses
- Pallor
- Fatigue
- Dyspnea
- Infection (usually bacterial)
- Fanconi anemia is associated with a characteristic phenotype, including short stature, hyper- or hypopigmentation, café-au-lait spots, abnormal kidneys (either absent, duplicated, or horseshoe), and skeletal anomalies (especially of the thumb and radius)

DIFFERENTIAL DX

- Leukemia
- Myelodysplastic syndrome
- Immunodeficiency
- Paroxysmal nocturnal hemoglobinuria
- Infections (EBV, HIV, viral hepatitis, parvovirus)
- Autoimmune disease
- Severe congenital neutropenia (Kostmann)
- Glycogen storage disease 1b

DIAGNOSTIC EVALUATION

- Peripheral blood smear reveals anemia, leukopenia, and thrombocytopenia and may reveal macrocytosis
- Bone marrow aspirate reveals reduced cellularity with fat spaces occupying more than 75% of the marrow
  - Send aspirate for flow cytometry and cytogenetics
- The workup of aplastic anemia should also include:
  - Antinuclear antibody (ANA) for systemic lupus erythematosus
  - Liver function tests
  - Appropriate viral serologies (eg, cytomegalovirus, Epstein-Barr virus, parvovirus, hepatitis)
  - Vitamin B_{12} and folate levels
  - CD 55 and 59 or Ham test for paroxysmal nocturnal hemoglobinuria
  - Diepoxybutane or mitomycin C incubation tests for chromosomal breakage analysis of peripheral blood lymphocytes (both are DNA cross-linking agents)
  - Chromosome analysis (eg, telomere length examination for dyskeratosis congenita)
  - Fetal hemoglobin level, usually via high-performance liquid chromatography (HPLC), without associated hemoglobinopathy

TREATMENT & MANAGEMENT

- Mild to moderate cases can be observed without specific treatment if not transfusion-dependent
- Transfusions should be minimized to prevent development of alloimmunization
- Aplastic anemia patients with moderate disease and requirements for transfusion should receive immunotherapy with cyclosporine A, antithymocyte globulin, steroids, and hematopoietic growth factors (granulocyte colony-stimulating factor or granulocyte/monocyte colony-stimulating factor)
- For severe aplastic anemia, stem-cell transplantation from an HLA-matched sibling is the first line of therapy; however, 75% of children with severe aplastic anemia do not have an HLA-matched sibling
- Antithymocyte globulin side effects can be severe and include serum sickness

PROGNOSIS & COMPLICATIONS

- Unless spontaneous recovery or successful intervention occurs, this disorder results in inexorable bone marrow failure and death (usually within 3 months) due to bleeding or infection
- The 2-year survival rate is 50–80% with immunotherapy, but 40% of patients will relapse
- The risk of clonal disease (AML, PNH, or MDS) is increased in survivors (18–30% at 10 years); thus, transplant is the treatment of choice when a matched sibling donor is available
- The 2-year survival rate increases to more than 80% with a successful HLA-matched sibling stem-cell transplantation
- Risk factors for graft rejection after stem-cell transplantation include many previous blood transfusions and an idiopathic type of aplastic anemia

Sickle Cell Anemia

INTRODUCTION

- Disorders of hemoglobin result in either quantitative and qualitative deficits
- Sickle cell disease is an inherited, qualitative disorder resulting in defective hemoglobin; the defective hemoglobin occurs due to a substitution of valine for glutamic acid at the sixth amino acid of the beta-globin chain
- Presents in several different forms depending on abnormalities of the paired globin gene:
  - HgbS trait: One beta[6] gene paired with normal beta gene
  - Hemoglobin SS disease (homozygous): Two abnormal beta[6] genes
  - Hemoglobin SC disease: One sickle gene paired with hemoglobin C gene
  - Sickle beta-thalassemia: One sickle gene paired with thalassemic beta gene

ETIOLOGY, EPIDEMIOLOGY, & RISK FACTORS

- The defective hemoglobin in sickle cell disease has diminished solubility in the deoxygenated form, resulting in sickle-shaped red blood cells that have difficulty traversing the microvasculature
- This results in occlusions and infarcts of the spleen, brain, kidney, lung, and other organs
- The spleen removes these abnormal cells, resulting in hemolytic anemia
- Homozygotes have full-blown sickle cell disease
- Heterozygotes are carriers for the sickle cell trait
- Autosomal recessive transmission
- Very common in blacks: Nearly 10% are heterozygous for the sickle cell trait; about 0.3% are homozygous
- The sickle cell defect may be combined with other hemoglobinopathies, such as thalassemia (as above)

PATIENT PRESENTATION

- Signs of hemolysis:
  - Anemia (pallor, fatigue, decreased exercise tolerance, murmur)
  - Jaundice
  - Cholelithiasis
  - Aplastic crises
- Signs of microvascular occlusion:
  - Dactylitis (swelling of fingers)
  - Priapism
  - Pulmonary, cerebral, and splenic emboli, resulting in pulmonary hypertension, stroke, and autosplenectomy
  - Retinal vessel obstruction and blindness
  - Painful vaso-occlusive crises (skeletal pain and fever)
  - Acute chest syndrome (fever, chest pain, dyspnea, pulmonary infiltrate)

DIFFERENTIAL DX

- Beta-thalassemia
- Iron deficiency anemia
- Leukemia
- Glucose-6-phosphatase dehydrogenase deficiency
- Pyruvate kinase deficiency
- Paroxysmal nocturnal hemoglobinuria
- Hereditary spherocytosis
- Hereditary elliptocytosis

DIAGNOSTIC EVALUATION

- Most cases are now identified by newborn screening
- Hemoglobin electrophoresis is the definitive test
  - HbS (sickled hemoglobin) will be greater than HbA (normal adult hemoglobin)
  - Patients with sickle cell disease have nearly 100% sickled cells (or HbS); carriers have 50% sickled cells
- Complete blood count with peripheral smear reveals microcytic, hypochromic anemia and sickled-appearing cells
- Hemolytic anemia with elevated bilirubin
- Elevated reticulocyte count; a depressed reticulocyte count in a known patient may herald an aplastic crisis, usually due to parvovirus or other viral insult
- Routine surveillance should include baseline pulse oximetry and renal and hepatic function testing
- Chest X-ray is indicated if the patient is dyspneic (to rule out acute chest syndrome) or pulse oximetry is below baseline
- Pain score should be assessed to direct therapy at baseline, at regular visits, and frequently during vaso-occlusive crises
- Blood and urine cultures during crises to rule out infection
- Supplemental oxygen should not be used unless the patient is significantly hypoxic, as oxygen shuts off reticulocytosis and can acutely worsen anemia

TREATMENT & MANAGEMENT

- Preventive and expectant management is crucial
- Bacteremia from encapsulated organisms (due to functional asplenia) is common; daily prophylactic penicillin should be started upon diagnosis to prevent sepsis
- Febrile patients should undergo prompt medical evaluation and receive broad-spectrum IV antibiotics while awaiting culture results
- Aggressive management of pain crises, including hydration and routine (not PRN) administration of analgesics; a combination of opioids and NSAIDs is most effective during severe vaso-occlusive pain crises
- Routine immunizations, especially for *Haemophilus influenzae* and *Pneumococcus*
- Routine screening with transcranial Doppler to identify patients at risk for stroke
- Assiduous dental and ophthalmologic follow-up
- Echocardiography and EKG screening, particularly to evaluate for pulmonary hypertension
- Antisickling agents (eg, hydroxyurea) increase production of fetal hemoglobin (which does not sickle), thereby increasing oxygen delivery
- Blood transfusions as needed for aplastic crises, splenic sequestration, strokes, and acute chest syndrome (ACS) (chronic transfusion programs may be necessary)
- Erythrocytopheresis for high-risk patients to lower the percentage of sickled hemoglobin

PROGNOSIS & COMPLICATIONS

- Acute and chronic injury to the spleen, lungs, and brain are responsible for most of the morbidity and mortality in children with sickle cell disease
- Prophylactic penicillin, timely immunizations, and aggressive management of febrile illness help to prevent morbidity and mortality from infections
- By adolescence, chronic microvascular obstruction leads to an enlarged, hypertrophic heart
- Many adults succumb to congestive heart failure due to progressive myocardial damage
- On average, patients live into their 40s or 50s
- Life-threatening crises: splenic/hepatic sequestration, stroke, aplastic crisis, severe ACS
- Patients with recurrent pain crises often have "target" organs or sites of pain, but this is a diagnosis of exclusion, and each episode must be evaluated individually

Iron Deficiency Anemia

INTRODUCTION

- Iron deficiency anemia is the most common cause of hematologic disease in infants and young children
- Two-thirds of the total body iron content is found in the hemoglobin of red blood cells
- Many enzymes also contain iron (eg, cytochromes, catalase, peroxidase, cytochrome C reductase and oxidase, nicotinamide adenine dinucleotide oxidase, xanthine oxidase), which is crucial for oxidative metabolism
- Anemia can be classified according to pathophysiologic mechanism (decreased red blood cell production, increased red blood cell destruction, blood loss) or by the size of circulating red blood cells (microcytic, normocytic, or macrocytic)

ETIOLOGY, EPIDEMIOLOGY, & RISK FACTORS

- The pathophysiologic classification groups anemia disorders based on decreased red blood cell production, increased red blood cell destruction (hemolysis), or blood loss
  - Decreased production may occur due to marrow infiltration or injury, nutritional (eg, iron deficiency) or erythropoietin deficiency (eg, renal disease), or ineffective erythropoiesis
- The most common cause in children is poor iron intake; premature infants at increased risk due to low iron endowment at birth
- Iron deficiency occurs in children with large amounts of cow's milk consumption, poor intake of iron-enriched foods, cow's milk protein intolerance, chronic blood loss (eg, excessive menses), malabsorption (eg, inflammatory bowel disease), and intense exercise
  - Cow's milk causes iron deficiency in several ways: (1) slow, continuous GI bleeding due to intolerance to milk protein; (2) "competition" with iron-rich foods (milk is low in iron and its iron is poorly absorbed, and children drink milk excessively to the exclusion of other foods rich in iron); (3) cow's milk binds iron and prevents absorption from other sources
- Most common between the ages of 9 and 24 months
- Only 7–10% of dietary iron is absorbed, usually in the duodenum
- Breast milk iron is highly bioavailable (50% absorption vs. 5–10% iron-fortified formula)
- Vegetarians at particular risk: poor oral intake of iron plus high phosphate intake

PATIENT PRESENTATION

- Pallor
- Fatigue, weakness, malaise
- Palpitations
- Pagophagia (compulsive ice craving) or pica of other substances
- Clinical stigmata of poor nutrition (eg, obesity, underweight for age)
- Neurologic or intellectual dysfunction
- Severe iron deficiency may present with irritability, tachycardia, cardiac murmurs, mouth soreness (cheilosis), difficulty swallowing, and spooning/curling of nails (koilonychia)
- Can lead to concomitant lead intoxication (due to pica)

DIFFERENTIAL DX

- Other microcytic, hypochromic anemias (eg, lead poisoning, thalassemia, anemia of chronic disease)
- Hemoglobinopathies (eg, sickle cell anemia)
- Infection
- Connective tissue disease
- Malignancy
- Stress
- Postoperative state

DIAGNOSTIC EVALUATION

- Iron deficiency occurs in 3 stages:
  - Depletion of iron stores, which results in low serum ferritin
  - Iron-deficient erythropoiesis, which results in low ferritin and transferrin saturation
  - Frank iron deficiency anemia, which results in low hemoglobin and low MCV
- Iron studies usually reveal low serum iron, low transferrin saturation, low ferritin, and elevated total iron-binding capacity (TIBC)
- Complete blood count usually reveals low hemoglobin, low MCV, low mean corpuscular hemoglobin (MCH), and elevated red cell distribution width (RDW)
- Low reticulocyte count indicates that marrow is unable to mount a hematopoietic response without sufficient iron
- Stool for occult blood to assess for a gastrointestinal source of iron loss
  - Supplemental oral iron intake should not cause a false-positive result
- Celiac disease can cause iron deficiency anemia that is unresponsive to supplemental iron
- Differentiate between other hypochromic, microcytic anemias:
  - Lead poisoning will present with basophilic stippling of RBCs, elevated lead level, and elevated free erythrocyte protoporphyrin level
  - Thalassemia will have a normal RDW
  - Anemia of chronic disease: increased transferrin, decreased TIBC, elevated ferritin levels
- Best test of iron deficiency is complete resolution upon a therapeutic trial of iron supplementation

TREATMENT & MANAGEMENT

- Treat the underlying cause, if necessary (eg, malabsorption syndromes)
- Iron supplementation: Need 3 mg/kg/d for mild cases and 6 mg/kg/d for moderate-to-severe cases; recheck hemoglobin and reticulocyte count in 1 week to assess response
- Monitor for reticulocytosis and elevated iron stores after 1 month
- Increase intake of iron-rich foods (eg, liver, pork, beef, veal, navy beans, lima beans, soybeans, lentils, prune and tomato juices, oatmeal, bran flakes, raisins, cream of wheat, spinach, collards, sweet potatoes, strawberries)
- Continue therapeutic iron supplementation for 2 or more months after resolution of abnormal iron indices
- Blood transfusions are usually not indicated
- Parenteral iron is rarely indicated
- Prevention of iron deficiency is the best treatment: Breastfeed for at least the first 6 months of life, use iron-fortified formula and infant cereal, and limit cow's milk to 18–24 oz/d after 1 year of age

PROGNOSIS & COMPLICATIONS

- Prognosis is generally favorable; however, outcome may be limited by inability to take iron supplements
- Be sure to properly diagnose iron deficiency anemia (IDA) rather than hemoglobinopathies or other causes due to the possibility of creating an iron overload state
- If hematologic parameters do not respond favorably within 3 months of treatment, other causes of anemia should be considered
- Untreated IDA is a reversible, significant cause of learning impairment (even with mild deficiency), decreased work performance, exercise intolerance, and impaired immunity
- Reversal of anemia does not always reverse mental and motor impairment; thus, avoidance of iron deficiency is key

Thalassemia

INTRODUCTION

- Hemoglobin is a tetramer of four globular chains (globins) and four heme groups
- Disorders of hemoglobin are classified as quantitative or qualitative
- The thalassemias are a group of quantitative genetic disorders of hemoglobin resulting in decreased amounts of functional hemoglobin
- Decreased production of either alpha or beta globins results in an imbalance between the two; when one chain is in excess of the other, the abnormal hemoglobin molecule precipitates and causes damage to the red blood cell (RBC) membrane
- Defective RBCs are then consumed by the reticuloendothelial system, resulting in ineffective erythropoiesis and hemolysis

ETIOLOGY, EPIDEMIOLOGY, & RISK FACTORS

- Mature adult hemoglobin (HbA) is a tetramer of two alpha and two beta chains (a_2b_2)
  - Fetal hemoglobin is normally replaced by adult hemoglobin within the first year of life
- Alpha-thalassemia: Deletion of alpha-globin gene(s) results in an excess of alpha-globin chains
  - Deletion of all four alpha genes is incompatible with life
  - Deletion of three alpha genes results in alpha-thalassemia (thalassemia intermedia)
  - Deletion of one or two alpha genes is carrier state only (thalassemia minor)
- Beta-thalassemia: Defective beta-globin gene(s) results in an excess of beta chains
- Thalassemias are the most common genetic disorder worldwide
- They are especially common where malaria is endemic
- Up to 15% of Mediterranean and Southeast Asian populations are affected
- The severity of anemia is based on the number of globin chains affected
  - Thalassemia minor: Mild anemia, asymptomatic trait state
  - Thalassemia intermedia: Moderate anemia, intermittent transfusion
  - Thalassemia major: Severe anemia, transfusion dependence

PATIENT PRESENTATION

- Anemia (pallor, fatigue, decreased exercise tolerance)
- Alpha-thalassemia
  - Deletion of all four alpha genes: In utero death from hydrops fetalis
  - Deletion of three alpha genes (hemoglobin H disease): Severe anemia with signs of hemolysis
  - Deletion of two alpha genes: Mild anemia
  - Deletion of one alpha gene: Asymptomatic carrier state
- Beta-thalassemia major: Severe anemia and bone changes, chipmunk face, frontal bossing, copper-colored skin, hemolysis (jaundice, icterus, hepatosplenomegaly)
- Beta-thalassemia minor: Generally asymptomatic

DIFFERENTIAL DX

- Other microcytic, hypochromic anemias (eg, iron deficiency, lead poisoning, anemia of chronic disease)
- Hemoglobinopathies (eg, sickle cell anemia)
- Leukemia (M6 type)
- Myelodysplastic syndromes

DIAGNOSTIC EVALUATION

- Complete blood count with peripheral smear revels hypochromic, microcytic anemia
  - The degree of anemia depends on the specific mutation present
  - A lower mean corpuscular volume (MCV) usually occurs than is typically seen in iron deficiency anemia or lead toxicity (often less than 70)
  - Signs of hemolysis (eg, fragmented RBCs) are present
- Hemoglobin electrophoresis is diagnostic
  - Normal: 97% HbA (a_2b_2); 3% HbF (a_2g_2) or HbA$_2$ (a_2d_2)
  - Alpha-thalassemia: Decreased HbA, with increasing percentage of HbH (depending on the severity)
  - Beta-thalassemia: Absent or diminished HbA, which is replaced by HbF or HbA$_2$

TREATMENT & MANAGEMENT

- Supportive therapy for anemia
- Genetic counseling (antenatal testing is available)
- Transfusions as needed to maintain hemoglobin over 10
  - Note that frequent blood transfusions may result in hemosiderosis and the need for iron chelation therapy
- Splenectomy may be indicated if there is an increasing need for transfusions or if there are clinical signs of hemolysis
  - Folic acid supplementation and aggressive surveillance for iron overload are necessary in patients who are treated with splenectomy
  - Stem-cell transplantation may be curative for thalassemia major if done before iron-induced organ damage occurs
- Patients may have concomitant iron deficiency
  - Iron studies are necessary to demonstrate true iron deficiency in order to avoid iatrogenic iron overloaded from unnecessary supplementation

PROGNOSIS & COMPLICATIONS

- Patients are often initially treated for iron deficiency anemia to the point of iron overload
  - Iron overload is multisystem disease requiring awareness, early diagnosis, and chelation therapy
- Alpha-thalassemia carriers have a benign course; genetic counseling should be offered
- Alpha-thalassemia disease (HbH disease) often results in severe hemolysis; splenectomy should be offered
- Hydrops fetalis results in death in utero
- Beta-thalassemia major usually results in severe anemia with a fatal course (by age 30) unless stem-cell transplantation is performed
- Beta-thalassemia minor results in mild anemia and is generally asymptomatic

Hemophilia

INTRODUCTION

- Hemophilia is a congenital bleeding disorder resulting from deficient or defective coagulation factors
- Hemophilia A is the most common form; it occurs due to a deficiency of coagulation factor VIII and accounts for 80–85% of hemophilia cases
- Hemophilia B (Christmas disease) is deficiency of coagulation factor IX
- Hemophilia is classified on the basis of severity: Severe (less than 1% of normal coagulation factor level), moderate (1–5% of normal coagulation factor level), or mild (6–40% of normal coagulation factor level)

ETIOLOGY, EPIDEMIOLOGY, & RISK FACTORS

- Hemophilia A is usually severe
- Both forms have X-linked inheritance
  - Female carriers are asymptomatic
  - However, females can have hemophilia through lionization of a normal X chromosome, Turner syndrome (XO), or a father with hemophilia and mother as carrier
- Hemophilia A affects 1 in 10,000 males
- Hemophilia B affects 1 in 100,000 males
- The severity of disease depends on the degree of coagulation factor deficiency
  - Severe disease results in spontaneous bleeding
  - Moderate disease predisposes to bleeding from minor trauma or surgery and occasional joint bleeds
  - Mild disease results in rare joint bleeding but significant bleeding upon major trauma or surgery
- Platelet function is normal; affected patients can still form a platelet plug, but they are unable to stabilize the platelet plug

PATIENT PRESENTATION

- Hemophilia A and B are clinically indistinguishable
- Delayed bleeding after trauma or surgery
- Delayed bleeding into closed spaces may result in compartment syndrome or venous congestion and may be mistaken for a mass or tumor
- Deep soft tissue bleeding and spontaneous hemarthrosis (blood in the synovial joint following trauma) are hallmarks of disease
- CNS bleeding may occur with/without trauma
- Oropharyngeal bleeding, possibly requiring intubation
- Newborns may have cephalohematoma, delayed separation or bleeding upon separation of the umbilical cord, or bleeding during circumcision
- Infants may have tongue or frenulum bleeding (especially as the teeth develop), and soft tissue bleeding of the forehead, forearms (while crawling), or immunization sites

DIFFERENTIAL DX

- Hemophilia A
- Hemophilia B
- Von Willebrand disease (a deficiency of von Willebrand factor, which stabilizes coagulation factor VIII)
  - Particularly type 2N (Normandy)
- Factor XI deficiency
- Factor XII deficiency
- Acquired coagulation disorders, including disseminated intravascular coagulation (DIC), vitamin K deficiency, and liver disease
- Leukocyte adhesion disorder
- Hypofibrinogenemia or dysfibrinogenemia

DIAGNOSTIC EVALUATION

- Evaluate bleeding studies and assays for coagulation factors VIII and IX
  - Prolonged partial thromboplastin time (PTT) occurs, but prothrombin time (PT), platelet count, and bleeding time are usually normal
- Prenatal testing is available
- Joint disease develops in 90% of patients with severe hemophilia
  - Repeated hemarthroses (4 bleeds/joint within 6 months or 20 bleeds/joint in a lifetime) can lead to joint damage and muscular atrophy with associated contractures and bony cysts
  - Joint pain and swelling should be treated as bleeding even if X-ray is normal

TREATMENT & MANAGEMENT

- Preventive measures include prevention of trauma (eg, avoid traumatic sports, give immunizations subcutaneously instead of intramuscularly) and avoidance of aspirin and other antiplatelet drugs
- Treat with coagulation factor replacement: The percent correction depends on the severity of injury
  - Factor VIII: 1 unit/kg raises factor VIII levels by 2% (half-life is 12 hours)
  - Factor IX: 1 unit/kg raises factor IX levels by 1% (half-life is 24 hours)
  - Cryoprecipitate, fresh frozen plasma, and recombinant factor VIIa (Novo7) may be indicated for life-threatening bleeds or bleeding unresponsive to correction of the specific coagulation factor
- Other treatments may include desmopressin (DDAVP), which releases von Willebrand factor from endothelial cells and increases platelet adhesion (useful in mild cases); antifibrinolytics (aminocaproic acid or tranexamic acid), which may be used to stabilize clot formation; and fibrin sealant
- Nonpharmacologic interventions include avoidance of prolonged splinting of joints and RICE therapy (rest, ice, compression, elevation) for minor injuries

PROGNOSIS & COMPLICATIONS

- Complications of therapy are common, including transfusion-related infections and chronic liver disease; however, recombinant coagulation factors virtually eliminate these risks
- Coagulation factor administration may result in IgG4 that inactivates factor VIII
  - Inhibitors are much more common in severe factor VIII deficiency (15–30% of cases) than in mild or moderate disease or factor IX deficiency
  - Inhibitors can be treated using bypassing products (activated prothrombin concentrates or recombinant factor VIIa), porcine factor VIII, or immune tolerance therapy
- Intracranial, retropharyngeal, and retroperitoneal hemorrhages may be life threatening
- Intra-abdominal or intragluteal hemorrhage can go unrecognized and lead to shock

von Willebrand Disease

INTRODUCTION

- von Willebrand disease (vWD) is a group of disorders of the von Willebrand factor (vWF), a protein that allows platelets to adhere to damaged endothelium to form a platelet plug
- The most common inherited bleeding disorder
- Clinical manifestations are highly variable

ETIOLOGY, EPIDEMIOLOGY, & RISK FACTORS

- vWF is a large, multimeric protein stored in platelets and endothelial cells; it mediates the adhesion of platelets to sites of vascular injury via platelet glycoprotein Ib
- von Willebrand disease may result from congenital absence of vWF or abnormalities in its structure or function
- vWF also functions as a carrier protein for coagulation factor VIII, protecting it from rapid clearance from the plasma; the absence of vWF creates a secondary deficiency of coagulation factor VIII
- Type 1 disease is most common: vWF is functionally and structurally normal but reduced in quantity; usually results in mild-to-moderate clinical disease
- Type 2: vWF is qualitatively abnormal; has multiple variant forms (2A, 2B, 2M, 2N); type 2B is associated with thrombocytopenia
- Type 3 is most severe: No detectable vWF exists, resulting in markedly decreased coagulation factor VIII activity; may resemble hemophilia
- Affects 1 in 200–500 children (1–3% of the general population)
- Typically inherited in an autosomal dominant manner
- Males and females are similarly affected; all racial groups are affected

PATIENT PRESENTATION

- Delayed bleeding
- Superficial bleeding due to failure to form a platelet plug
  - Skin: Petechiae, purpura, easy bruising
  - Mucous membranes: Gingival bleeding (especially with tooth brushing), epistaxis, gastrointestinal bleeding
  - Genitourinary bleeding: Menorrhagia
- Postoperative bleeding (typically after a tooth extraction or tonsillectomy)

DIFFERENTIAL DX

- Liver disease
- Leukemia
- Aplastic anemia
- Connective tissue disease
- Vitamin K deficiency
- Qualitative platelet dysfunction
- Idiopathic thrombocytopenic purpura
- Deficiency of coagulation factors VIII, IX, XI, or XII
- Disseminated intravascular coagulation (DIC)

DIAGNOSTIC EVALUATION

- Detailed patient and family history is of primary importance
- Complete blood count may reveal thrombocytopenia; platelets, PT, and activated PTT may be normal
- von Willebrand disease should be suspected in patients with a prolonged PTT (due to the effect of vWF deficiency on coagulation factor VIII) or a prolonged bleeding time (due to secondary platelet dysfunction)
  - Bleeding time is now measured through PFA-100 (platelet function assay), also called PFT (platelet function test)
- von Willebrand factor assays
  - Ristocetin cofactor assay: Tests vWF function by inducing vWF binding to platelets using the antibiotic ristocetin
  - von Willebrand factor antigen level
  - von Willebrand factor levels may be affected by many conditions (eg, inflammation, pregnancy, oral contraceptive use, thyroid status, blood type, stress, age, diabetes, malignancy)
  - Coagulation factor VIII clotting activity, a functional measurement of factor VIII, will show decreased activity in patients with von Willebrand disease
  - Multimeric analysis: Identifies quantitative abnormalities in von Willebrand factor and determines the subtype of disease

TREATMENT & MANAGEMENT

- Desmopressin (DDAVP) is used to induce the release of von Willebrand factor from storage sites; it is the treatment of choice for most bleeding episodes (causes a 2- to 4-fold increase in vWF and coagulation factor VIII levels within 15–30 minutes of administration)
  - DDAVP is the treatment of choice for type 1
  - DDAVP has variable response for type 2
  - DDAVP is contraindicated for type 2B because it worsens thrombocytopenia
  - DDAVP is ineffective for type 3
- Epistaxis is one of the most common symptoms and can usually be controlled with local pressure and one dose of DDAVP
- Menorrhagia may be reduced by use of oral contraceptives
- A patient undergoing a laceration repair or tooth extraction must receive DDAVP prior to the procedure plus an antifibrinolytic agent (eg, aminocaproic acid) for 7–10 days afterwards
- For more severe bleeding episodes or surgeries, plasma-derived von Willebrand factor concentrate may be administered
- All patients should avoid aspirin-containing products

PROGNOSIS & COMPLICATIONS

- 80% of patients have type 1 disease
- Clinical manifestations are much less severe than those of hemophilia; the disease generally only becomes a problem during severe trauma or surgery
- However, type 3 disease may be problematic even during menses or minor trauma; sequelae are similar to hemophilia, with joint bleeding and development of inhibitors after coagulation factor replacement therapy (refer to Hemophilia entry)
- Bleeding episodes resulting in significant morbidity are uncommon

Idiopathic Thrombocytopenic Purpura

INTRODUCTION

- Thrombocytopenia may occur due to decreased platelet production, increased platelet destruction (immune or nonimmune causes), or platelet sequestration (usually) in the spleen
- Idiopathic thrombocytopenic purpura (ITP) is an acquired, quantitative, usually transient, immune-mediated disorder that results in accelerated destruction of platelets
- Platelet destruction results in a primary hemostatic disorder, with immediate bleeding into the skin and mucous membranes
- ITP is the most common acquired bleeding disorder in children

ETIOLOGY, EPIDEMIOLOGY, & RISK FACTORS

- Autoantibodies, usually IgG, attach to platelet membranes, inappropriately signaling them for destruction by macrophages and monocytes in the spleen and liver
- Two-thirds of cases occur several weeks after a preceding infectious illness (especially Epstein-Barr virus)
  - May rarely be the initial presentation of HIV or systemic lupus erythematosus
- Acute ITP is more common in children and adolescents
  - Peak incidence at 4–8 years
  - Males and females have equal incidence
- Chronic ITP is more likely to develop in adolescents and young adults, especially adolescent females

PATIENT PRESENTATION

- The typical presentation is a child who develops petechiae and bruising with no other signs or symptoms
- Superficial bleeding
  - Skin: Easy bruising, petechiae, purpura
  - Mucous membranes: Nose (epistaxis), mouth, and gastrointestinal bleeding
  - Genitourinary: Menorrhagia, hematuria
- Splenomegaly may be present in cases of splenic sequestration
- Intracranial hemorrhage is possible but very uncommon
- Lack of other positive exam and laboratory findings

DIFFERENTIAL DX

- Leukemia (virtually never presents with isolated thrombocytopenia)
- Congenital thrombocytopenia (eg, thrombocytopenia absent radius syndrome)
- Aplastic anemia
- Collagen vascular disease
- Acute infection
- HIV
- Drugs
- Wiskott-Aldrich syndrome
- Hemolytic-uremic syndrome
- Evans syndrome (thrombocytopenia and hemolytic anemia)
- Gray platelet syndrome
- Bernard-Soulier syndrome
- Hermansky-Pudlak

DIAGNOSTIC EVALUATION

- A diagnosis of exclusion
- A history of viral illness or upper respiratory tract infection may be present
- Complete blood count with peripheral smear reveals very low platelets (typically <20,000)
  - Normal hemoglobin and white blood cell counts
  - Normal differential cell counts
  - Normal morphology, except for large platelets
- Bone marrow biopsy may be used to rule out other diagnoses (eg, leukemia) but is not necessary if clinical and laboratory features are classic for ITP
  - Bone marrow is normal in ITP
  - Indicated in patients with lymphadenopathy, hepatomegaly, protracted systemic symptoms (eg, fever, bone pain), or other abnormal findings on CBC
  - Should also be done prior to steroid therapy, prior to splenectomy, or in cases that do not respond to therapy
- Consider antinuclear antigen (ANA) or HIV testing in selected, high-risk patients

TREATMENT & MANAGEMENT

- Specific treatment is not necessary if platelet count is >30,000; observation and activity restriction are sufficient
- For children with platelet counts <30,000, treatment is based on the presence and severity of bleeding symptoms
  - Corticosteroids reduce the production of antiplatelet antibodies
  - Intravenous immunoglobulin (IVIG) blocks receptors on platelets, thereby decreasing destruction
  - Anti-RhD immunoglobulin (WinRho) decreases platelet destruction; used only for Rh-positive patients
  - Platelet transfusions are only indicated if the platelet count is severely depressed with ongoing bleeding or significant risk of intracranial bleeding
- Chronic ITP may require splenectomy in severe cases
  - Other treatment modalities include pulse steroids, IVIG, IV anti-D, rituximab, or combination chemotherapy
- Emergency management of life-threatening hemorrhage may include platelet transfusions, IV steroids (30 mg/kg, maximum dose of 1 gram for up to three doses), IVIG (1 g/kg, repeat daily as clinically indicated for up to 5 doses), or emergency splenectomy

PROGNOSIS & COMPLICATIONS

- Nearly 90% of patients recover within a few months with or without treatment
- Less than 5% of patients with acute ITP develop recurrent, acute thrombocytopenia
- About 10% of patients develop chronic ITP (defined as thrombocytopenia lasting longer than 6 months)
- Risk of collagen vascular disease or other underlying pathology is higher in cases of chronic ITP
- The major form of morbidity is intracranial hemorrhage; risk is negligible if platelet count is above 10,000

G6PD Deficiency

INTRODUCTION

- Glucose-6-phosphatase dehydrogenase (G6PD) is an enzyme that helps protect red blood cells (RBCs) from oxidative damage
- G6PD deficiency is the most common red cell enzyme disorder worldwide, causing intrinsic hemolytic anemia
- G6PD deficiency results in decreased production of NADPH, which results in inability to maintain necessary levels of reduced glutathione
- Anemia resulting from G6PD deficiency may be acute after exposure to an oxidant or may be mild and chronic

ETIOLOGY, EPIDEMIOLOGY, & RISK FACTORS

- Exposure to oxidative stress results in episodes of hemolytic anemia
- Hemolytic anemia is defined by increased destruction of red blood cells and compensatory increase in red blood cell production
- Oxidative agents include infections, fava beans, mothballs (due to naphthalene), and various medications (eg, primaquine, sulfonamides, nitrofurans, vitamin K analogs, methylene blue, dimercaprol, probenecid)
- X-linked recessive transmission affecting only males
- 8–10% of black males are affected
- Prevalence is highest in Africa, the Mediterranean, and Southeast Asia
- The geographic distribution of G6PD deficiency matches the distribution of malaria
  - Heterozygous females and hemizygous males are afforded protection from malaria

PATIENT PRESENTATION

- Patients have signs and symptoms of acute hemolytic anemia
- Pallor
- Jaundice, icterus
- Hepatosplenomegaly
- Abdominal pain
- Vomiting
- Diarrhea
- Low-grade fever
- Hemoglobinuria (cola-colored urine)
- Fatigue
- Gallstones

DIFFERENTIAL DX

- Autoimmune hemolytic anemia
- Hemolytic-uremic syndrome
- Malaria-induced hemolysis
- Other red blood cell enzyme disorders (eg, pyruvate kinase deficiency)
- Hereditary spherocytosis
- Hereditary elliptocytosis
- Hereditary stomatocytosis
- Paroxysmal nocturnal hemoglobinuria
- Paroxysmal cold hemoglobinuria
- Wilson disease

DIAGNOSTIC EVALUATION

- A screening test for G6PD deficiency is included in the extended newborn screen
  - Less than 30% of normal G6PD activity is considered a positive test
- The diagnosis is confirmed with a quantitative assay
- Assay must be done only after resolution of acute hemolytic crisis because reticulocytes contain five times more G6PD than mature RBCs (so the assay can be falsely normal)
- G6PD electrophoresis should be performed to determine the specific disease variant
- Lab testing during hemolytic episodes includes:
  - Complete blood count (leukocytosis, anemia)
  - Reticulocyte count (elevated)
  - Peripheral smear: reticulocytosis, anisocytosis, bite cells (RBCs with areas bitten off by splenic macrophages), Heinz bodies (denatured hemoglobin)
  - Elevated unconjugated bilirubin
  - Decreased haptoglobin
  - Urinalysis positive for bilirubin and urobilinogen

TREATMENT & MANAGEMENT

- Patient education is paramount
- Remove or avoid inciting agents
- In severe cases, hydration with IV fluids is necessary to prevent clogging of the renal tubules
- Folic acid supplementation may be given during periods of hemolytic anemia (some authorities recommend lifetime administration)
- Packed red blood cell transfusions are only necessary in cases of severe anemia resulting in cardiovascular compromise

PROGNOSIS & COMPLICATIONS

- Most patients are asymptomatic until exposed to an inciting agent; acute hemolysis then develops within 24–48 hours of exposure
- In most cases, hemolytic episodes are mild and self-limiting
- Recovery from the acute episode occurs within 48–72 hours
- Anemia usually resolves within 3–6 weeks
- Patients should wear medical ID bracelets and carry a card that lists medications to avoid

Dermatology

Atopic Dermatitis (Eczema)

INTRODUCTION

- Atopic dermatitis, or eczema, is a chronic, itchy disease that is very common in young children
- Affected children also usually have a tendency to have asthma and/or hay fever; the presence of all three is often referred to as the "atopic triad"
- The rash consists of rough erythematous patches, with the distribution generally determined by the patient's age
- Although the rash can be very pruritic and develop secondary complications, most children outgrow the disease by 2 years of age

ETIOLOGY, EPIDEMIOLOGY, & RISK FACTORS

- Chronic superficial inflammation of the skin occurs; it is a pruritic dermatitis induced by specific triggers
- Patients often have a personal or family history of asthma or hay fever
- It is postulated that an ineffective epidermal barrier allows irritants through cracks in the skin, resulting in dermatitis
- Secondary bacterial infections are common
- 5% of children under age 5 are affected
- 70% of affected children have a first-degree relative with atopic dermatitis, asthma, or environmental allergies
- Early onset occurs in many cases (60% of affected children develop disease by age 1)
- Rare after age 30
- Increased incidence in urban areas

PATIENT PRESENTATION

- The infantile form begins on the cheeks and scalp and progresses to the trunk and the extensor surfaces of the extremities; parents may report a history of poor sleep or increased irritability, which is a reflection of the infant's pruritus
- The childhood form is common on flexor surfaces (antecubital, popliteal, wrists, neck, feet, and hands)
- The adolescent form predominantly occurs on the hands but may be on the face or flexor surfaces
- Acute eczema results in erythematous, weeping, edematous patches
- Chronic eczema results in scaly, lichenified, erythematous patches that can develop hyper- or hypopigmentation
- Pruritus is always present and can be severe during exacerbations

DIFFERENTIAL DX

- Contact dermatitis
- Drug reaction
- Seborrheic dermatitis
- Photodermatitis
- Nummular eczema
- Psoriasis
- Wiskott-Aldrich syndrome
- Tinea corporis
- Diaper dermatitis
- Candidiasis
- Varicella
- Folliculitis
- Urticaria
- X-linked agammaglobulinemia

DIAGNOSTIC EVALUATION

- History and physical examination
  - There is usually a personal or family history of atopic diseases
  - History of exposure to triggers (eg, soap, pets, clothing, foods)
  - The rash is of typical morphology and distribution; it is always pruritic
- There are many minor criteria, including dry eyes, elevated IgE, and evidence of hypersensitivity to triggers
- Allergy testing is indicated in patients with food allergies or with severe reactions to airborne allergens (eg, asthma, rhinitis)
- Histologic examination may be indicated if uncertainty exists

TREATMENT & MANAGEMENT

- Avoid irritants, harsh soaps, and rough or tight clothing
- Lubricate with petroleum jelly, ointments, or creams to keep the skin moisturized
- Hydrocortisone cream or stronger topical steroids may be used when needed
- Topical immune modulators (eg, Protopic, Elidel)
- Rarely, systemic steroids or other immunosuppressants are needed for severe exacerbations
- Oral antihistamines as needed for pruritus
- Topical or oral antibiotics for superinfected lesions

PROGNOSIS & COMPLICATIONS

- Follows a chronic relapsing and remitting course
- Most children improve within 5 years of onset
- If not controlled, patients can develop secondary bacterial or viral infections
- Often resolves or lessens in severity and frequency by adolescence or early adulthood

Acne Vulgaris

INTRODUCTION

- Acne vulgaris is the most common skin condition worldwide; it affects nearly 100% of individuals at some point during their lifetime
- 85% of adolescents develop some form of acne
- Children may be affected by a combination of comedones, nodules, and pustules
- Typically begins at puberty and resolves by adulthood, although some adults will have persistent or even new lesions

ETIOLOGY, EPIDEMIOLOGY, & RISK FACTORS

- Lesions result from follicular obstruction with a keratinous plug in the lower infundibulum
- Multifactorial etiology involving hormones, inflammation, and skin lipid composition
  - Androgen hormones play a role; boys are more prone to severe acne than girls due to their higher androgen levels
  - Altered skin lipid composition (excess sebum)
  - Inflammation, most likely initiated by *Propionibacterium acnes* bacteria
- Oil-based cosmetics may result in acne cosmetica
- Friction caused by tight-fitting helmets, clothes, or sports equipment is common (acne mechanica)
- Certain medications (eg, steroids, lithium, some antiepileptics, iodides) can promote acne
- Average age of onset is 10–12 years
- Family history may help predict severity

PATIENT PRESENTATION

- Initial lesions are frequently comedonal
  - Open comedones (blackheads): papules with a dilated central opening filled with blackened keratin
  - Closed comedones (whiteheads): yellowish papules
- Nodules
- Lesions can become inflamed, resulting in an erythematous or pustular appearance
- In severe cases, scarring may occur
- Areas affected are those with increased concentrations of sebaceous glands (face, neck, chest, and back)
- May be pruritic

DIFFERENTIAL DX

- Rosacea
- Miliaria
- Keratosis pilaris
- Molluscum contagiosum
- Nevus comedonicus
- Polycystic ovarian syndrome
- Adenoma sebaceum (tuberous sclerosis)
- Folliculitis

DIAGNOSTIC EVALUATION

- A clinical diagnosis
- Patients often know the diagnosis and are seeking forms of treatment that are not available over the counter
- In females with irregular menses and hirsutism, DHEA-S and testosterone levels can be evaluated to rule out an endocrine disorder

TREATMENT & MANAGEMENT

- Topical retinoic acid (Retin-A) and adapalene (Differin gel)
- Topical antibiotics (eg, clindamycin, erythromycin, benzoyl peroxide)
- Oral contraceptives may be used in females to suppress endogenous androgen hormones
- Systemic antibiotics may be used for severe, inflammatory acne (eg, tetracycline, erythromycin, doxycycline)
- Oral retinoids, including isotretinoin (Accutane), are used only for severe or recalcitrant cystic acne
  - These are potent teratogens; they should be used with extreme caution in adolescent females (oral contraceptives may be a better choice)
- Dietary changes may be effective; however, no evidence exists to prove benefit
- Surgical comedone extraction in extreme cases

PROGNOSIS & COMPLICATIONS

- Often self-limited
- May take up to 2 months to see results from medical treatment
- Lesions can heal with hyper- or hypopigmentation
- Severe cystic acne may lead to permanent scarring of the face and trunk; therefore, it is important to treat it aggressively
- Isotretinoin is a teratogen; must screen for pregnancy and warn patients of the risks of conception while using this drug
- Dry skin is a complication of many acne drugs

Psoriasis

INTRODUCTION

- Psoriasis is a chronic inflammatory skin disorder that is characterized by erythematous plaques often covered by silvery, white scales
- It can affect people of all ages and can have variable symptoms

ETIOLOGY, EPIDEMIOLOGY, & RISK FACTORS

- Psoriasis is an inflammatory disease that results in abnormal epidermal differentiation and hyperproliferation
- Psoriatic epithelial cells have a faster cell cycle than normal cells, and they take 5–6 days to migrate to the skin surface from the basal layer in order to be exfoliated (vs. nearly 30 days in normal cells)
- 1–2% of the entire population is affected
- 50–75% of patients have a positive family history
- One-third of cases present while the patient is under 18 years old
- The guttate variant can be triggered by an acute infection, such as a streptococcal pharyngitis
- 10% of patients with psoriasis develop psoriatic arthritis
  - A seronegative arthritis associated with HLA-B27
  - Often begins in the DIP joints
  - Swelling of fingers occurs ("sausage digits")
  - Flares and remissions coincide with skin lesions
- Some drugs can induce psoriasis flares (eg, beta-blockers, lithium, systemic steroids)

PATIENT PRESENTATION

- Plaque psoriasis is most common: Presents with well-demarcated erythematous plaques with overlying silvery scales; often involves the scalp and extensor surfaces
- Guttate psoriasis: 2- to 5-mm lesions appear abruptly after an infection
- Pustular psoriasis: "Lakes" of pus occur; patients can be very ill; pruritus may or may not be present
- Auspitz sign: Pinpoint bleeding where a scale is removed due to dilated dermal capillaries
- Koebner phenomenon: Lesions appear at sites of injury
- Can affect the nails with random pitting, yellow discoloration, or distal lifting (onycholysis)
- Involved joints are tender and swollen

DIFFERENTIAL DX

- Reiter syndrome
- Lichen planus
- Eczema
- Pityriasis rosea
- Pityriasis rubra pilaris
- Tinea corporis
- Dermatomyositis
- Subacute cutaneous lupus erythematosus
- Drug reactions
- Seborrheic dermatitis

DIAGNOSTIC EVALUATION

- History and physical examination of lesions
- Skin biopsy will demonstrate epidermal proliferation with collections of neutrophils
- Throat or perianal culture in patients with guttate psoriasis
- Microscopic exam with KOH prep and fungal cultures to distinguish from fungal infection
- X-rays for suspected psoriatic arthritis

TREATMENT & MANAGEMENT

- Skin emollients and ointments should be used prophylactically
- Corticosteroid ointments or steroids are used during flare-ups
- Keratolytic shampoos for scalp lesions
- Calcipotriol cream (a vitamin D analog)
- Anthralin or tar preparations
- Phototherapy: UVA, UVB, or PUVA (UVA plus oral 8-methoxypsoralen) is particularly effective for cases of guttate psoriasis
- Systemic immunosuppressants (eg, methotrexate, cyclosporine) may be necessary for severe disease
- Oral acitretin (a retinoid) must be used with caution in women of childbearing potential
- Biologic agents (eg, etanercept, efalizumab, alefacept, infliximab, adalimumab)

PROGNOSIS & COMPLICATIONS

- Relapsing and remitting chronic course, without a definitive cure
- Exacerbations last an average of 8 weeks
- Flare-ups tend to occur during winter months and during times of stress
- Emotional consequences are often much greater than physical consequences
- Early onset and family history are associated with a worse prognosis

Birthmarks

INTRODUCTION

- Birthmarks are skin lesions that appear at or shortly after birth; they are extremely common, occurring in 99% of newborns
- They usually consist of abnormally placed melanocytes or blood vessels but can also come from other tissue
- Most birthmarks are benign; some will regress with age

ETIOLOGY, EPIDEMIOLOGY, & RISK FACTORS

- Most birthmarks are hamartomas (collections of normal types of cells)
- Lesions are characterized as vascular (eg, vascular malformations, hemangiomas) or melanocytic (eg, nevus, Mongolian spot, café-au-lait macule)
- Some birthmarks are inherited, but most are sporadic
- Infantile hemangiomas are the most common type of vascular birthmark and the most common benign tumor of childhood; one-third are present at birth
- Mongolian spots are the most common hyperpigmented lesions; they are more common in Asian and black infants

PATIENT PRESENTATION

Vascular Birthmarks
- Infantile hemangioma: Red papules or nodules with rapid growth during first year
- Capillary malformations: Pink-red macule present at birth
  - "Stork bite" on nape of neck
  - "Angel's kiss" found over eyelids
- Port-wine stains: Deep red or purple vascular lesions; often unilateral

Melanocytic Birthmarks
- Café-au-lait spots: Tan, round macules
- Mongolian spots: Irregular blue patches located on the trunk
- Nevus depigmentosus: Irregular, unilateral, hypopigmented patch

DIFFERENTIAL DX

- Port-wine stains from hemangiomas
- Nevus depigmentosus must be distinguished from vitiligo, nevus anemicus, and ash-leaf spots

DIAGNOSTIC EVALUATION

- Diagnosis is made by visual inspection
- No specific laboratory tests are necessary
- In rare cases, biopsy or imaging may be necessary to distinguish a benign hemangioma from a malignant vascular growth
- Children with six or more café-au-lait macules larger than 5 mm should be evaluated for neurofibromatosis type 1
- Children with a port-wine stain in the ophthalmic division of the trigeminal nerve should be evaluated for Sturge-Weber syndrome, which can also affect the eye and nervous system
- Children with large segmental facial hemangiomas should be evaluated for PHACES syndrome, which can affect the central nervous system, heart, and arteries

TREATMENT & MANAGEMENT

- Most hemangiomas (90%) will undergo partial or complete involution without intervention
  - Rapidly growing lesions may require treatment to prevent scarring or impingement on vital structures, such as the airway; these cases may be treated with intralesional or oral corticosteroids
  - Avoid intralesional steroid injections near the eye due to the risk of ophthalmic artery occlusion
  - Interferon has been used to treat life-threatening or large hemangiomas, such as those that cause airway compromise
- Port-wine stains may be treated with pulsed dye laser at wavelengths that target hemoglobin
- Pigmented lesions are not usually treated, except for giant congenital nevi, which are excised because of the risk for malignant transformation

PROGNOSIS & COMPLICATIONS

- Capillary malformations resolve spontaneously in most cases
- Hemangiomas often regress spontaneously but can leave hypopigmentation, telangiectasias, excess skin, or fibrofatty residual tissue
- Ulcers are the most frequent complication of hemangiomas, especially in the diaper area
- Port-wine stains do not resolve with time
- Nevus depigmentosus lesions grow commensurately with the patient

Impetigo

INTRODUCTION

- Impetigo is a contagious bacterial infection that most commonly affects infants and children
- A common cause of pediatric office visits; accounts for 10% of office visits for skin complaints
- Although it usually originates in injured skin, it can also occur as a primary condition
- The infection is seldom serious, but complications can occur
- Treatment can sometimes be difficult given the development of antibiotic resistance

ETIOLOGY, EPIDEMIOLOGY, & RISK FACTORS

- The infection is caused by group A β-hemolytic streptococci or *Staphylococcus aureus*
- Bullous impetigo is always caused by coagulase-positive *S. aureus*
- Abrasions, lacerations, bites, burns, dermatitis, or excoriated lesions serve as a portal of entry of the bacteria into the skin
- The disease is highly contagious
- The nonbullous form accounts for 70% of cases

PATIENT PRESENTATION

Nonbullous Impetigo
- Tiny vesicles rupture and classically become honey-colored, crusted lesions
- Most common on the face or extremities
- Not painful, sometimes pruritic

Bullous Impetigo
- Large, flaccid bullae that rupture, leaving an erythematous moist base with a collarette of the blistered skin
- Most common on the perineum, buttocks, trunk, extremities, or face
- Lesions usually develop on intact skin
- Local lymphadenopathy is common in both forms
- Not usually associated with fever

DIFFERENTIAL DX

- Nonbullous impetigo: tinea corporis, scabies
- Bullous impetigo: epidermolysis bullosa, pemphigus, burns
- Vesicular impetigo: herpes simplex, varicella, herpes zoster
- Nonaccidental trauma

DIAGNOSTIC EVALUATION

- The diagnosis is usually clinical; history and physical exam reveal predisposing factors and signs of bacterial infection
- A honey-colored crust on an eroded base is virtually diagnostic
- Diagnosis can be confirmed by Gram stain and bacterial culture with antibiotic sensitivities

TREATMENT & MANAGEMENT

- Localized, small lesions may be treated with topical antibiotic ointments (eg, bacitracin, mupirocin)
- Multiple lesions or moderate to severe disease requires systemic treatment with a first- or second-generation cephalosporin or amoxicillin-clavulanate
  - Clindamycin or erythromycin can be used in penicillin allergy

PROGNOSIS & COMPLICATIONS

- Most infections resolve with a 7- to 10-day antibiotic course
- Usually resolve without scar formation
- Culture is recommended if poor response to therapy
- Cellulitis may complicate nonbullous impetigo
- Other complications include osteomyelitis, septic arthritis, sepsis, pneumonia, endocarditis, lymphadenitis, and lymphangitis
- Acute poststreptococcal glomerulonephritis or staphylococcal scalded skin syndrome may occur
- Rheumatic fever *does not* result from impetigo

Candidiasis

INTRODUCTION

- Candidiasis is a fungal infection caused by any of the *Candida* yeast species
- When present in the mouth, it is referred to as thrush
- The clinical presentations vary with the site of involvement, but the infection is usually found in exposed and moist body sites
- Systemic disease can occur in severely immunocompromised patients

ETIOLOGY, EPIDEMIOLOGY, & RISK FACTORS

- Most commonly caused by overgrowth of *Candida albicans*, which is part of the normal oral and intestinal flora
- Thrush may be precipitated by illness, stress, medication use, and immune disorders
- Diaper dermatitis may be caused by *Candida* in the anogenital region; possible contributors include friction from the diaper material, extended exposure to urine or feces, and antibiotic use
- Candidiasis is most often seen in infants but may affect people of all ages
- Candidiasis occurs with increased frequency in immunocompromised patients

PATIENT PRESENTATION

- Candidiasis can be extremely painful

Diaper Dermatitis
- Initially presents as an erythematous, erosive patch
- Red papules appear as satellite lesions in the skin folds, sometimes pus-filled with raised borders
- Collarette-like scaling occurs at the margins of the rash

Thrush
- Extensive "cottage cheese–like" plaques that reveal a reddened, friable, tender area when removed
- Found on the dorsum of the tongue, buccal mucosa, palate, and pharynx

DIFFERENTIAL DX

Diaper Dermatitis
- Contact dermatitis
- Psoriasis
- Irritant dermatitis
- Seborrheic dermatitis
- Impetigo
- Allergic dermatitis
- Perianal streptococcal disease
- "Mixed dermatitis" (candidal, bacterial, irritant)

Thrush
- Oral hairy leukoplakia
- Milk accumulation
- Lichen planus
- Bite irritation

DIAGNOSTIC EVALUATION

- Usually a clinical diagnosis
- The diagnosis may be confirmed by microscopic examination with KOH prep revealing pseudohyphae and budding yeast
- Fungal culture is of limited use due to the ubiquitous nature of *Candida*

TREATMENT & MANAGEMENT

Diaper Dermatitis
- Keep the affected skin dry and clean
- Antifungal creams (eg, nystatin, clotrimazole, ketoconazole, miconazole) should be applied to the rash at least four times a day

Thrush
- Treat with oral nystatin or clotrimazole prior to feeds
- If the infant is breastfed, it is important to also treat the mother's nipples with applications of a topical antifungal
- For bottle-fed infants, bottle nipples and pacifiers should be frequently changed until the infection is cleared
- Gentian violet or fluconazole (Diflucan) may be used in persistent cases

PROGNOSIS & COMPLICATIONS

- With proper treatment, candidiasis should resolve within 2 weeks
- Complications are rare but may include malnutrition (secondary to pain), spread of *Candida* to other areas, and secondary infection
- Candidiasis in infants is not uncommon and is not usually associated with other diseases

Tinea

INTRODUCTION

- Tinea, or "ringworm," is a contagious fungal infection caused by any dermatophyte fungus
- It is classified according to the body site involved
- Infections are usually responsive to treatment
- Presents in people of all ages and races

ETIOLOGY, EPIDEMIOLOGY, & RISK FACTORS

- There are three dermatophyte genera: *Microsporum*, *Trichophyton*, and *Epidermophyton*
- All dermatophytes live on keratinized structures (eg, hair, nails, stratum corneum)
- Transmitted from contact with soil, animals, or humans
- Especially common in immunocompromised states, diabetes, antibiotic use, and steroid use
- Warm, moist environments are most conducive to infection
- Tinea capitis is the most common dermatophyte infection in children, especially in African-American patients

PATIENT PRESENTATION

- Tinea corporis (ringworm) affects the torso and extremities; may be asymptomatic or pruritic; may present as a papular, pustular, vesicular, scaly, or eczematous rash
- Tinea capitis (ringworm of scalp): Asymptomatic patches of hair loss and "black dots" (broken hairs); may cause an inflammatory reaction (kerion); can have swollen lymph nodes
- Tinea pedis (athlete's foot): Pruritic, scaly, pink rash along sides of feet, on soles, and between toes; may also affect the hand (tinea manuum)
- Tinea cruris (jock itch): Pruritic, annular erythematous lesion on the inner thigh and groin (does not affect the scrotum)
- Tinea unguium (onychomycosis): Yellow discoloration, thickening, and scaling of the nail plate, not involving every nail

DIFFERENTIAL DX

- Tinea corporis: Eczema, psoriasis, pityriasis rosea, seborrheic dermatitis, erythema chronicum migrans, tinea versicolor (tinea versicolor is not a true tinea infection)
- Tinea capitis: Traction alopecia, dry scalp, psoriasis, seborrheic dermatitis, and alopecia areata
- Tinea pedis: Dyshidrotic eczema
- Tinea cruris: Candidal infection, intertrigo

DIAGNOSTIC EVALUATION

- Clinical appearance and history
- Microscopic examination with KOH prep reveals branching hyphae
- Fungal culture if necessary; however, diagnosis is specific to the location of infection rather than the specific organism
- Infected broken-off hairs in tinea capitis may fluoresce green under a Wood's lamp (called ectothrix as the fungus invades the outside of the hair shaft); however, most cases do not fluoresce (called endothrix as the fungus invades inside the hair shaft)

TREATMENT & MANAGEMENT

- Tinea corporis: Topical clotrimazole cream
- Tinea capitis: Oral griseofulvin and selenium sulfide shampoo for at least 6–8 weeks
- Tinea pedis: Topical clotrimazole
- Tinea cruris: Topical clotrimazole
- Tinea unguium: Oral Lamisil or Diflucan
- Oral treatment is indicated if hair or nails are involved; must be given for 6 weeks for tinea capitis and 3 months for tinea unguium

PROGNOSIS & COMPLICATIONS

- The virulence of the dermatophyte strain, the patient's previous response to a tinea infection, and the condition of the skin prior to infection all play a role in predicting the severity of disease
- More severe disease occurs in immunocompromised or immunosuppressed patients and diabetics
- Skin infections tend to clear within 4 weeks with topical treatments, without scarring
- Hair infections may take 6 weeks or longer to clear
- Nail infections often take more than 3 months to clear

Viral Exanthems

INTRODUCTION

- Erythema infectiosum (or "fifth disease") is a common childhood viral infection caused by parvovirus B19; it presents with a characteristic, three-stage course and usually resolves without any complications
- Roseola infantum is the most common cause of viral exanthems in children; it usually presents with high fevers and occasionally febrile seizures, followed by a rash; most patients recover completely, unless immunocompromised

ETIOLOGY, EPIDEMIOLOGY, & RISK FACTORS

Erythema Infectiosum

- Due to parvovirus B19 infection, which induces immune complex formation and deposition in joints and skin
- The virus is transmitted primarily by aerosolized respiratory secretions; vertical transmission may also occur
- Occurs in all ages, but most common in school-age children
- More prevalent in late winter and early spring
- Cases may be subclinical

Roseola Infantum

- A common, self-limited, often benign viral exanthem due to human herpesvirus 6 (HHV-6) infection
- A common cause of acute febrile illness
- Occurs in otherwise well-appearing children ages 6 months to 3 years
- The most common cause of viral exanthem
- It is contagious via respiratory fluids or saliva
- Febrile seizures occur in 5–10% of cases

PATIENT PRESENTATION

Erythema Infectiosum

- Prodrome with low fever, malaise, headache, and coryza beginning 7 days after exposure
- Presents in 3 stages:
  - "Slapped cheek" appearance (bright erythema, edema) that resolves in 2–4 days
  - Morbilliform rash on extremities
  - Reticular erythema lasting 3 wk and worsened by sun exposure, heat, exercise, stress
- No longer contagious by the time rash appears

Roseola Infantum

- High, spiking fever lasting an average of 4 days
- An erythematous, nonpruritic, rose-colored, maculopapular rash appears several days later; it begins on the trunk and spreads peripherally
- May have associated vomiting and/or diarrhea
- Pharyngeal injection without exudates
- Cervical lymphadenopathy

DIFFERENTIAL DX

- Measles
- Rubella
- Drug reaction
- Streptococcal pharyngitis, scarlet fever
- Lyme disease
- Rheumatoid arthritis
- Systemic lupus erythematosus
- Meningitis
- Urinary tract infection
- Kawasaki disease
- Bacterial sepsis

DIAGNOSTIC EVALUATION

Erythema Infectiosum
- A clinical diagnosis made by history of a viral prodrome followed by characteristic rash
- If the diagnosis is questionable, antiparvovirus IgM or IgG titers can be measured
- Eosinophilia may be present

Roseola Infantum
- History of fever without other symptoms preceding the onset of a rash and without possible bacterial source of illness
- May have early leukopenia and neutropenia

TREATMENT & MANAGEMENT

- Supportive care, including antipyretics for fever
- In cases of erythema infectiosum, antihistamines may be used for pruritis

PROGNOSIS & COMPLICATIONS

- Erythema infectiosum follows a benign, self-limited course; the disease is mild in otherwise healthy children
  - Rarely, aplastic crisis results from replication of the virus in erythroid progenitor cells; this is most dangerous in patients who have underlying chronic anemia or immunosuppression
  - In utero infection is associated with hydrops fetalis, which carries a 5% mortality rate (most dangerous in the first trimester of pregnancy)
- Roseola infantum is usually benign and self-limited in immunocompetent individuals
  - The fever typically resolves once the rash appears
  - The rash disappears in 2–5 days
  - The most common complication is febrile seizures

Erythema Multiforme

INTRODUCTION

- Erythema multiforme (EM) is a self-limited skin disease that typically occurs as a reaction to an infection (most commonly HSV-1) or medication
- Most common in young adults but can affect anyone
- In addition to a characteristic rash, there may be mucosal involvement
- Severe cases can be life-threatening

ETIOLOGY, EPIDEMIOLOGY, & RISK FACTORS

- A hypersensitivity reaction manifested by a polymorphous skin eruption
- EM minor: A self-limited illness usually lasting 2 weeks that heals without complications
- EM major: Stevens-Johnson syndrome and toxic epidermal necrolysis
- Common causes include medications (eg, antibiotics, anticonvulsants, barbiturates, allopurinol), infections (eg, herpes simplex, *Mycoplasma*, histoplasmosis), and immunologic disorders (eg, inflammatory bowel disease, SLE, graft-versus-host disease)
- A specific cause found in only half of cases
- 20% of cases occur in childhood; most cases occur in people aged 20–40
- 25–30% of cases are recurrent

PATIENT PRESENTATION

- There is a wide spectrum of severity
- EM minor: Develops as a symmetric eruption of red, round macules, edematous papules, and target lesions of varying sizes; most common on the dorsa of the hands and forearms
- Stevens-Johnson syndrome: Symmetric erythematous macules that spread from the head and neck to the lower body and progress to bullae with large areas of skin necrosis and denudation; severe erosions of at least two mucosal surfaces (eg, eyes, nose, mouth) covering less than 10% of body surface area
- Toxic epidermal necrolysis: Begins with a generalized, sunburn-like erythroderma followed by widespread necrosis and skin sloughing; more than 30% of the body surface area is affected
- Stevens-Johnson syndrome and toxic epidermal necrolysis may overlap (10–30% of body surface)

DIFFERENTIAL DX

EM Minor
- Urticaria
- Fixed drug eruption
- Erythema chronica migrans
- Erythema annulare centrifugum
- Subacute cutaneous lupus erythematosus

EM Major
- Staphylococcal scalded skin syndrome
- Pemphigus, pemphigoid
- Linear IgA dermatosis

DIAGNOSTIC EVALUATION

- Clinical examination reveals a targetoid rash with history of exposure to an etiologic agent
- Skin biopsy is diagnostic
- Erythrocyte sedimentation rate (ESR), white blood cell count, and platelet count may be elevated
- Nikolsky sign (gentle pressure on a bulla leads to epidermal shearing and lateral extension of the bulla) occurs in cases of toxic epidermal necrolysis

TREATMENT & MANAGEMENT

- Recurrent EM minor is treated with a 6-month course of acyclovir if herpes simplex virus is involved
- EM major is treated as a burn because of the loss of epidermal barrier
  - Correct fluid and electrolyte imbalances
  - Monitor urine output; consider urology evaluation
  - Protection from secondary infection is important; periodic cultures of the skin, eyes, and mucosal sites should be performed
  - Ophthalmologic evaluation to prevent conjunctival and corneal complications
  - Early skin grafting or biologic dressings for large, denuded areas is recommended
  - Intravenous immunoglobulin (IVIG) in severe cases
- Systemic steroids are contraindicated due to risk of secondary infections

PROGNOSIS & COMPLICATIONS

- EM minor tends to recur in crops for 2–4 weeks, while individual lesions heal in 7–10 days
  - Postinflammatory pigmentary changes are common
  - 25–30% of adults have recurrent episodes
  - Often spontaneous resolution
- EM major may result in as high as 30% mortality rate
  - Follows a protracted course lasting 4–6 weeks
  - May develop high fevers, myalgias, arthralgias, sore throat, and headache
  - Complications include sepsis, stress ulcers, and pyoderma
  - Mucosal adhesions can occur

Conditions of the Newborn

Perinatal Asphyxia

INTRODUCTION

- Perinatal asphyxia is an insult to various fetal or infant organs, including the brain, due to hypoxia (lack of oxygen) and/or ischemia (lack of perfusion) around the time of birth
- Permanent damage to the brain can result in cerebral palsy, mental retardation, or death
- Features suggesting an intrapartum insult is responsible for neonatal brain injury include:
  - Evidence of fetal distress (cord blood gas pH <7 and base deficit >12)
  - Depression at birth (Apgar score ≤ 3 for >5 minutes)
  - Overt neurologic signs in the first few hours and days of life
  - Evidence of hypoxic-ischemic damage to other major organ systems
- Incidence of perinatal asphyxia is about 1–1.5% of all live births

ETIOLOGY, EPIDEMIOLOGY, & RISK FACTORS

- Perinatal asphyxia accounts for 20% of all perinatal deaths
- Etiologies are based on the timing of the insult:
  - Combination of antepartum and intrapartum insults (20%) include major uterine bleeding and severe hypotension and placental insufficiency
  - Intrapartum insults (35%) include traumatic delivery (eg, breech extraction, shoulder dystocia), prolonged labor with transverse arrest, cord prolapse and compression, and meconium aspiration
  - Antepartum insults (35%) are similar to intrapartum insults
  - Postnatal insults (10%) include severe recurrent apneic spells, severe cardiac failure, and severe pulmonary disease
- Predisposing factors for placental insufficiency include maternal diabetes, preeclampsia, maternal infection, and postmaturity
- Causes for major uterine bleeding include placenta previa and abruptio placentae

PATIENT PRESENTATION

- The neurologic syndrome that accompanies serious perinatal asphyxia is known as hypoxic-ischemic encephalopathy (HIE); the severity of this neurologic syndrome depends on the extent of brain injury and is classified into three stages (Sarnat stages):
- Stage 1: Hyperalert, irritable, normal tone or hypertonia, exaggerated neonatal reflexes, dilated reactive pupils, regular respiration, tachycardia
- Stage 2: Lethargy, hypotonia, seizures, incomplete Moro reflex, constricted reactive pupils, periodic breathing, bradycardia
- Stage 3: Coma, flaccid tone, absent neonatal reflexes, variable or fixed pupils, ataxic respirations, apnea, bradycardia, hypotension

DIFFERENTIAL DX

- Maternal drug abuse
- Maternal anesthetic agents
- Acute intracranial bleeding
- CNS malformation
- Genetic disorder
- Neuromuscular disorder
- Infection
- Inborn errors of metabolism

DIAGNOSTIC EVALUATION

- Cord arterial blood gas will reveal metabolic acidosis with low pH and high base deficit
- Arterial blood gas will demonstrate acidosis, high or low PCO_2, low pO_2, and low pH
- Lactic acid provides a measure of end-organ perfusion
- Serum, urine, and meconium toxicology screening to assess confounding causes
- Evidence for target organ injury can be confirmed by:
  - Liver: Elevated AST/ALT, abnormal coagulation studies (PT/PTT)
  - Kidney: Elevated BUN and creatinine
  - Heart: Elevated creatine kinase-MB
  - Bone marrow: Neutropenia, thrombocytopenia
  - Brain: Elevated serum and/or cerebrospinal fluid CPK-BB (not routinely done)
- Cranial ultrasound may reveal intraventricular hemorrhage and/or periventricular leukomalacia in premature infants
- CT scan of the head reveals cerebral edema 2–4 days after the insult
  - Multifocal hypodense areas suggest infarcted areas
  - Cerebral atrophy, cystic encephalomalacia, and porencephalic cysts may occur later
- MRI of the brain reveals increased signals in the cerebral cortex, basal ganglia, and white matter within 2–4 days
- EEG: Stage 1 is normal; stage 2 has low-voltage slow waves, periodic pattern, and seizure activity; stage 3 is isoelectric
- Amplitude integrated EEG (aEEG) helps to monitor cerebral function and prognosis

TREATMENT & MANAGEMENT

- Supportive management is directed toward maintaining systemic homeostasis
  - Maintain adequate oxygenation and ventilation
  - Maintain acid-base balance, normocalcemia, and normoglycemia
  - Maintain adequate blood pressure (dopamine, dobutamine)
  - Total parenteral nutrition is necessary until adequate gut perfusion is ensured
  - Maintain normal body temperature
  - Antibiotics if infection is suspected
- Acute renal failure and SIADH can be managed by restricting fluid intake
- Seizures can be treated with phenobarbital, phenytoin, or lorazepam
- Minimize abrupt changes in blood pressure and serum pH (avoid fluid boluses and sodium bicarbonate infusions) to prevent intraventricular hemorrhage
- Investigational neuroprotective strategies include:
  - Selective head cooling and whole-body hypothermia
  - Phenobarbital used both antenatally and postnatally, even in the absence of seizures
  - Glutamate receptor antagonists (eg, dextromethorphan, ketamine)
  - Calcium channel blockers (eg, nimodipine, nicardipine)
  - Free-radical scavengers (vitamin E) and vasodilators (eg, prostacyclin)

PROGNOSIS & COMPLICATIONS

- Multisystem organ failure usually resolves if the infant survives
- Overall mortality is 10–20%
- Neurologic outcome: Stage 1, nearly 100% have normal brain function; stage 2, 80% of cases are normal; stage 3, 50% die and 50% have severe impairment
- Early complications include cerebral edema, SIADH, intraventricular hemorrhage, acute tubular necrosis, DIC, persistent pulmonary hypertension, and necrotizing enterocolitis
- Late complications include cerebral palsy, mental retardation, epilepsy, and ADHD
- Poor prognostic indicators are early onset seizures (<12 hr), elevated intracranial pressure, abnormal MRI, absent Moro reflex, and abnormal neurologic exam on discharge

Birth Trauma

- Birth trauma is defined as impairment of an infant's body or structure due to adverse influences that occurred at birth
- Significant birth injury is still a major cause of neonatal deaths and stillbirths in the U.S.
- Birth injury is responsible for 3.7 deaths per 100,000 live births

ETIOLOGY, EPIDEMIOLOGY, & RISK FACTORS

- Head and neck injuries: Caput succedaneum, cephalohematoma, subgaleal hemorrhage, intracranial hemorrhages, ocular injury, congenital muscular torticollis
- Nerve injuries: Brachial plexus injury (Erb palsy, Klumpke palsy), facial nerve palsy, phrenic nerve palsy, recurrent laryngeal nerve palsy, spinal cord injury
- Fractures of the skull, clavicle, humerus, femur
- Intra-abdominal injuries: Liver, spleen, adrenals
- Soft tissue injuries: Abrasions, lacerations, petechiae, ecchymoses, fat necrosis
- Risk factors for birth injury include:
  - Large for gestational age (LGA) babies (birth weight >4000 g)
  - Breech or other abnormal fetal presentation
  - Forceps or vacuum-assisted delivery
  - Shoulder dystocia
  - Excessive traction during delivery
  - Prolonged labor; precipitous delivery
  - Prematurity
  - Fetal monitoring electrodes
  - Fetal anomalies

PATIENT PRESENTATION

- Caput succedaneum is a serosanguinous fluid collection above the periosteum with poorly defined margins and crossing suture lines
- Cephalohematoma is a subperiosteal collection of blood and hence does not cross suture lines
- Subgaleal hemorrhage is between the galeal aponeurosis of scalp and periosteum; it appears as a firm to fluctuant mass on the scalp a few hours after birth and progresses with potential for massive blood loss into the space
- Erb palsy presents with "waiter's tip" hand deformity and abnormal Moro reflex
- Klumpke palsy presents with weakness of intrinsic hand muscles and poor grasp reflex
- Torticollis presents with head tilt and a sternomastoid mass within 2–4 weeks of birth
- Ocular injury may present with corneal clouding, hyphema, or subconjunctival hemorrhage

DIFFERENTIAL DX

- Intracranial hemorrhage: Perinatal asphyxia, structural brain malformations
- Brachial plexus injury: Cerebral injury, Horner syndrome
- Long bone fractures: Osteogenesis imperfecta
- Facial nerve palsy: Mobius syndrome, Goldenhar syndrome, congenital absence of depressor anguli oris muscle
- Phrenic nerve palsy: Eventration of diaphragm
- Adrenal hemorrhage (flank mass): Neuroblastoma, Wilms' tumor

DIAGNOSTIC EVALUATION

- Assess maternal and delivery history to identify risk factors
- Perform a complete neonatal physical exam, including examination of the head, skin, face, clavicles, extremities, and abdomen
- Skull X-ray is indicated in cases of severe cephalohematoma
  - Linear skull fractures may be present in as many as 5% of cases
  - Depressed skull fractures show "ping pong ball" type of fractures due to the resilient neonatal bones
- Cranial ultrasound or head CT scan should be performed if suspect significant head injury
- Long bone films and chest X-ray to identify fractures
- Chest ultrasound or fluoroscopy can confirm paradoxical diaphragmatic movements in cases of phrenic nerve palsy
- Cervical spine X-ray for torticollis to rule out vertebral anomalies
- Abdominal ultrasound for subcapsular liver hematomas and splenic injury
- Serial hematocrit evaluation to assess continuing blood loss in cases of intra-abdominal hemorrhage and subgaleal hemorrhage

TREATMENT & MANAGEMENT

- Treatment is specific to the site and type of injury
  - Caput succedaneum requires no treatment and resolves over a few days
  - Uncomplicated cephalohematomas resolve spontaneously and do not require intervention; occasionally, they calcify and cause a hard bony swelling lasting for months
  - Packed red cell transfusion in cases of massive subgaleal hemorrhage
  - Depressed skull fracture management is controversial; options include neurosurgical elevation, digital pressure, and negative pressure suction with breast pump or vacuum extractor
  - Early and prolonged physiotherapy for congenital muscular torticollis; surgical correction should be considered if there is no improvement after 6 months
  - Clavicle fractures are treated by pinning the sleeve of the affected arm to the shirt to immobilize for 7–10 days
  - Brachial plexus injury is managed initially with immobilization of the arm across the chest for 1 week to avoid discomfort, followed by passive range-of-motion exercises, which should begin after 1 week
  - Plication of the diaphragm may be required in patients with phrenic nerve palsy
  - Tracheostomy may be required for severe or bilateral recurrent laryngeal nerve palsy
  - Volume replacement, packed red cell transfusion, and correction of coagulopathy for intra-abdominal bleeding

PROGNOSIS & COMPLICATIONS

- Cephalohematomas resolve within weeks, with occasional calcifications
- Mortality rate from subgaleal hematomas range from 14–22% with greatest risk in patients who experience greater than 25% drop in hematocrit and associated birth asphyxia
- Clavicle fractures heal completely between 2–4 months
- Approximately 90% of brachial plexus injuries resolve spontaneously; infants without recovery by 3 months should be considered for surgical exploration
- Residual long-term deficits from brachial plexus injury may include progressive bony deformities, muscle atrophy, joint contractures, and weakness of shoulder girdle
- Facial nerve palsy resolves spontaneously in 90% of patients

Meconium Aspiration Syndrome

INTRODUCTION

- Meconium aspiration syndrome (MAS) is defined as respiratory distress in an infant born through meconium-stained amniotic fluid whose symptoms cannot be otherwise explained
- Meconium is the first gastrointestinal discharge and contains epithelial cells, fetal hair, mucus, and bile
- MAS occurs when passage of meconium occurs prior to delivery (into the amniotic fluid) and is aspirated by the fetus
- Approximately 13% of all live births are complicated by meconium-stained amniotic fluid
- Only 5% of neonates born through meconium-stained amniotic fluid develop MAS

ETIOLOGY, EPIDEMIOLOGY, & RISK FACTORS

- Meconium aspiration syndrome can be classified as:
  - Mild MAS: Disease requiring <40% supplemental oxygen for <48 hours
  - Moderate MAS: Disease requiring >40% oxygen for >48 hours without air leak
  - Severe MAS: Disease requiring assisted ventilation for >48 hours
- Meconium-stained amniotic fluid is rare prior to 37 weeks of gestation
- The incidence of MAS is declining due to reduction in births beyond 41 weeks of gestation
- Meconium staining of amniotic fluid: Associated w/fetal acidosis, abnormalities in fetal HR, and low Apgar scores, suggesting hypoxia as stimulant for passage of meconium in utero
- The mechanisms of lung injury in MAS include:
  - Mechanical obstruction of airways: A "ball-valve" effect, resulting in air trapping
  - Chemical pneumonitis: Direct toxic effect mediated by inflammation
  - Vasoconstriction of pulmonary vessels
  - Inactivation of surfactant, leading to atelectasis and decreased lung compliance
  - Activation of complement and release of cytokines
- Risk factors for MAS include postterm pregnancy, preeclampsia, maternal hypertension, maternal diabetes, chronic maternal respiratory and cardiovascular diseases, heavy smoking, intrauterine growth retardation, and thickened, "pea soup" meconium-stained amniotic fluid

PATIENT PRESENTATION

- Yellow staining indicates old meconium; green staining indicates a more recent exposure
- Meconium staining of the skin, hair, umbilicus, and nails is noticed upon delivery
- Classic signs of postmaturity including:
  - Dry, cracked, peeling, loose, wrinkled skin
  - Malnourished appearance
  - Decreased subcutaneous tissue
  - Long yellow-stained nails
- Signs of respiratory distress occur within a few hours of birth and include tachypnea, nasal flaring, intercostal retractions, increased anterior-posterior chest diameter, cyanosis, grunting, and rales or crackles on auscultation
  - Air leaks may occur due to damaged alveolar epithelium; causes include pulmonary interstitial emphysema, pneumothorax, pneumomediastinum, and pneumopericardium

DIFFERENTIAL DX

- Other causes of respiratory distress
  - Pneumonia
  - Pneumothorax
  - Perinatal asphyxia
  - Neonatal respiratory distress syndrome
  - Persistent pulmonary hypertension of the newborn

DIAGNOSTIC EVALUATION

- Monitoring should include continuous pulse oximetry and preductal and postductal oxygen saturation to detect pulmonary hypertension
- Frequent arterial blood gas monitoring
  - Hypoxemia is common
  - Respiratory alkalosis is seen in patients who are hyperventilating
  - Hypercapnia and respiratory acidosis is seen in moderate to severe cases
  - Metabolic acidosis is seen in severe cases
- Chest X-ray reveals coarse, irregular pulmonary infiltrates; patchy areas of atelectasis and consolidation; hyperinflation of lung fields, flattened diaphragms, and a tubular heart
  - Pneumothorax and pneumomediastinum are common in severe cases
  - Cardiomegaly might be seen, indicating underlying hypoxemic insult
  - The extent of X-ray findings might not correlate with clinical severity
- EKG to rule out ischemic changes
- Echocardiogram may reveal pulmonary hypertension with right-to-left shunting at the ductus arteriosus and/or foramen ovale and is also helpful in assessing cardiac function
- Blood glucose and calcium to check for hypoglycemia and hypocalcemia

TREATMENT & MANAGEMENT

- Intrapartum management includes:
  - Monitor fetal heart rate tracing and, if required, fetal scalp pH
  - Fetal pulse oximetry, if available (investigational)
  - Amnioinfusion may be considered (infusion of sterile isotonic solution into the amniotic cavity through a catheter to dilute the meconium and relieve cord compression)
- There is no advantage of nasal and oropharyngeal suctioning at the perineum prior to delivery of the shoulder; this is no longer recommended by American Academy of Pediatrics
- If the baby is vigorous at birth, endotracheal suctioning is not required; however, if the baby is depressed with heart rate less than 100 bpm or poor respiratory effort, immediate endotracheal intubation and suctioning should be done
- Subsequent management includes:
  - Supportive respiratory therapy to correct hypoxemia and respiratory acidosis, including supplemental oxygen and mechanical ventilation
  - High-frequency ventilation may be successful in patients with severe disease
  - Nitric oxide therapy and extracorporeal membrane oxygenation (ECMO) may be required for severe cases with persistent pulmonary hypertension
  - Management usually includes broad-spectrum antibiotics to treat presumed bacterial pneumonia or sepsis

PROGNOSIS & COMPLICATIONS

- MAS has a mortality rate of up to 40%
- Persistent pulmonary hypertension of the newborn (PPHN) is a common complication
- Use of inhaled nitric oxide therapy and ECMO for PPHN has reduced mortality
- The risk for pneumothorax is estimated to be 15–35%
- Air leaks are more common in patients requiring mechanical ventilation
- Chronic lung disease or bronchopulmonary dysplasia may result from oxygen toxicity and prolonged ventilation
- Long-term prognosis depends more on the associated perinatal asphyxia than the pulmonary disease
- Those with significant asphyxia may demonstrate neurologic sequelae

Transient Tachypnea of the Newborn

INTRODUCTION

- A relatively mild, self-limited respiratory disorder resulting from delayed resorption of fetal lung fluid
- Lung fluid is produced actively in utero by a chloride pump that causes influx of chloride and water from the interstitium into the alveolar space
- Approximately 2–3 days before delivery, lung liquid starts to clear due to transformation of the pulmonary epithelium
- Delayed resorption of this fluid increases airway resistance and decreases lung compliance

ETIOLOGY, EPIDEMIOLOGY, & RISK FACTORS

- Retained fluid in the peribronchial lymphatics and bronchovascular spaces cause compression and collapse of the bronchioles
- Another explanation for the delayed clearance of fluid in Caesarean (C) section deliveries is absence of the "thoracic squeeze" that the baby is usually subjected to during vaginal delivery
- May also occur secondary to mild surfactant deficiency
- Incidence of approximately 11 cases per 1000 live births
- Risk factors include elective C-section delivery, precipitous delivery, male sex, macrosomia, excessive maternal sedation, excessive intravenous fluid administration to mothers during labor, prolonged labor, birth asphyxia, and multiple gestations

PATIENT PRESENTATION

- Term or near-term infants with tachypnea (>60 breaths/min)
- Mild to moderate respiratory distress with nasal flaring and subcostal retractions
- "Barrel chest" appearance with increased anteroposterior diameter
- Expiratory grunting is common
- Good air entry with widespread crackles
- Usually persists for 12–24 hours

DIFFERENTIAL DX

- Pneumonia
- Congenital heart disease
- Respiratory distress syndrome
- Neonatal sepsis
- Central hyperventilation associated with birth asphyxia
- Meconium aspiration syndrome
- Persistent pulmonary hypertension
- Polycythemia
- Total anomalous pulmonary venous return

DIAGNOSTIC EVALUATION

- Arterial blood gas reveals mild respiratory acidosis, hypoxemia, and hypercarbia
- Chest X-ray shows:
  - Prominent perihilar streaking representing engorged perihilar lymphatics involved in alveolar fluid clearance
  - Fluid in the minor interlobar fissure and mild pleural effusions
  - Patchy infiltrates due to fluid-filled alveoli that clear within 48 hours
  - Hyperexpansion of the lung fields with flattening of the diaphragm due to air trapping may be seen
  - Mild to moderately enlarged heart
- Complete blood count with differential to assess for sepsis and rule out polycythemia
- Blood cultures should be performed if sepsis is suspected

TREATMENT & MANAGEMENT

- Management is mainly supportive
- Supplemental oxygen to maintain oxygen saturation greater than 90%
- Continuous positive airway pressure (CPAP) may be helpful for lung expansion
- Intubation and mechanical ventilation may be considered in the most severe cases
- Feeding via an orogastric tube and IV fluids should be considered because there is a high risk of aspiration and subsequent respiratory distress
- A course of antibiotics (ampicillin and gentamicin) may be started for suspected sepsis; discontinue if the blood culture is negative after 48 hours

PROGNOSIS & COMPLICATIONS

- Self-limited; generally lasts 12–24 hours
- Occasionally can last for 2–3 days in persistent cases
- Increased risk of air leaks and pneumothorax
- Prognosis is excellent without any long-term consequences

Apnea

INTRODUCTION

- Apnea is defined as cessation of spontaneous breathing for longer than 20 seconds or for a shorter duration if associated with bradycardia (<100 beats/min) and/or cyanosis
- Apnea is a common problem in premature infants and is called idiopathic apnea of prematurity if it occurs in the absence of identifiable factors
- Apnea can be classified as:
  - Central: Absence of inspiratory effort due to decreased central nervous system stimuli
  - Obstructive: Absent airflow secondary to obstruction despite the presence of respiratory effort
  - Mixed (most common): A combination of poor respiratory drive and airway obstruction

ETIOLOGY, EPIDEMIOLOGY, & RISK FACTORS

- Incidence of apnea varies inversely with gestational age: Approximately 25% of infants born earlier than 34 weeks of gestation and almost all infants born before 28 weeks have apnea
- Apnea of prematurity is due to immaturity of infant's neurologic and respiratory system
- Collapse of the pharyngeal airway due to poor muscle tone, usually during sleep, may be the initial event that precipitates obstructive apnea
- The frequency of apnea increases with REM sleep
- Apnea causes chemoreceptor-induced inhibition of heart rate leading to bradycardia
- Apneic episodes are rare in term infants and require immediate diagnostic evaluation
- Common causes for apnea in term infants include birth asphyxia, intracranial hemorrhage, seizures, depression from sedative medications, and structural brain malformations
- Gastroesophageal reflux has been historically linked to obstructive or mixed apnea, which may be related to aspiration or vagally mediated laryngospasm
  - Recently, this association has been called into question as impedance monitoring and pH probe studies have not consistently demonstrated an association
  - Reflux is more likely if the event occurs while awake, after a feed, or with vomiting

PATIENT PRESENTATION

- Apnea is uncommon on the first day of birth and usually signifies underlying illness
- In premature babies, apnea usually occurs from the second to seventh days of life
- Persistent chest wall motion with absent air entry on auscultation may be noticed in obstructive apnea
- Cyanosis, pallor, hypotension, and bradycardia may be noted if apnea is prolonged
- Apnea starting after the second week of life usually suggests underlying disease in an otherwise normal premature infant
- Signs of increased intracranial pressure, abnormal heart sounds or rhythms, inadequate chest wall movement, abdominal distension, and pallor (anemia) may be present

DIFFERENTIAL DX

- Exclude the following prior to diagnosing apnea of prematurity:
  - CNS: Intraventricular hemorrhage, seizures, drugs, hypoxic injury, Ondine curse
  - Respiratory: Pneumonia, upper airway obstruction, hyaline membrane disease
  - Cardiovascular: Patent ductus arteriosus, congestive cardiac failure, anemia, hypovolemia
  - Infectious: Sepsis, meningitis, respiratory syncytial virus
  - Gastrointestinal: Gastroesophageal reflux, necrotizing enterocolitis
  - Metabolic: Hypoglycemia, hypocalcemia, hypothermia

DIAGNOSTIC EVALUATION

- Complete history and physical examination
- Continuous pulse oximetry and nasal impedance apnea monitoring should be performed during the hospital course
- Laboratory studies include:
  - Complete blood count may suggest infection, anemia, or polycythemia
  - Blood culture
  - Serum electrolytes, calcium, and glucose to rule out a metabolic abnormality
  - Arterial blood gas to rule out acidosis, hypoxia, hypercapnia
  - Urine, meconium, and/or serum toxicology screen
  - Cerebrospinal fluid examination if meningitis is suspected
- Chest X-ray to rule out pneumonia and atelectasis
- EKG and/or echocardiography if congenital heart disease is suspected
- Abdominal X-ray to detect necrotizing enterocolitis
- Cranial ultrasound to detect intraventricular hemorrhage
- EEG if seizures or encephalopathy are suspected
- Pneumocardiogram with esophageal pH probe is occasionally done in refractory cases

TREATMENT & MANAGEMENT

- Most apneic episodes respond to tactile stimulation
- Maintain oxygen saturation
  - Position the neck to avoid extreme flexion or extension
  - Administer supplemental oxygen by nasal cannula or face mask, if necessary
  - Continuous positive airway pressure (CPAP) via nasal cannula if other therapies fail
  - Mechanical ventilation if apnea persists despite nasal CPAP
- Maintain a neutral thermal environment
- Reflux precautions (head up, prone position, small volume feeds, pharmacologic treatments) for infants with gastroesophageal reflux might be helpful
- Methylxanthines (eg, caffeine, theophylline) stimulate the brainstem respiratory center and reduce the incidence and severity of apneic episodes; they also decrease the need for mechanical ventilation
- Doxapram (a respiratory stimulant) is very rarely used for refractory apnea
- If an underlying cause is identified, specific therapy should be instituted:
  - Phenobarbital for seizures
  - Antibiotics for suspected sepsis or pneumonia
  - Glucose supplementation for hypoglycemia
  - Calcium supplementation for hypocalcemia

PROGNOSIS & COMPLICATIONS

- Prognosis varies depending on the etiology of apnea
- Apnea of prematurity does not alter the prognosis of prematurity unless it is severe and refractory to therapy
- Gradual decrease in frequency is noted in the first few weeks as the premature infant grows and matures
- Most premature infants grow out of apnea by 40 weeks after conception
- CNS etiologies carry higher risk to long-term development
- Discharging patients on home apnea monitors is controversial
- Most neonatologists allow a 5- to 10-day apnea-free period after discontinuation of drug therapy before sending a premature infant home without a monitor

Congenital Diaphragmatic Hernia

INTRODUCTION

- Congenital diaphragmatic hernia (CDH) is a defect in the diaphragm that leads to herniation of the abdominal viscera into the thorax
- It usually occurs due to failure of closure of the pleuroperitoneal canal during the 8th week of gestation
- Most common on the left side through the posterolateral lumbocostal triangle, called the "foramen of Bochdalek"
- Defects can vary from several centimeters to complete absence of the hemidiaphragm
- Herniation of the viscera can lead to pulmonary hypoplasia and intestinal obstruction
- Other rare types of CDH are through the foramen of Morgagni and pars sternalis

ETIOLOGY, EPIDEMIOLOGY, & RISK FACTORS

- Most cases are sporadic; some cases have been reported with autosomal dominant inheritance
- Incidence is about 1 in 3000–5000 live births; however, CDH can be detected in 1 in 2200 prenatal ultrasound studies, which indicates that some fetuses never reach the treatment stage
- Overall mortality rate is reported as high as 75% due to associated anomalies, severe pulmonary hypoplasia, and persistent pulmonary hypertension
- Associated anomalies are seen in 20–50% of cases and in 95% of stillborn infants; these include congenital heart defects, extralobar sequestrations, renal agenesis, hydronephrosis, anencephaly, spina bifida, hydrocephalus, trisomy (21, 18, and 13), intestinal atresia, and malrotation of the intestines
- 10–20% of cases occur in association with chromosomal anomalies
- Bilateral diaphragmatic hernias are uncommon (1%)

PATIENT PRESENTATION

- Severe respiratory distress and cyanosis within minutes after birth
- Displacement of the mediastinal structures, resulting in decreased or absent breath sounds on affected side and shifting of heart sounds to the opposite side
- Scaphoid abdomen secondary to dislocation of the abdominal viscera through the defect and into the chest
- Bowel sounds on chest auscultation
- Worsening respiratory distress and cyanosis occurs with bag-mask ventilation
- Small hernias and right-sided hernias have more subtle presentation with feeding problems and mild respiratory distress
- Approximately 5% of affected patients present later in life with signs of intestinal obstruction, including vomiting and abdominal pain

DIFFERENTIAL DX

Prenatal
- Congenital cystic adenomatoid malformation
- Bronchogenic cysts
- Cystic mediastinal teratoma
- Extrapulmonary sequestration
- Neurogenic tumors

Postnatal
- All of the above plus:
- Respiratory distress syndrome
- Pneumothorax
- Complex congenital heart disease with dextrocardia
- Congenital pneumonia

DIAGNOSTIC EVALUATION

- Prenatal diagnosis can be made by prenatal ultrasound as early as 15 weeks of gestation
  - Diagnostic features include presence of viscera above the level of inferior margin of scapula or at the level of the four-chamber view of the heart
  - Development of polyhydramnios later in pregnancy is an indication for fetal ultrasound
  - Maternal serum alpha-fetoprotein (MS-AFP) is low, particularly in patients with trisomies
- Postnatal diagnosis:
  - Chest X-ray reveals bowel gas pattern in chest with displacement of mediastinum
  - Chromosomal studies
  - Echocardiogram to rule out congenital heart defects
  - Abdominal ultrasound to rule out renal agenesis and hydronephrosis

TREATMENT & MANAGEMENT

- Prenatal therapies include:
  - Antenatal steroid therapy to improve lung maturity
  - Fetal corrective surgery may be performed if the liver is below the diaphragm
  - Temporary occlusion of fetal trachea to allow lung development has been investigated
- Delivery should be in a tertiary care center, if possible:
  - Avoid bag-mask ventilation if the diagnosis is known
  - All cases with respiratory distress should be electively intubated immediately after delivery
  - A large orogastric tube should be inserted to decompress the stomach and should be attached to continuous suction
- Preoperative management includes:
  - Gentle ventilation to provide adequate oxygenation and avoid lung injury
  - Inhaled nitric oxide and high-frequency ventilation have proven effective
  - Extracorporeal membrane oxygenation (ECMO) may be required 72–96 hours prior to hernia repair to stabilize the infant
  - Most centers delay repair for a few days to stabilize the patient and reduce pulmonary vasoreactivity
- The hernia is then surgically reduced, and the defect is repaired using either diaphragmatic tissue or a prosthetic patch

PROGNOSIS & COMPLICATIONS

- Poor prognostic signs on prenatal ultrasound include polyhydramnios, detection at early gestation (less than 24 weeks), and herniation of the left lobe of the liver or stomach
- Patients who present with symptoms after 8 hours of life have sufficient pulmonary development and better survival
- Prognosis also depends on associated anomalies and severity of pulmonary hypoplasia
- Survival with excellent tertiary care varies from 40–80%
- Severely affected infants may develop chronic lung disease
- Neurologic follow-up is needed to assess for hearing deficits and CNS injury
- Feeding difficulties, gastroesophageal reflux, and growth failure are common
- Scoliosis and chest wall deformities (eg, pectus excavatum) are common

Persistent Pulmonary Hypertension of the Newborn

INTRODUCTION

- Persistent pulmonary hypertension of the newborn (PPHN) is defined as a failure of normal pulmonary vascular relaxation at or shortly after birth
- After birth, normally pulmonary vascular resistance (PVR) falls rapidly with the first breath and lung expansion, and the systemic vascular resistance increases rapidly with umbilical cord clamping as the low-resistance placenta is cut off from the circuit
- Normally, PVR decreases in newborns due to increasing oxygen tension and prostacyclin and nitric oxide synthesis, combined with decreased production of vasoconstrictor substances, such as endothelin-1; failure of decrease in PVR leads to right-to-left shunting of deoxygenated blood through patent ductus arteriosus and foramen ovale, resulting in cyanosis

ETIOLOGY, EPIDEMIOLOGY, & RISK FACTORS

- Because of the presence of these fetal shunts, this condition was also incorrectly referred to in the past as persistent fetal circulation
- Incidence of 1–2 cases per 1000 live births; more common in term and postterm infants
- Risk factors include meconium-stained amniotic fluid, chorioamnionitis, maternal exposure to NSAIDs, perinatal hypoxia, and acidosis
- The most common causes for PPHN include meconium aspiration syndrome (50%), pneumonia or sepsis (20%), and respiratory distress syndrome (5%)
  - Idiopathic in 20% of cases
  - Other causes include congenital diaphragmatic hernia, pulmonary hypoplasia, perinatal asphyxia, maternal diabetes, polycythemia, and alveolar-capillary dysplasia
- Mechanisms for PPHN include:
  - Pulmonary vasospasm due to hypoxia, acidosis, and inflammation
  - Pulmonary hypoplasia, as occurs in oligohydramnios, renal agenesis, and congenital diaphragmatic hernia
  - Pulmonary vascular remodeling with increased muscle thickness of the tunica media of arteries and extension of muscularization into nonmuscular intra-acinar arteries

PATIENT PRESENTATION

- Infant becomes ill within the initial 12 hours of life
- Cyanosis worsens with time and minimal stimulation
- Prominent precordial impulse
- Single second heart sound due to early closure of the pulmonary valve
- Right ventricular heave secondary to increased pulmonary vascular resistance
- Systolic murmur consistent with tricuspid or mitral regurgitation secondary to papillary muscle dysfunction
- Tachypnea, grunting, nasal flaring, and retractions
- Signs of respiratory distress may be minimal initially, especially if not due to pulmonary cause
- Signs of multiorgan failure (eg, oliguria, edema, jaundice, lethargy, hypotension, shock) may follow as the disease progresses

DIFFERENTIAL DX

- Severe parenchymal lung disease (unaccompanied by PPHN)
  - Respiratory distress syndrome
  - Meconium aspiration syndrome
  - Severe pneumonia
  - Congenital diaphragmatic hernia
- Pulmonary hemorrhage
- Sepsis
- Total anomalous pulmonary venous return
- Tricuspid atresia
- Transposition of the great arteries
- Critical pulmonic stenosis
- Hypoplastic left ventricle
- Coarctation of aorta

DIAGNOSTIC EVALUATION

- PPHN should be considered routinely in evaluating a cyanotic newborn
- Simultaneous preductal and postductal oxygen saturation monitoring will reveal greater than 10% difference (preductal greater than postductal)
- Laboratory studies include complete blood count to rule out polycythemia, blood culture to rule out sepsis, and blood glucose to rule our hypoglycemia
- Arterial blood gas shows hypoxemia (pO_2 <60 mmHg) and metabolic acidosis
- Preductal (right radial artery) and postductal (umbilical artery) blood gases will reveal a difference in pO_2 of at least 20 mmHg
- Hyperoxia test (exposure to 100% oxygen) may distinguish between pulmonary hypertension and cyanotic congenital heart disease
- Chest X-ray is usually normal, but may reveal:
  - Parenchymal disease (eg, pneumonia, meconium aspiration syndrome)
  - Pulmonary vascular markings are minimal because pulmonary blood flow is diminished
  - Mild cardiomegaly due to myocardial hypoxemia
  - Hypoxemia is usually out of proportion to the X-ray findings
- EKG commonly shows right ventricular predominance and may show changes of myocardial ischemia
- Echocardiography is indicated to determine right-sided pressures, evaluate right-left shunting, determine ventricular function, and rule out structural heart disease

TREATMENT & MANAGEMENT

- Avoid unnecessary interventions because these children tend to become hypoxemic following even minimal handling
- Sedation, analgesia, and paralysis may be required to reduce catecholamine release
- Be sure to correct hypoglycemia, hypoxia, acidosis, hypotension, and polycythemia because these accentuate shunting
- Primary goals of treatment are to reverse hypoxemia and reduce elevated pulmonary vascular resistance
- Administer supplemental oxygen up to 100% to maintain pO_2 >80 mmHg and normal PCO_2 (35–45 mmHg)
  - Provide mechanical ventilation if hypoxemia persists despite 100% oxygen
  - Inhaled nitric oxide (a pulmonary vasodilator) can be provided with mechanical ventilation
- Metabolic alkalosis reduces pulmonary vascular resistance, but hyperventilation and use of sodium bicarbonate infusions to achieve metabolic alkalosis are controversial
- Dopamine or dobutamine may be required to counter systemic hypotension
- 5–10% of patients fail conventional therapy and require extracorporeal membrane oxygenation (ECMO), which is a form of cardiopulmonary bypass that augments systemic perfusion and provides gas exchange

PROGNOSIS & COMPLICATIONS

- Survival and prognosis vary with underlying diagnosis
- Survivors of PPHN have a high incidence (40–50%) of major neurodevelopmental impairment
- Infants requiring high levels of ventilator support may develop bronchopulmonary dysplasia
- The availability of inhaled nitric oxide therapy and ECMO has reduced the mortality from as high as 50% in the past to as low as 10% today
- Inhaled nitric oxide therapy has reduced the need for ECMO significantly; methemoglobinemia and bronchial hyperreactivity that occur due to toxic levels of nitrogen dioxide are potential side effects of inhaled nitric oxide therapy

Gastroschisis

INTRODUCTION

- Gastroschisis is a full-thickness defect in the abdominal wall, usually located just to the right of the umbilical cord
- Rarely, it is located in the mirror-image position to the left of the umbilical cord
- The defect occurs between 10 and 12 weeks of gestation
- As a result, the intestines and other abdominal organs become herniated outside the abdominal wall with no covering membrane or sac
- Incidence is increasing and ranges between 0.43 cases per 10,000 births

ETIOLOGY, EPIDEMIOLOGY, & RISK FACTORS

- Eviscerated contents that herniated through the gastroschisis may include the small bowel, stomach, and proximal colon
- Gastroschisis has a very strong association with young maternal age, with most of the affected mothers being younger than 20 years; other risk factors include maternal exposure to cigarette smoking, illicit drugs, vasoactive over-the-counter drugs (eg, pseudoephedrine), and environmental toxins
- Unlike omphalocele, the incidence of associated anomalies is low (10–20%)
- Approximately 10% of cases are associated with intestinal atresia or stenosis; other less common associated anomalies include undescended testes, Meckel diverticulum, and intestinal duplications
- The exposed bowel is vulnerable to injury, including volvulus and loss of the entire midgut due to twisting of the bowel around the mesenteric vascular pedicle
- Exposure to amniotic fluid causes an inflammatory "peel" or serositis that can make the bowel loops indistinguishable from one another

PATIENT PRESENTATION

- Diagnosis can be made by prenatal ultrasound
- The defect is lateral to the umbilical cord
- At birth, edematous and matted-appearing intestinal bowel loops that have been exposed to amniotic fluid for many weeks are seen
- The herniated bowel may appear thickened and foreshortened with segments of ischemia, necrosis, stenosis, and atresia
- Because the bowel herniates before normal rotation and fixation has occurred, malrotation is present

DIFFERENTIAL DX

- Omphalocele

DIAGNOSTIC EVALUATION

- Prenatal diagnosis can be made as early as 12 weeks of gestation by prenatal ultrasound
- Prenatal ultrasound can accurately distinguish omphalocele from gastroschisis by the location of the defect (to the right of the umbilicus), absence of a peritoneal sac, normal insertion of the cord, and absence of other anomalies
- Elevated maternal serum alpha-fetoprotein (very high levels) occurs

TREATMENT & MANAGEMENT

- Prenatal management may include early delivery of the fetus to avoid unpredictable fetal death; additionally, amniotic fluid exchange transfusion replacing amniotic fluid with saline has been reported
- Delivery room management includes the following:
  - Secure the airway; in case of respiratory distress, mechanical ventilation may be necessary
  - Place an orogastric tube to decompress the bowel
  - Inspect the exposed viscera and avoid twisting of the mesenteric vascular pedicle
  - Protect the viscera and minimize fluid and heat loss by placing the lower half of the infant along with the viscera into a sterile plastic bowel bag
- Subsequent management includes the following:
  - The umbilical artery and vein may be cannulated, if needed, during resuscitation
  - Primary surgical closure can be done immediately
  - Another approach is to use a prefabricated, spring-loaded silastic silo placed in the defect to cover the exposed bowel at the bedside; the size of the silo is progressively reduced over 5–10 days; delayed primary closure is done once the bowel moves into the abdominal cavity
- Monitor fluids and electrolytes (closely monitor urine output); the neonate may require twice the maintenance fluid volumes

PROGNOSIS & COMPLICATIONS

- Prognosis depends on the condition of the vulnerable bowel
- Overall survival is excellent (90–95%)
- Gastroschisis is associated with an increased risk of intrauterine growth retardation, unpredictable fetal death, and premature delivery
- Oligohydramnios is present in up to 25% of cases
- Poor feeding tolerance is common; patients need parenteral nutrition for weeks to months
- Postoperative necrotizing enterocolitis is not uncommon when feeds are being advanced and should be suspected if bloody stools are observed
- Intestinal dysmotility is common
- 5–10% have intestinal obstruction later in life

Omphalocele

INTRODUCTION

- An omphalocele is a midline abdominal wall defect of variable size; in contrast to gastroschisis, abdominal viscera herniates through the defect but is covered by a membrane and contained within the peritoneal sac
- The membrane covering consists of peritoneum on the inner surface, amnion on the outer surface, and Wharton's jelly between the layers
- The umbilical vessels insert into the membrane but not the body wall
- The intestines and liver remain morphologically and functionally normal
- Omphalocele is also known as exomphalos

ETIOLOGY, EPIDEMIOLOGY, & RISK FACTORS

- The abdominal wall is formed by infolding of the cranial, caudal, and lateral embryonic folds; normal folding leads to an intact umbilical ring by 5 weeks of gestation
- The intestines migrate outside the abdominal cavity through this umbilical ring and into the umbilical cord during the sixth week of gestation
- An intact abdominal wall is formed after the intestines return to the abdominal cavity by 10–12 weeks
- Partial or complete arrest of the return of the intestines into the abdominal cavity leads to an omphalocele with herniation of the midgut organs
- Failure of the cranial folds to fuse leads to pentalogy of Cantrell: omphalocele, anterior diaphragmatic hernia, sternal clefts, pericardial defects, and cardiac defects
- Failure of caudal folds to fuse leads to bladder or cloacal exstrophy and a lower omphalocele
- The incidence of omphalocele ranges from 1.5–3 per 10,000 births
- Advancing maternal age (over 30 years) is a major risk factor
- In contrast to gastroschisis, patients with omphalocele have a very high (up to 50–70%) incidence of associated anomalies, including chromosome anomalies (notably trisomies 13, 14, 15, 18, and 21), which are present in up to 30% of cases

PATIENT PRESENTATION

- Often diagnosed by prenatal ultrasound
- At birth, the umbilical herniation of abdominal viscera within the peritoneal sac is visible
- Because a membranous sac is present, the bowel is well protected
- The membrane might be ruptured, resulting in exposure of the abdominal organs to the outside
- Features of associated anomalies, if present, include:
  - Ectopia cordis
  - Features of trisomies
  - Anterior diaphragmatic hernia
  - Bladder or cloacal exstrophy
  - Beckwith-Wiedemann syndrome, consisting of macroglossia, organomegaly, and hypoglycemia

DIFFERENTIAL DX

- Gastroschisis

DIAGNOSTIC EVALUATION

- Prenatal diagnosis via prenatal ultrasound can accurately distinguish omphalocele from gastroschisis by visualizing a defect through the umbilicus rather than the abdominal wall; the umbilical cord inserts into the sac, and there may be associated fetal anomalies
- Elevated maternal serum alpha-fetoprotein occurs
- High-resolution ultrasound may be indicated to assess for other structural defects
- Chromosomal studies may be indicated

TREATMENT & MANAGEMENT

- Unlike gastroschisis, there is usually no reason to consider early delivery
- Avoid hypothermia; heat loss from the exposed viscera is a common problem
- Gastric decompression by orogastric tube insertion and continuous suction
- Secure the airway; mechanical ventilation may be necessary if respiratory distress occurs
- Start broad-spectrum prophylactic antibiotics
- Inspect the defect to make sure that the covering membrane is intact
- Apply nonadherent dressings to stabilize the sac and to prevent trauma
- If the sac is ruptured, protect the viscera and minimize fluid and heat loss by placing the lower half of the infant and the viscera into a sterile bowel bag
- Avoid placement of umbilical arterial and venous lines
- Surgical repair is not emergent unless the sac is ruptured
  - Small omphaloceles (<6 cm) can be repaired in a single-stage procedure
  - Primary closure includes excision of the omphalocele membrane, reduction of the herniated viscera, and closure of the fascia and skin
  - Larger defects require gradual reduction into the abdominal cavity and healing by epithelialization of the membrane
- Administer maintenance IV fluids; evaporative fluid losses are not as great as in gastroschisis since the peritoneal sac envelops the viscera

PROGNOSIS & COMPLICATIONS

- Prognosis primarily depends on the severity of the associated anomalies rather than the abdominal wall defect
- There is a high risk of fetal deaths and stillbirths due to associated anomalies
- Cardiac defects are seen in 30–50% of patients
- Mortality rate of 30–40% due to high incidence of serious associated malformations

Necrotizing Enterocolitis

INTRODUCTION

- Necrotizing enterocolitis (NEC) is an acquired neonatal disorder of unknown etiology that results in acute intestinal necrosis
- NEC is predominantly a disorder of premature infants
- It is hypothesized that, when enteral feeds are started, partially digested formula provides a substrate for bacterial proliferation; associated hypoxia, poor gut perfusion, and other factors cause tissue injury
- After mucosal invasion, bacterial proliferation and release of toxins lead to transmural necrosis, perforation, and peritonitis
- The terminal ileum and proximal colon are most commonly affected

ETIOLOGY, EPIDEMIOLOGY, & RISK FACTORS

- The overall incidence of NEC is up to 10% of all neonatal intensive care admissions
- NEC has a high mortality rate and accounts for at least 1000 deaths annually in the U.S.
- NEC occurs in 4–13% of all very low birth weight babies (<1500 g)
- Approximately 10–25% of those affected are term infants
- The age of onset of NEC is inversely related to birth weight and gestation
- Term infants present earlier (<7 days) versus preterm infants (14–20 days)
- Prematurity is the only definite risk factor identified to date
- Other potential risk factors include enteral feeding (NEC is rare in unfed infants); high feeding volumes, timing of enteral feeding, and overly rapid advancement of feeding; hyperosmolar formulas and medications; polycythemia (causes reduced sluggish blood supply and poor perfusion to the gut); perinatal asphyxia; poor cardiac output states (eg, congestive cardiac failure, patent ductus arteriosus); and indomethacin and steroids (reduce gastrointestinal perfusion)
- Breastfeeding significantly lowers the risk for NEC

PATIENT PRESENTATION

- The clinical presentation of NEC is highly variable; it ranges from mild feeding intolerance or abdominal distension to fulminant shock and death
- The classic description involves abdominal distention (most frequent), microscopic or grossly bloody stools, increased gastric residuals, and localizing abdominal signs
- Other features include bilious gastric aspirate, abdominal wall erythema or induration, persistent localized abdominal mass, ascites, apnea and bradycardia, temperature instability, irritability, poor feeding, lethargy, hypotension, oliguria, and poor perfusion

DIFFERENTIAL DX

- Sepsis
- Malrotation with midgut volvulus
- Intestinal duplication
- Mesenteric vessel thrombosis
- Incarcerated inguinal hernia
- Isolated intestinal perforation
- Paralytic ileus
- Infectious enterocolitis
- *Campylobacter* diarrhea
- Allergic colitis
- The differential diagnosis for occult blood in stool includes:
  - Anal fissure
  - Swallowed maternal blood
  - Trauma from nasogastric tube
  - Gastric stress ulcers
  - Other hemorrhagic diatheses
  - Allergic colitis

DIAGNOSTIC EVALUATION

- CBC reveals high white cell count with a high bands, neutropenia, and thrombocytopenia
- Blood culture for aerobes and anaerobes and urine culture are indicated
- Arterial blood gas shows metabolic acidosis
- Basic metabolic panel reveals severe refractory hyponatremia, low CO_2, and elevated BUN
- Stool examination for occult blood
- Abdominal X-ray (perform both AP and cross-table lateral or left lateral decubitus views)
  - Pneumatosis intestinalis (presence of gas within the bowel wall) is pathognomonic for NEC and is caused by hydrogen gas produced by bacteria
  - Portal venous gas is seen in 10–30% of cases and may indicate severe disease
  - Other findings include abnormal bowel gas pattern, bowel wall edema, fixed loop of bowel on serial X-rays, ileus, free peritoneal air, and pneumobilia
- Bell staging of NEC (based on clinical and X-ray findings):
  - Stage I (suspected NEC): Nonspecific clinical signs, feeding intolerance, occult blood in stools, normal or nonspecific radiologic signs
  - Stage II (definite NEC): Abdominal distension, abdominal wall edema with or without abdominal mass, pneumatosis intestinalis, ileus
  - Stage IIIA (advanced NEC): Impending intestinal perforation, hypotension, oliguria, fixed intestinal loop on X-ray
  - Stage IIB (perforated NEC): Shock, disseminated intravascular coagulation (DIC), perforated bowel, pneumoperitoneum

TREATMENT & MANAGEMENT

- Discontinue feeding and ensure bowel rest until resolution (usually 10–14 days)
- Gastric decompression with nasogastric tube and continuous suction
- Antibiotics based on local resistance patterns (eg, ampicillin, gentamicin, clindamycin)
- Monitoring includes vital signs, abdominal girth, fluid intake and output, electrolytes, and pH; perform serial abdominal X-rays (every 6–8 hours) to monitor disease progression
- Correct thrombocytopenia, anemia, and DIC, if present
- Ensure central venous access and vigorous fluid resuscitation
- Respiratory support with intubation and mechanical ventilation is often required
- Low-dose dopamine (3–5 μg/kg) may be used to optimize splanchnic blood flow
- Total parenteral nutrition should be instituted as early as possible
- Surgical consultation for impending or obvious intestinal perforation
- Basic surgical procedures include resection of necrotic bowel, diversion of proximal healthy bowel with a stoma (secondary reanastomosis is performed electively after an adequate period of healing), and peritoneal drainage without laparotomy in unstable babies smaller than 1000 g with severe NEC
- Strategies for prevention may include probiotics, prophylactic oral antibiotics, gastric acidification, immunoglobulin (IgA and IgG), and glutamine and arginine supplementation

PROGNOSIS & COMPLICATIONS

- NEC with perforation has a mortality of 20–40%
- Intestinal strictures and stenosis may form as early as 2 weeks
- Partial strictures may present as recurring episodes of sepsis and feeding intolerance
- Malabsorption and short gut syndrome are common with extensive intestinal resection
- Infants undergoing surgical resection require long-term parenteral nutrition (PN)
- Cholestasis associated with total PN is a common complication of long-term PN
- 6% of infants who develop NEC experience a recurrence
- Infants without short gut syndrome may achieve normal growth by the end of the first year
- Extraintestinal complications include increased risk of bronchopulmonary dysplasia, sepsis, and neurodevelopmental delay

Neonatal Sepsis

INTRODUCTION

- A clinical syndrome that occurs during the first month of life and is characterized by systemic signs of infection accompanied by a positive blood culture
- "Early-onset" sepsis occurs from birth to 7 days of life and is primarily caused by vertical transmission
- "Late-onset" sepsis occurs beyond 7 days of life and is acquired postnatally or by nosocomial transmission
- Neonatal sepsis is a major cause of mortality and morbidity in newborns
- Clinical signs may be subtle but can rapidly progress to life-threatening disease

ETIOLOGY, EPIDEMIOLOGY, & RISK FACTORS

- The most common organisms include:
  - Early and late onset: Group B streptococci (also known as GBS or *Streptococcus agalactiae*), Gram-negative enteric organisms (eg, *Escherichia coli*), and *Listeria monocytogenes*
  - Late onset: Coagulase-negative *Staphylococcus*, *Staphylococcus aureus*, *Candida*, and *Pseudomonas*
- Less common organisms include *Enterococcus*, other streptococci, *Klebsiella*, anaerobes, and *Haemophilus*
- Risk factors include premature onset of labor, premature and/or prolonged rupture of membranes, maternal chorioamnionitis, maternal GBS colonization, peripartum maternal fever, invasive procedures (eg, scalp monitoring), prematurity, and low birth weight
- The incidence rate is 1–4 cases per 1000 live births
  - Incidence is 3- to 10-fold higher in premature and low birth weight infants
- Meningitis accompanies sepsis in approximately 25% of infants with sepsis
- The mortality rate approaches 50% in some populations, with the highest rates in premature infants and cases of Gram-negative sepsis

PATIENT PRESENTATION

- Temperature irregularity
- Gastrointestinal signs include feeding intolerance, vomiting, poor feeding, abdominal distension, and jaundice
- Respiratory signs include tachypnea, respiratory distress, and apnea
- Cardiovascular signs include tachycardia, hypotension, poor perfusion, mottling, cyanosis
- Neurologic signs include lethargy, hypotonia, hyporeflexia, seizures, high-pitched cry, and a full fontanel
- Unexplained metabolic acidosis, hypoglycemia, or hyperglycemia may occur
- Hepatosplenomegaly and petechiae are late manifestations of severe sepsis
- Focal manifestations may include cellulitis, abscesses, omphalitis, otitis media, conjunctivitis, osteomyelitis

DIFFERENTIAL DX

- Intraventricular hemorrhage
- Necrotizing enterocolitis
- Neonatal asphyxia
- Drug withdrawal
- Congenital cyanotic heart disease
- Congenital viral infections
- Inborn errors of metabolism

DIAGNOSTIC EVALUATION

- Blood cultures are diagnostic but may be negative if antibiotics were administered to the mother
- Urine cultures via transurethral catheter or suprapubic aspiration specimen
- CSF analysis for protein, glucose, cell count, and cultures
- CBC with differential
  - May reveal leukocytosis (WBC count >20,000/mm^3) or severe leukopenia (WBC count <500/mm^3)
  - Immature-to-total neutrophil ratio (I:T) >0.2 should raise suspicion of sepsis
  - Anemia and thrombocytopenia are nonspecific indicators
- Further testing includes chest X-ray to assess for pneumonia, basic metabolic panel to assess for hypoglycemia and metabolic acidosis, cultures of tracheal aspirates, and diagnostic needle aspiration of appropriate body fluids
- Less commonly performed testing includes acute-phase reactants (eg, C-reactive protein, fibrinogen), cytokine measurements (eg, IL-6, IL-8, GM-CSF, TNF-α, IL-1), erythrocyte sedimentation rate (ESR), buffy coat microscopic examination for bacteria, histopathology of placenta for chorioamnionitis and inflammation of the umbilical cord (funisitis), and urine latex agglutination test (for GBS)

TREATMENT & MANAGEMENT

- Preventive measures can significantly reduce the incidence of neonatal sepsis
  - Testing for GBS at 35–37 weeks of gestation via vaginal and rectal cultures
  - Maternal intrapartum antibiotics (at least 4 hours prior to delivery) for GBS-colonized mothers and cases of chorioamnionitis
- Blood, urine, and CSF cultures should be obtained from all infants with suspected sepsis
- Antibiotics should be started empirically on minimal suspicion
  - Presumptive antibiotic therapy for early-onset sepsis includes ampicillin and an aminoglycoside (eg, gentamicin)
  - First-line antibiotics for late-onset sepsis depend on the circumstances; the most commonly used antibiotics are cefotaxime (for Gram-negative organisms), vancomycin (for coagulase-negative *Staphylococcus*), ceftazidime (for *Pseudomonas*), nafcillin (for *Staphylococcus aureus*), and amphotericin (for *Candida*)
  - Antibiotics can be discontinued after 48–72 hours if cultures are negative
- Duration of treatment varies according to the degree of illness and suspicion of sepsis
- Most bloodstream infections are treated for a total of 7–10 days
- Adjunctive therapy is occasionally used and includes granulocyte, G-CSF, and GM-CSF infusions; intravenous immunoglobulin (IVIG); and double-volume exchange transfusions

PROGNOSIS & COMPLICATIONS

- Prognosis is very good if promptly and adequately treated
- Gram-negative sepsis has a high mortality rate
- Bacteremia may cause endocarditis, septic emboli, abscess, and bone or joint destruction
- Immediate complications associated with meningitis, cerebritis, ventriculitis, subdural effusion, and cerebral abscess
- Late complications include hearing loss, cerebral palsy, and developmental delay

Congenital Infections

INTRODUCTION

- A few pathogens that women are exposed to during pregnancy possess the ability to infect the placenta and damage the developing fetus
- These pathogens were traditionally grouped as the "TORCH" infections (**T**oxoplasmosis, **O**ther agents, **R**ubella, **C**ytomegalovirus, and **H**erpes simplex); however, a better terminology is "transplacental intrauterine infections"
- Other transplacental infections include syphilis, varicella zoster, parvovirus B19, enteroviruses, congenital malaria, and Chagas disease
- Most infants with transplacental infections are asymptomatic; however, these infections are important causes of deafness, vision loss, and behavioral or neurologic disorders

ETIOLOGY, EPIDEMIOLOGY, & RISK FACTORS

- ***Toxoplasma gondii*** is an obligate intracellular protozoan
  - Humans acquire *Toxoplasma* by ingesting undercooked meat containing bradyzoites or fruits, vegetables, and other foodstuffs that are contaminated by oocysts
  - Incidence varies from 1 in 1000 to 1 in 10,000 live births
- **Cytomegalovirus** (CMV) is a common virus that infects nearly 100% of the population by adulthood
  - Of the women who acquire primary CMV infection during pregnancy, 40% transmit CMV to their fetuses, and 10% of the infected infants develop CMV disease
  - Incidence is about 1 in 1000 live births
- **Herpes simplex-2** (HSV-2) infects as many as 2% of pregnant women
  - Congenital HSV-2 infection of the fetus is rare; less than 50 cases have been described
  - Neonatal disease is more common when mothers have genital HSV infection near the time of delivery
  - Presents with skin vesicles, encephalitis, or disseminated illness
- Congenital **rubella** syndrome (CRS) has become rare due to widespread vaccination
  - Less than 1–3 cases occur annually, mostly in immigrants

PATIENT PRESENTATION

- Features in congenital infections include:
  - Optic: Chorioretinitis, cataracts, glaucoma, optic atrophy, and microphthalmos
  - Hematologic: Anemia, bleeding diathesis
  - CNS: Seizures, intracranial calcifications, microcephaly, hydrocephalus
  - GI: Jaundice, diarrhea, hepatosplenomegaly
  - Systemic: Fever, lymphadenopathy, hydrops, intrauterine growth restriction
  - Respiratory: Pneumonitis
  - Cardiac: Myocarditis
  - Skin: Petechiae, purpura, vesicles
- Features based on etiology include:
  - *Toxoplasma*: Hydrocephalus, chorioretinitis
  - Rubella: Cataracts, heart defects
  - CMV: Sensorineural deafness
  - Varicella: Limb hypoplasia
  - Parvovirus: Anemia, hydrops

DIFFERENTIAL DX

- Aicardi syndrome
- Warburg syndrome
- Incontinentia pigmenti
- Neonatal Graves disease
- Cerebral malformations

DIAGNOSTIC EVALUATION

- **Toxoplasmosis** is usually diagnosed by the presence of both *Toxoplasma* IgG and IgM in the serum
  - Urine or CSF IgG and IgM is also diagnostic
  - *Toxoplasma* may be isolated from the placenta or peripheral blood
- **CMV**: Urine culture using the shell vial assay is the gold standard for the diagnosis
  - CMV-specific IgG or IgM in the infant's serum has much lower sensitivity
  - Polymerase chain reaction (PCR) can detect CMV DNA in urine and other body fluids
- **HSV-2**: Skin vesicle fluid, CSF, and swabs of the conjunctiva, rectum, and oropharynx for herpes virus culture or PCR is diagnostic
- Congenital **rubella**: Virus present in nasal secretions, urine, or CSF is diagnostic of congenital rubella syndrome
  - Rubella virus–specific IgM in infant serum is also diagnostic
- Other general investigations for transplacental infections:
  - Cranial ultrasound and head CT scan may demonstrate characteristic intracranial calcifications
  - Long bone films may show metaphyseal lucency and irregularity of the epiphyseal plates
  - CSF may show pleocytosis or elevated protein
  - CBC may reveal anemia, thrombocytopenia, or eosinophilia
  - Liver enzymes may be elevated with direct hyperbilirubinemia

TREATMENT & MANAGEMENT

- Toxoplasmosis:
  - Pregnant women can reduce exposure by avoiding cats and undercooked meat
  - Infected mothers can be treated with spiramycin or pyrimethamine-sulfadiazine
  - Treat infants with a prolonged (1-year) course of sulfadiazine and pyrimethamine
  - Obstructive hydrocephalus is treated with ventriculoperitoneal shunting
  - Corticosteroids are used for chorioretinitis or if CSF protein is elevated
- CMV
  - Pregnant women can reduce their risk of CMV infection by avoiding direct contact with the urine and saliva of toddler-aged children
  - Ganciclovir may improve sensorineural hearing loss and CMV pneumonia
- Herpes simplex
  - Acyclovir has little or no beneficial effect in transplacental infection
  - Neonatal-acquired infections are treated with acyclovir for 3 weeks
- Rubella
  - CRS cannot be treated effectively by postnatal antiviral therapy
  - If termination of pregnancy is not an option, immunoglobulin can be considered

PROGNOSIS & COMPLICATIONS

- Infants with symptomatic transplacental infections can develop epilepsy, cerebral palsy, visual impairment, deafness, and mental retardation
- Treated infants with toxoplasmosis have much lower rates of the same complications
- Approximately 15% of children with asymptomatic CMV infection will manifest later with varying degrees of sensorineural hearing loss
- Children with congenital rubella syndrome have an increased risk of growth failure or diabetes mellitus
- Efficacy of antenatal varicella zoster immunoglobulin (VZIG) in preventing the fetal varicella syndrome or postnatal acyclovir in treating the same is unproven

Congenital Syphilis

INTRODUCTION

- Congenital syphilis usually results from transplacental transmission
- The infection can also be acquired by contact with genital lesions during delivery
- The organs most severely affected include bone, brain, liver, lung, and the skeletal system
- Congenital syphilis is classified into early and late disease
  - Early congenital syphilis represents active infection and inflammation; features are seen before 2 years of age
  - Late congenital syphilis reflects the body's response to persistent inflammation; manifestations occur beyond 2 years of age
- Approximately two-thirds of live-born cases are asymptomatic

ETIOLOGY, EPIDEMIOLOGY, & RISK FACTORS

- Treponemes (*Treponema pallidum*) are microaerophilic, Gram-negative bacteria visualized by dark-field or phase-contrast microscopy
- Transplacental transmission during maternal spirochetemia can occur as early as 9 -10 weeks of gestation and at any subsequent time during pregnancy
- The rate of fetal transmission depends on the stage of maternal disease:
  - 100% transmission rate during primary maternal disease
  - 90% transmission during maternal secondary syphilis
  - 30% transmission during maternal latent syphilis
- The prevalence of seropositivity in pregnancy is between 0.02–4.5% in the U.S.; however, only a small proportion of these pregnancies will result in congenital syphilis
- The incidence of congenital syphilis is 11 cases per 100,000 live births in the U.S.
- Abortion, intrauterine growth retardation, stillbirth, nonimmune hydrops, neonatal death, and prematurity are common with transplacental transmission of the infection
- Risk factors associated with acquisition of syphilis include poverty, inadequate prenatal care, cocaine use, trading sex for drugs and money, and infection with HIV

PATIENT PRESENTATION

- Early congenital syphilis presents with:
  - Hepatosplenomegaly, lymphadenopathy
  - Skeletal: Pseudoparalysis
  - Mucocutaneous: Maculopapular rash, palmar and plantar bullae, condyloma lata, mucous patches, rhinitis (snuffles), petechiae, jaundice
  - Central nervous system: Aseptic meningitis
  - Ocular: Uveitis, chorioretinitis, glaucoma
- Untreated late manifestations appear after 2 yr:
  - Skeletal: Frontal bossing, short maxilla, high palatal arch, saddle nose, saber shins, scaphoid scapula, Clutton joints (painless hydrarthrosis)
  - Dental: Mulberry molars, Hutchinson teeth (notched incisors), enamel dystrophy
  - Neurologic: Eighth nerve deafness, mental delay, convulsive disorders, paresis, paralysis
  - Ocular: Interstitial keratitis, uveitis, glaucoma

DIFFERENTIAL DX

- Sepsis
- Congenital toxoplasmosis
- Congenital rubella
- Congenital cytomegalovirus infection
- Herpes simplex infection
- Parvovirus B19 infection
- HIV infection
- Neonatal varicella

DIAGNOSTIC EVALUATION

- Begin with serologic tests
  - Quantitative nontreponemal antibody tests (VDRL, RPR) are used as the initial screening test on the infant's serum; shows titers that are 4-fold higher than maternal serum
  - If screening is positive, treponemal serologic tests are indicated: fluorescent treponemal antibody-adsorption test (FTA-ABS), microhemagglutinin assay for *T. pallidum* (MHA-TP)
  - Nontreponemal tests become negative after treatment (as opposed to treponemal tests)
  - FTA-ABS IgM distinguishes neonatal from maternal disease
- Dark-field exam or direct fluorescent antibody of exudates or tissue is diagnostic
- Laboratory testing includes CBC (reveals Coombs negative hemolytic anemia and thrombocytopenia) and liver function tests (reveal elevated AST, ALT, and bilirubin)
- Cerebrospinal fluid findings are considered suggestive of neurosyphilis if WBC count is $>25/mm^3$ (up to 200 mononuclear cells/mm^3), protein level is >150 mg/dL (>170 mg/dL in premature infants), or positive CSF VDRL
- X-ray of long bones may reveal osteitis, osteochondritis, periostitis, and Wimberger sign (tibial osteochondritis); late manifestations include Higoumenaki sign (sternoclavicular thickening) and saber shin (tibial bowing)
- Chest X-ray may occasionally show pneumonitis (pneumonia alba)
- Examination of the placenta reveals a large placenta thickened with hypercellular villi and acute and chronic inflammation; the umbilical cord contains abscess-like necrotic foci (necrotizing funisitis) around the vessels

TREATMENT & MANAGEMENT

- Universal precautions are necessary for patients with suspected or proven syphilis until therapy has been initiated for 24 hours
- Treat with IV aqueous crystalline penicillin G for 10–14 days
  - Indications for treatment include physical or radiologic evidence of disease, positive dark-field or FTA-ABS tests, nontreponemal titer at least 4 times higher than the mother's titer, abnormal CSF examination or reactive CSF VDRL, inadequate maternal therapy, or in any infant at risk for congenital syphilis when a full workup cannot be performed
  - IM procaine penicillin G can be administered for 10 days as alternative therapy
- Neonates may experience Jarisch-Herxheimer reactions (fever, tachypnea, hypotension, tachycardia, skin rash, and even death) during treatment
- Some authorities treat all infants who have a positive VDRL; this is because it may be difficult to document that mother had adequate treatment with serial titers, low titers may be present in latent maternal syphilis, infected infants may have no clinical signs at birth, and follow-up may be difficult in populations at risk
- All seropositive infants should have a repeat VDRL or RPR test every 2–3 months until the test becomes negative or the titers decrease 4-fold
- CSF analysis is repeated every 6 months in infants with neurosyphilis until it becomes normal

PROGNOSIS & COMPLICATIONS

- If asymptomatic, infants treated at birth have good outcomes without sequelae
- Mental retardation, hydrocephalus, cranial nerve palsies, and deafness are complications of neurosyphilis
- Nonimmune hemolytic anemia can occur and persist for weeks after effective treatment
- Hydrops fetalis due to anemia is a potentially lethal complication
- Failure to thrive, pancreatitis, nephritis, nephrotic syndrome, myocarditis, ileitis, malabsorptive gastrointestinal fibrosis, testicular masses, alopecia, nail exfoliation, and pituitary gumma are known complications

Intraventricular Hemorrhage

INTRODUCTION

- Intraventricular hemorrhage (IVH) occurs when the fragile network of blood vessels in the subependymal germinal matrix rupture into the lateral ventricles
- Germinal matrix is a periventricular structure located between the caudate nucleus and the thalamus at the level of the foramen of Monro
- The matrix contains pluripotent neuronal and glial precursor cells
- It is highly vascular and has weakly supported stroma; thus, it is prone to rupture upon even minimal fluctuations in cerebral blood flow
- The matrix is prominent between 26 and 34 weeks of gestation and then undergoes spontaneous regression by term; as a result, IVH is principally found in premature infants

ETIOLOGY, EPIDEMIOLOGY, & RISK FACTORS

- Occurs in 15–20% of infants born at less than 32 weeks of gestation; rare after 32 weeks of postconceptional age
- Incidence and severity are inversely proportional to gestational age
- 90% of cases occur within the first 3 days of life; they may progress in severity during the first few days to weeks of life
- New-onset IVH is rare after the first week of life
- Risk factors include anything that causes fluctuations in cerebral blood flow (eg, birth asphyxia, need for rigorous resuscitation at birth, seizures, pneumothorax, mechanical ventilation, tracheal suctioning, patent ductus arteriosus)
- Classification system:
  - Grade I: Isolated germinal matrix hemorrhage
  - Grade II: Intraventricular hemorrhage without ventricular dilation
  - Grade III: Intraventricular hemorrhage with ventricular dilation
  - Grade IV: Intraventricular hemorrhage with parenchymal involvement

PATIENT PRESENTATION

- IVH is usually asymptomatic unless it is severe
- Some infants present with subtle features, including decreased level of consciousness, abnormal eye movements, apnea, and bradycardia
- Rarely, infants present with ominous signs, including severe neurologic impairment and paralysis, severe hypotonia, severe metabolic acidosis and shock, seizures, or bulging and tense anterior fontanel
- Severe IVH (grades III and IV) may be complicated by posthemorrhagic hydrocephalus and present with increasing head circumference and bulging anterior fontanel

DIFFERENTIAL DX

- Cerebral hemorrhage or infarct
- Choroid plexus cyst
- Perinatal asphyxia
- Sepsis
- Meningitis
- Metabolic disorders
- Bleeding disorders (eg, hemophilia, factor V Leiden)

DIAGNOSTIC EVALUATION

- Cranial ultrasound through the anterior fontanel is diagnostic and is indicated if IVH is suspected clinically
  - Routinely used as a screening tool for all infants with birth weight less than 1500 g or younger than 32 weeks of gestation
  - Ultrasound at 1 week of life will detect more than 90% of all hemorrhages
  - If initial screening is negative, no further ultrasounds are needed to detect hemorrhage
  - If IVH is present on initial screening, serial ultrasounds at weekly intervals are needed to follow-up progression of the bleed and assess for the development of hydrocephalus
  - In a very sick infant or extremely premature baby, consider an ultrasound within the first 24 hours to look for severe bleeding
- Examination of the CSF may show elevated red and white blood cells and elevated protein but may be normal in 20% of affected patients
- A sudden drop in hematocrit and metabolic acidosis may be seen in severe IVH
- Head CT scan and MRI of brain may be indicated to delineate the extent of damage

TREATMENT & MANAGEMENT

- Preventive measures include:
  - Avoid premature delivery or prolong pregnancy, if possible
  - Administer antenatal steroids to the mother (betamethasone or dexamethasone)
  - Low-dose, prophylactic indomethacin administered to the premature infant within 3 days significantly reduces the incidence of severe IVH; however, it has no effect on existing IVH
  - Maintain normal blood volume and stable acid-base balance
  - Avoid rapid fluid bolus infusions, if possible
  - Avoid infusion of hyperosmolar solutions (eg, sodium bicarbonate)
  - Avoid large fluctuations in blood pressure
- There is no specific therapy available; supportive management includes providing stable cerebral perfusion and correcting thrombocytopenia and coagulation disturbances promptly
- Treatment of posthemorrhagic hydrocephalus:
  - Serial ventricular drainage via ventricular reservoir or lumbar punctures done every 1–3 days to remove 10–20 mL of CSF with each draw for 3–4 weeks
  - Serial ultrasound measurements of ventricular size
  - Ventriculoperitoneal shunt placement if ventricular dilatation is progressive
  - Drugs, including acetazolamide to decrease CSF production and glycerol for hyperosmolar therapy, have been tried with varying degrees of success

PROGNOSIS & COMPLICATIONS

- Prognosis varies with the severity of bleeding and presence of complications
- Small IVH (grades I and II) usually resolve spontaneously without neurologic sequelae
- 50–80% of infants with severe IVH (grades III and IV) manifest major developmental disabilities, including spastic diplegia and hemiparesis
- Long-term outcome also depends on extent and location of associated parenchymal injury
- Periventricular leukomalacia (ischemic infarction of the white matter adjacent to the lateral ventricles) may be associated with IVH and results in worse prognosis
- Posthemorrhagic hydrocephalus arrests or regresses in 65% of patients
- Progressive hydrocephalus leading to shunt placement worsens prognosis
- Ventriculoperitoneal shunt malfunctions or infections are known complications

Neonatal Seizures

INTRODUCTION

- Neonatal seizures occur due to sudden, abnormal synchronous depolarization of a group of neurons in the central nervous system
- In most cases, neonatal seizures are indicators of significant underlying neurologic disease
- Clinical features and EEG characteristics differ significantly from seizures in children
- The immature brain is more susceptible to epileptiform activity
- Neonatal seizures are poorly classified, underrecognized, and difficult to treat
- Prompt recognition, diagnosis, and intervention are indicated to minimize morbidity because seizures may have deleterious effects on developing brain
- Incidence is 0.2–1.4% of all newborns and is only rarely idiopathic

ETIOLOGY, EPIDEMIOLOGY, & RISK FACTORS

- The most common cause of neonatal seizures is hypoxic-ischemic encephalopathy (50–60% of cases); other causes include:
  - Intracranial infections (10% of cases): Bacterial infections include group B *Streptococcus*, *Listeria*, and *E. coli*; nonbacterial causes include toxoplasmosis, cytomegalovirus, herpes simplex, and rubella
  - Intracranial hemorrhage (10% of cases): Intraventricular hemorrhage is most common, as well as subarachnoid and subdural hemorrhages
  - Metabolic disturbance (eg, hypoglycemia, hypocalcemia, hypomagnesemia, hyponatremia)
  - Drug withdrawal (eg, cocaine, heroin, barbiturates)
  - Inborn errors of metabolism are relatively rare causes
  - Pyridoxine dependency is a rare condition but presents in the neonatal period
  - Cerebral dysgenesis and brain malformations
- Four distinctive neonatal seizures include: (1) familial neonatal convulsions, which are benign seizures starting the second or third day of life into infancy; (2) "fifth day fit," which may be due to zinc deficiency; (3) Ohtahara syndrome, which involves brief repetitive tonic spasms that carry a poor prognosis; and (4) early myoclonic encephalopathy, which is a refractory myoclonus with poor prognosis

PATIENT PRESENTATION

- Subtle seizures such as bicycling movements, lip smacking, roving eye movements, and apnea are more commonly seen in preterm infants
- Clonic seizures can either be focal or multifocal and are more typically seen in term infants
  - Focal: rhythmic, slow, jerking movements involving face and extremities on one side of body
  - Multifocal: several body parts seize together; newborns will not exhibit a classic Jacksonian march or a partial seizure with secondary generalization
- Tonic seizures (focal or generalized) are more common in premature infants with tonic posturing of neck, trunk, and upper extremities
- Myoclonic seizures (focal, multifocal, or generalized) are single or multiple, rapid, nonrhythmic jerks

DIFFERENTIAL DX

- Jitteriness (abolished by passive restraint)
- Benign sleep myoclonus
- Stimulus-evoked myoclonus
- Hyperekplexia or stiff man syndrome
- Apnea
- Drug withdrawal
- Sandifer syndrome
- Alternating hemiplegia of childhood
- Decerebrate or decorticate posturing
- Tetany from hypocalcemia

DIAGNOSTIC EVALUATION

- Obtain a careful history, including maternal history of drug use, intrauterine infection, and genetic or metabolic conditions, and physical examination, including blood pressure and evaluation for skin lesions and hepatosplenomegaly
- Neurologic examination should include level of alertness, cranial nerve testing, motor function, neonatal reflexes, and papillary exam, and should assess the fontanel
- Initial laboratory investigations should address potentially treatable causes and include serum chemistries (glucose, calcium, sodium, magnesium), arterial blood gas to determine pH and rule out metabolic acidosis, and lumbar puncture to identify subarachnoid hemorrhage or infection
- Further investigations include cranial ultrasound to rule out intraventricular hemorrhage; head CT scan and/or MRI of the brain to assess infarction, intracranial hemorrhage, calcifications, and cerebral malformations; and EEG to confirm and characterize the seizure activity
- Additional screening if these studies are negative includes serum ammonia, amino acids, lactate, pyruvate, and urine organic acids for metabolic diseases; serum, meconium, and urine toxicology screening; follow-up of routine expanded newborn screening results; urine for CMV and serum antibody titers for CMV and toxoplasmosis; and continuous EEG monitoring and video EEG monitoring

TREATMENT & MANAGEMENT

- Stabilize vital functions:
  - Secure the airway, which may require endotracheal intubation
  - Breathing: Supplemental oxygen, bag-mask ventilation
  - Circulation: Ensure IV access
- Correct metabolic disturbances:
  - Hypoglycemia: 10% dextrose IV (2 mL/kg) bolus followed by dextrose infusion
  - Hypocalcemia: 5% calcium gluconate IV (4 mL/kg) under cardiac monitoring
  - Hypomagnesemia: 50% magnesium sulfate IM (0.2 mL/kg)
- Anticonvulsant therapy:
  - Phenobarbital IV 20 mg/kg loading dose, followed by repeat doses of up to 40 mg/kg
  - Lorazepam IV (0.1 mg/kg)
  - Phenytoin IV (20 mg/kg) or phosphenytoin IV
- Pyridoxine IV (50–100 mg/kg) with continuous EEG monitoring
- Other anticonvulsants rarely used include primidone, lamotrigine, thiopentone, and carbamazepine
- Duration of anticonvulsant therapy depends on the etiology of seizures
- Early withdrawal of phenobarbital can be considered if the infant has a normal neurologic examination on discharge and repeat EEG is normal

PROGNOSIS & COMPLICATIONS

- Overall prognosis for survival in neonatal seizures is 85%
- Prognosis for long-term neurodevelopmental outcome is poor in half of cases
- Recurrent seizures, mental retardation, and motor dysfunction are common
- The most important determinant of outcome is the etiology of the seizures
- Metabolic disturbances, such as hypoglycemia and hypocalcemia, generally have a good prognosis
- Early onset of seizures, frequent or prolonged seizures, and seizures that are refractory to multiple anticonvulsants are associated with poor prognosis
- Neonatal seizures in infants younger than 32 weeks of gestation portend a poor prognosis

Neonatal Hypoglycemia

INTRODUCTION

- There is controversy over the definition of a "safe" blood glucose concentration (ie, a value below which there is risk of long-term neurodevelopmental impairment); a rigid definition of hypoglycemia relevant to all clinical situations cannot be made
- An operational definition of hypoglycemia is plasma glucose level of less than 40 mg/dL, below which further evaluation is required
- In clinical practice, hypoglycemia is most commonly seen in premature infants, small for gestational age infants, or infants of diabetic mothers
- Basal glucose utilization rates in newborn infants are 4–6 mg/kg/min, almost twice the weight-specific rates as adults

ETIOLOGY, EPIDEMIOLOGY, & RISK FACTORS

- Neonatal hypoglycemia is usually due to failure to adapt from the fetal state of continuous transplacental glucose consumption to the extrauterine pattern of intermittent nutrient supply
- Once the umbilical cord is clamped, glucose levels drop to a nadir within 1–2 hours
- The infant usually responds to this fall in glucose levels with glycogenolysis, gluconeogenesis, and utilization of glucose from feeds
- Glucose levels usually stabilize by 3–4 hours of life
- The overall incidence is 1–5 per 1000 live births but varies based on the definition
- Occurs in 8% of large for gestation babies and 15% of small for gestation babies
- Causes for hypoglycemia include:
  - Decreased stores (eg, prematurity, intrauterine growth retardation)
  - Hyperinsulinism states (eg, infant of diabetic mother, Beckwith-Wiedemann syndrome, erythroblastosis fetalis, islet cell hyperplasia, insulin-secreting tumors)
  - Perinatal stress (eg, sepsis, asphyxia, hypothermia, heart failure, respiratory distress)
  - Decreased glucose production (eg, glycogen storage disorders, galactosemia, adrenal insufficiency, hypopituitarism, hypothyroidism, cortisol deficiency, glucagon deficiency)
  - Reduced glucose supply (eg, delayed onset of feeding, inadequate caloric intake)
  - Iatrogenic factors (eg, glucose infusions in labor, maternal use of β-sympathomimetics)

PATIENT PRESENTATION

- Symptoms attributed to hypoglycemia are non-specific and may include:
  - Temperature instability
  - Sweating
  - Poor feeding
  - Vomiting
  - Apnea or irregular respirations
  - Tachypnea
  - Grunting
  - Cyanosis
  - Tachycardia
  - Hypotonia, limpness
  - Weak or high-pitched cry
  - Tremors
  - Jitteriness
  - Irritability
  - Seizures
  - Lethargy or stupor; coma

DIFFERENTIAL DX

- Hypocalcemia
- Sepsis
- Perinatal asphyxia
- Intracranial hemorrhage
- Drug withdrawal
- Inborn errors of metabolism
- Early necrotizing enterocolitis
- Aminophylline toxicity
- Hypomagnesemia
- Hyponatremia
- CNS malformations

DIAGNOSTIC EVALUATION

- Serial blood glucose levels should be routinely measured with reagent strips in high-risk infants, starting within 1–2 hours of birth
- Confirmatory laboratory plasma glucose (preferably by venous or arterial blood draw) should be performed if reagent strip level is less than 40 mg/dL
- Suggested investigations for persistent or severe hypoglycemia include:
  - Serum electrolytes, liver functions, serum ketones, and acid-base status
  - Serum ammonia, plasma amino acids, lactate, pyruvate, and free fatty acids
  - Insulin and C peptide, growth hormone, cortisol, and thyroid hormones
  - Other blood tests include galactosemia screen, alanine, glycerol, total and free carnitine, and acylcarnitine profile
  - Urine for ketones, organic acids, and reducing substances (galactosemia)
  - Other investigations include ophthalmic examination (septo-optic dysplasia) and either cranial ultrasound scan or brain MRI (pituitary and hypothalamic anomalies)
  - Blood samples for additional testing should be drawn during a hypoglycemic episode

TREATMENT & MANAGEMENT

Prevention
- Avoid excessive maternal glucose infusion during labor and neonatal hypothermia
- All healthy and mature infants should be fed as soon as possible after birth
- Near-term infants too immature to suckle should be given supplementary feeds either by cup or by gavage; sick infants should be started on 10% dextrose infusion prophylactically

Management
- Moderate, asymptomatic hypoglycemia should first be treated by adjusting the enteral feeding regimen (eg, frequent feeding, supplementing with additional calories)
- Indications for IV therapy include failure of enteral feeding, symptomatic hypoglycemia, severe hypoglycemia (<25 mg/dL), and sick infants in whom enteral feeds are contraindicated
- Emergency management should be with bolus of 10% dextrose solution (2 cc/kg)
- This is followed by a glucose infusion at a rate of 6–8 mg/kg/min
- Increase rate of glucose infusion as needed to maintain normal glucose levels; monitor glucose levels every hour until stable; taper IV fluids gradually as enteral feeding is resumed
- If glucose infusion rate of 16–20 mg/kg/min is needed to maintain normoglycemia, look for underlying endocrine disorders
- For severe, persistent hypoglycemia, consider IV hydrocortisone and oral diazoxide
- Other drugs used include glucagon (IM or IV), somatostatin, and octreotide

PROGNOSIS & COMPLICATIONS

- Most hypoglycemia will resolve within 2–3 days
- Transient asymptomatic hypoglycemia in a healthy neonate has a good prognosis
- There is no evidence that low blood glucose concentrations among healthy breastfed term babies are detrimental to outcome
- Prognosis depends on the etiology, severity, and persistence of hypoglycemia
- Data on long-term neurologic damage due to hypoglycemia in neonates is inconclusive
- Hypoglycemic seizures suggest increased risk for long-term developmental problems
- Hypoglycemia may contribute to abnormal neurodevelopmental outcomes in infants who have other risk factors for brain injury, such as prematurity or hypoxic-ischemic brain injury

Neonatal Jaundice

INTRODUCTION

- Jaundice or hyperbilirubinemia implies an excessive level of serum bilirubin
- Neonatal jaundice is a common condition; the cause is most often developmental, and the course is usually benign
- Severe, indirect (unconjugated) hyperbilirubinemia is potentially neurotoxic
- Direct (conjugated) hyperbilirubinemia usually signifies liver disease or systemic illness
- Acute bilirubin encephalopathy describes the clinical central nervous system findings caused by bilirubin toxicity to the basal ganglia and various brainstem nuclei
- The term "kernicterus" should be reserved for the chronic and permanent clinical sequelae of bilirubin toxicity

ETIOLOGY, EPIDEMIOLOGY, & RISK FACTORS

- Bilirubin is derived from the breakdown of hemoglobin in senescent or hemolyzed RBCs
- Factors that predispose to physiologic hyperbilirubinemia in newborn infants include: increased bilirubin production from high red cell load, decreased red cell survival, and ineffective erythropoiesis; decreased uptake, conjugation, and excretion of bilirubin by the liver due to immaturity; and increased enterohepatic circulation of bilirubin due to the absence of anaerobic flora in the neonatal intestines that normally conjugates bilirubin
- Physiologic jaundice is usually visible by the second or third day, peaks at 5–6 mg/dL between the third and fourth day, and then drops below 2 mg/dL between the fifth and seventh day
- Jaundice is considered pathologic if onset is before 24 hours, if bilirubin is rising at greater than 0.5 mg/dL/hr, if it persists after 14 days, or if there are signs of underlying illness
- Early jaundice (1–2 days) is usually due to acute hemolytic conditions (eg, Rh or ABO incompatibility) or other unusual antibodies
- Jaundice between the third and tenth days may be due to physiologic jaundice, infant of a diabetic mother, cephalohematoma, infection, or asphyxia
- Late-onset or prolonged jaundice (beyond 14 days) may be due to biliary atresia, galactosemia, hepatitis, or infection

PATIENT PRESENTATION

- Jaundice is usually seen in the face first and progresses caudally to the trunk and extremities
- Other signs and symptoms may be present depending on the etiology (eg, large cephalohematoma, excessive bruising, pallor, petechiae, hepatosplenomegaly, omphalitis, dysmorphic features, microcephaly, chorioretinitis)
- Signs of acute bilirubin encephalopathy include:
  - Early phase (1–2 days): Poor suck, hypotonia, and lethargy
  - Intermediate phase (3–7 days): Moderate stupor, irritability, hypertonia, opisthotonos, retrocollis
  - Advanced phase (>7 days): Pronounced retrocollis-opisthotonos, shrill cry, no feeding, apnea, fever, deep stupor, coma, seizures
- Signs of kernicterus

DIFFERENTIAL DX

- Indirect hyperbilirubinemia:
  - Physiologic jaundice
  - ABO incompatibility
  - Breast milk jaundice
  - Rh isoimmunization
  - Neonatal sepsis
  - G6PD deficiency
  - Hereditary spherocytosis
  - Gilbert disease
  - Crigler-Najjar syndrome
- Direct hyperbilirubinemia:
  - Biliary atresia
  - Idiopathic neonatal hepatitis
  - Choledochal cyst
  - Neonatal (TORCH) infection
  - α_1-antitrypsin deficiency
  - Parenteral nutrition
  - Galactosemia

DIAGNOSTIC EVALUATION

- During pregnancy, test for ABO and Rh blood types and perform a serum screen for unusual isoimmune antibodies
- If a mother is Rh-negative (or if prenatal testing is not done), do a direct antibody test (direct Coombs test), blood type, and Rh type on the infant's cord blood
- If mother is type O and Rh-positive, test the cord blood for infant's blood type and DAT
- Indications for measuring transcutaneous bilirubin (TcB) or total serum bilirubin (TSB) in a term or near-term (>35 weeks of gestation) infant include: Jaundice during the first 24 hours or jaundice that appears excessive for the infant's age
- Bilirubin levels should be interpreted according to the infant's age in hours
- If the infant requires phototherapy or if jaundice is rising rapidly, test for blood type and Rh type, CBC with smear, and total and direct bilirubin
- If the infant is not responding to phototherapy or if bilirubin level is reaching exchange transfusion levels, perform a reticulocyte count, G6PD screen, and serum albumin level
- If direct bilirubin levels are elevated, then, in addition to the above, consider liver function tests, blood and urine cultures, TORCH screen, serum α_1-antitrypsin levels, urine for reducing substances (galactosemia), abdominal ultrasound (cholelithiasis, choledochal cysts), and radionuclide scan (to evaluate the biliary anatomy)

TREATMENT & MANAGEMENT

- Prevent severe jaundice by nursing infants at least 8–12 times per day for the first several days, and perform repeated systematic assessments during the neonatal period
- Treat with phototherapy according to AAP recommended nomograms
  - Phototherapy is most effective with blue light of 425- to 475-nm wavelength
  - Bilirubin absorbs this light from the skin surface and undergoes photoisomerization to a less toxic isomer that is excreted readily into bile, structural isomerization to lumirubin, which is rapidly excreted into bile and urine, and photo-oxidation to a more polar substance that is soluble in urine
  - Repeat testing for total serum bilirubin level in 4–24 hours, depending on the infant's age and bilirubin level; discontinue phototherapy when total serum bilirubin is less than 13–14 mg/dL
- Exchange transfusion is considered if total serum bilirubin is >25 mg/dL in a term infant, total serum bilirubin is >20 mg/dL in a sick or premature infant, or there is rapidly rising total serum bilirubin despite intensive phototherapy
- Intravenous immunoglobulin (IVIG) can be tried in patients who are close to requiring exchange transfusions
- Consider supplemental formula or IV fluids if weight loss less than 12% of birth weight

PROGNOSIS & COMPLICATIONS

- Use of intensive early screening and phototherapy has significantly decreased the need for exchange transfusions and the incidence of kernicterus
- Side effects of phototherapy include increased insensible water loss, watery diarrhea, hypocalcemia, and skin rashes
- There is a theoretical risk of retinal damage, mutations, DNA strand breaks, and sister chromatid exchange, and thus warrants eye and scrotal shielding during phototherapy
- Complications of exchange transfusion includes hypocalcemia, hypomagnesemia, hypoglycemia, acid-base imbalance, hyperkalemia, volume overload, blood-borne infections, thrombocytopenia, clotting factor deficiencies, and hemolysis
- Prognosis for direct hyperbilirubinemia depends on the etiology

Infant of Diabetic Mother

INTRODUCTION

- Infants of diabetic mothers (IDM) are at risk for hypoglycemia in the neonatal period
- Infants born to mothers with diabetes are also at significantly greater risk for spontaneous abortion, stillbirth, congenital malformations, and perinatal morbidity and mortality
- The pathologic conditions in an infant of a diabetic mother are the result of fetal hyperglycemia and/or hyperinsulinemia
- Macrosomia (birth weight >4000 g or 90th percentile) in these babies places them at greater risk for shoulder dystocia, birth trauma, and need for cesarean section delivery
- With appropriate management and good glycemic control, outcomes are comparable to the general population

ETIOLOGY, EPIDEMIOLOGY, & RISK FACTORS

- 3–10% of all pregnancies are affected by abnormal glucose regulation and control; of these, 80% are caused by gestational diabetes mellitus
- 30–40% of IDM have hypoglycemia after birth, and nearly 10% have congenital anomalies
- The Pedersen hypothesis suggests that maternal hyperglycemia results in fetal hyperglycemia because glucose readily traverses the placenta
- Before 20 weeks of gestation, the fetal islet cells are not capable of responsive insulin secretion, and hence the fetus is exposed to the detrimental effects of hyperglycemia
- After 20 weeks, unchecked fetal hyperglycemia results in hypertrophy of the fetal pancreatic islets and hyperinsulinemia
- The incidence of congenital anomalies is 4-fold higher with poor maternal glucose control in early gestation
- Hyperinsulinemia, a major anabolic hormone, and hyperglycemia, a major anabolic fuel, results in macrosomia during late gestation
- Abrupt cessation of placental glucose delivery accompanied by hyperinsulinemia leads to neonatal hypoglycemia

PATIENT PRESENTATION

- Signs and symptoms of hypoglycemia, hypocalcemia, and hypomagnesemia
- Macrosomia
- Intrauterine growth retardation due to maternal renovascular disease occurs in 5% of cases
- Respiratory distress due to transient tachypnea (TTN) and respiratory distress syndrome (RDS)
- Signs of cardiac failure due to cardiac anomalies or myocardial dysfunction
- Cyanosis due to cyanotic heart diseases
- Single umbilical artery
- Vomiting due to duodenal atresia
- Failure to pass meconium due to anorectal atresia or small left colon syndrome
- Hematuria due to renal vein thrombosis
- Brachial plexus injuries, clavicle fractures due to shoulder dystocia
- CNS abnormalities may occur

DIFFERENTIAL DX

Macrosomia
- Large for gestational age infant
- Beckwith-Wiedemann syndrome
- Sotos syndrome
- Simpson-Golabi-Behmel syndrome
- Weaver syndrome

Hypoglycemia
- Prematurity
- Sepsis
- Congenital hyperinsulinism
- Defects in counterregulatory hormones
- Metabolic disease

DIAGNOSTIC EVALUATION

- Prenatal investigations include: Prenatal ultrasound for diagnosis of macrosomic fetus or organ defects, biophysical profile, and maternal hemoglobin A_{1c} level
- Delivery room physical assessment should evaluate for congenital anomalies and birth injuries, size for dates, and respiratory distress
- Postnatal evaluation includes: Blood glucose estimation by glucometer at 0.5, 1, 2, 4, 8, 12, 24, 36, and 48 hours; calcium levels at 6, 24, and 48 hours to rule out hypocalcemia; magnesium levels should be checked if calcium is low; CBC to rule out polycythemia and thrombocytopenia; and bilirubin levels due to higher risk of hyperbilirubinemia
- Also consider the following tests based on clinical suspicions:
  - Chest X-ray for TTN and RDS
  - Blood gas to evaluate gas exchange and right-to-left shunting
  - Echocardiogram and EKG may show septal hypertrophy due to the growth effects of insulin
  - Renal ultrasound may show kidney and renovascular pathologies
  - Abdominal imaging, including X-rays, barium enema, and upper GI series, if suspect obstruction

TREATMENT & MANAGEMENT

- Asymptomatic infants with normal blood glucose levels should be started on enteral feeding as early as possible
- Consider infusion of 10% dextrose to maintain euglycemia (glucose >40 mg/dL) in infants with symptomatic hypoglycemia, failure of enteral feeding, sick infants, and infants <2000 g birth weight
- Maintain glucose infusion rates of 6–8 mg/kg/min, and increase as necessary
- Follow and correct electrolytes and calcium and magnesium disturbances as necessary
- Supplemental oxygen and mechanical ventilation for respiratory distress
- Monitor for signs of heart failure and hypoperfusion in cases of septal hypertrophy and cardiomyopathy
- Treat hyperbilirubinemia as necessary
- Partial exchange transfusion is occasionally required for polycythemia
- Poor feeding is a major problem, often in the absence of other problems, and is a major reason for prolonged hospital stay

PROGNOSIS & COMPLICATIONS

- Macrosomia usually resolves during infancy; however, there might be an increased incidence of diabetes mellitus and obesity in later life
- Neurodevelopmental sequelae also depend on the presence of anomalies, perinatal asphyxia, hypoglycemia, and metabolic acidosis
- Prognosis is improved if appropriate care is provided during the perinatal period
- Cardiovascular anomalies: Septal hypertrophy, cardiomyopathy, complex congenital heart disease; renal anomalies: hydronephrosis, renal agenesis, renal vein thrombosis, double ureter
- Neurologic: Agenesis of the lower spine (caudal regression syndrome), hemivertebrae, meningocele, anencephaly, and spina bifida
- Gastrointestinal: Small left colon syndrome

Sudden Infant Death Syndrome

INTRODUCTION

- Sudden infant death syndrome (SIDS) is defined as the sudden death of an infant less than 1 year old that cannot be explained by history and postmortem evaluation
- A thorough postmortem evaluation includes a complete autopsy, review of the death scene, and review of the clinical history
- Apparent life-threatening event (ALTE) is defined as an episode that is frightening to the observer and is characterized by some combination of apnea, color change, change in muscle tone, choking, or gagging
- "Aborted crib death" or "near-miss SIDS," used previously for ALTE, should be abandoned because these imply a misleadingly close association between ALTE and SIDS

ETIOLOGY, EPIDEMIOLOGY, & RISK FACTORS

- SIDS is the third leading cause of infant mortality, after congenital anomalies and disorders related to short gestation and low birth weight
- Peak incidence is between 2–4 months; 90% of cases occur within the first 6 months
- Incidence has decreased dramatically after adopting "back to sleep" recommendations in 1992
- SIDS rates are higher in the African-American population than in the Caucasian, Hispanic, and Asian populations, and it appears to be more common in male infants, premature and low birth weight infants, intrauterine growth restriction, and in multiple gestations
- Prone sleeping position has a higher risk for SIDS than other positions
- Environmental risk factors include lower socioeconomic status, crowded living conditions, winter season, soft mattresses, and bed sharing
- Maternal risk factors include smoking, drug abuse, young maternal age, higher parity, unmarried mothers, single parenthood, and lack of breastfeeding
- Apnea of prematurity is not a risk factor for SIDS
- Proposed mechanisms include accidental asphyxiation on bedding or clothing, developmental abnormalities of the cardiorespiratory center, undetected cardiac arrhythmias including prolonged QT interval, and impaired arousal responses during illness

PATIENT PRESENTATION

- Death scene investigation might reveal:
  - Prone or side-sleeping position
  - Soft sleeping surface
  - Unsafe sleeping environment
  - Poor heating or overheating, causing thermal stress
  - Parental drug use or smoking
  - Prematurity
  - Small for gestational age infant
  - Petechial hemorrhages
  - Frothy secretions at nose or mouth
  - Evidence of congenital anomalies
  - Recent illness or infection

DIFFERENTIAL DX

- Traumatic child abuse
- Unintentional injury (eg, suffocation due to a soft mattress, strangulation from toys, overlaying by a caregiver during sleep)
- Death due to natural causes (eg, infection and sepsis, congenital anomalies, cardiac arrhythmias, or metabolic disorders, such as medium-chain acyl-coenzyme A dehydrogenase deficiency, urea cycle disorders, and propionic and methylmalonic acidemias)

DIAGNOSTIC EVALUATION

- SIDS is a postmortem diagnosis of exclusion, and no pathology explains death
- Some common but subtle observations on autopsy consistent with SIDS include:
  - Petechial hemorrhages
  - Pulmonary edema
  - Hepatic erythropoiesis
  - Intrathoracic petechiae
  - Retention of periadrenal brown fat
  - Minor inflammatory changes in respiratory tract
  - Brainstem gliosis
  - Persistence of dendritic spines in the brainstem respiratory centers
  - Brainstem hypomyelination
  - Periventricular leukomalacia
- Pneumograms and polysomnographs cannot predict the risk for SIDS and should not be used for this purpose; they can be used judiciously in premature infants with apnea and patients with acute life-threatening events to clarify the details of the event and guide therapy
- Gastroesophageal reflux has not been convincingly linked to SIDS

TREATMENT & MANAGEMENT

- Preventive measures include:
  - Recommend supine sleeping position for healthy infants
  - Educate parents about the dangers of exposing babies to tobacco smoke
  - Recommend the use of firm crib mattress meeting federal standards
  - Avoid putting babies to sleep on sofas, bean bags, sheepskin, pillows, and other soft surfaces
  - Bed sharing may be hazardous, especially if parents smoke or abuse alcohol or drugs
  - Educate daycare providers of the risk factors for SIDS
  - Avoid overheating the bedroom and avoid overdressing infants
  - Encourage breastfeeding
  - The use of a pacifier during sleep may reduce risk
- Routine EKG screening of all infants to detect prolonged QT interval is not recommended
- Devices advertised to maintain sleep position or reduce risk of rebreathing are not recommended
- Home apnea monitors may be of value in selected patients with extreme instability (eg, premature babies with symptomatic apnea and bradycardia at the time of discharge, selected patients with acute life-threatening events)

PROGNOSIS & COMPLICATIONS

- Prevention campaigns have been successful in decreasing the incidence of SIDS internationally through the past decade
- Continued education of the public and scientific communities will reduce the incidence further; however, it is unlikely that this disorder will be eliminated completely

Respiratory Distress Syndrome

INTRODUCTION

- Neonatal respiratory distress syndrome (RDS) differs from adult RDS in that it is a disease of prematurity; it was previously called "hyaline membrane disease"
- Occurs due to insufficient production or activity of lung surfactant, which is a complex mixture of phospholipids and proteins that coats the inner surface of the alveoli, reducing alveolar surface tension to maintain alveolar stability
- Surfactant appears in the fetal lung at 23–24 weeks gestation, but adequate amounts are not secreted until at least 30–32 weeks of gestation; deficiency results in a marked decrease in lung compliance, leading to alveolar collapse, atelectasis, and intrapulmonary shunting
- Antenatal corticosteroids/exogenous surfactant replacement have improved outcome

ETIOLOGY, EPIDEMIOLOGY, & RISK FACTORS

- The most common cause of respiratory failure in premature infants
- Incidence/severity inversely proportional to gestational age: Occurs in 60–80% of infants born <28 weeks but 15–30% born at 32–36 weeks; other risk factors include: male, Caucasian, maternal diabetes, perinatal asphyxia, hypothermia, multiple gestation, and Caesarian section
- Factors that reduce the risk and severity of disease include chronic or pregnancy-induced hypertension, maternal opiate use, prolonged rupture of membranes, chronic congenital infections, and antenatal steroids
- Deficient surfactant synthesis causes profound atelectasis with resultant hypoxia, pulmonary edema, intra-alveolar vascular and lymphatic congestion, interstitial emphysema, and intra-alveolar hemorrhage
- The classic eosinophilic "hyaline membrane" that lines the terminal bronchioles and alveolar ducts appears as early as 6–8 hours after birth; it consists of a fibrinous matrix of material derived from blood and cellular debris from the injured epithelium
- Pathologic findings include atelectasis, pulmonary edema, intra-alveolar vascular and lymphatic congestion, interstitial emphysema, and intra-alveolar hemorrhage
- Exposure to high inspired oxygen concentration and mechanical ventilation cause further damage to the alveolar epithelial lining

PATIENT PRESENTATION

- Signs of respiratory distress occur within the first minutes to first hours of life: tachypnea, grunting, subcostal and sternal retractions, decreased breath sounds, fine rales or crackles on auscultation, cyanosis, hypercapnia
- Apnea and irregular respirations are ominous signs of respiratory failure and require immediate intervention
- Additional features include pallor, hypotension, peripheral edema, and poor perfusion
- Symptoms reach a peak within 3 days, after which there is gradual improvement, which is usually heralded by a phase of diuresis
- In severe cases, recovery may be delayed for days, weeks, or months

DIFFERENTIAL DX

- Transient tachypnea of the newborn
- Pneumonia
- Spontaneous pneumothorax
- Perinatal asphyxia
- Diaphragmatic hernia
- Early-onset sepsis
- Congenital heart disease or lung anomaly
- Persistent pulmonary hypertension
- Aspiration syndromes
- Anemia or polycythemia
- Pulmonary hypoplasia
- Congenital alveolar proteinosis
- Surfactant protein B deficiency

DIAGNOSTIC EVALUATION

- Prenatal prediction of lung maturity by amniocentesis:
  - Lecithin-sphingomyelin ratio in amniotic fluid for fetal lung maturity
  - Surfactant-albumin ratio in amniotic fluid is another index of fetal lung maturity
- History may reveal corresponding history of prematurity and other risk factors
- Clinical examination may reveal early respiratory distress with grunting, flaring, and retractions, as well as decreased air entry and fine rales throughout the lung fields
- Chest X-ray shows a characteristic pattern:
  - "Ground-glass" appearance with increased density and fine granularity of both lung fields
  - Air bronchograms (the outline of an air-filled bronchiole surrounded by fluid-filled parenchyma or air spaces)
  - Hypoinflation with elevation of the diaphragm
  - Complete "white-out" with complete loss of heart borders in severe cases
  - Pneumothorax and pneumomediastinum are common in severe cases
  - Cardiomegaly indicates underlying hypoxemic insult or patent ductus arteriosus
- Lab testing includes arterial blood gas (ABG), CBC, calcium, glucose, and blood cultures
  - Frequent ABG monitoring is required: Hypoxemia is common, hypercapnia and respiratory acidosis occur in moderate to severe cases, metabolic acidosis in severe cases
  - CBC and blood cultures to rule out early-onset neonatal sepsis
- Echocardiogram in selected cases may reveal a patent ductus arteriosus or pulmonary hypertension and is also helpful in assessing cardiac function

TREATMENT & MANAGEMENT

Preventive Measures

- Avoid prematurity by optimizing timing of Caesarean deliveries and appropriate management of high-risk pregnancies
- Estimate fetal lung maturity prior to delivery in high-risk cases
- Antenatal dexamethasone or betamethasone given to women at risk of preterm delivery accelerates fetal surfactant production and lung maturation

Postnatal Management

- Supplemental oxygen to maintain arterial pO_2 between 55–70 mmHg (may be the sole therapy for larger infants with minimal hypercarbia and mild to moderate hypoxemia)
- Nasal CPAP to reduce O_2 requirements and need for mechanical ventilation, prevent atelectasis, and improve gas exchange; endotracheal intubation and mechanical ventilation are required in severe cases; high-frequency ventilation may be successful in severe disease
- Administer exogenous surfactant via endotracheal tube (repeated doses may be required in severe cases); replacement is most effective when given at the time of delivery (prophylactic), rather than when symptoms develop (rescue)
- Broad-spectrum antibiotics to treat presumed bacterial pneumonia or sepsis
- Rapid correction of metabolic acidosis with sodium bicarbonate infusion should be avoided because it may increase the risk for intraventricular hemorrhage

PROGNOSIS & COMPLICATIONS

- In infants older than 32–33 weeks of gestation, lung function may normalize within 1 week
- In more premature infants, prolonged mechanical ventilation and oxygen will usually be required; bronchopulmonary dysplasia is the long-term complication of this and is common in most infants who weigh less than 1000 g at birth
- Complications may include barotrauma, patent ductus arteriosus, nosocomial infections, intraventricular hemorrhage, bronchopulmonary dysplasia, and retinopathy of prematurity
- If death occurs, it is usually due to associated pneumothorax, pulmonary hemorrhage, or intraventricular hemorrhage

Congenital/Genetic Diseases

Trisomy 21 (Down Syndrome)

INTRODUCTION

- Down syndrome is a well-recognized genetic disorder that arises from either a simple duplication of chromosome 21 (sometimes mosaic), a balanced translocation in either parent, or a de novo Robertsonian translocation
- Mental retardation and a characteristic facial appearance are the most-well known features, but the disorder may also include cardiac, orthopedic, head and neck, gastrointestinal, and immunologic abnormalities
- Extensive, cohesive, comprehensive care is required to meet the broad medical, developmental, and psychosocial needs of the patient and family

ETIOLOGY, EPIDEMIOLOGY, & RISK FACTORS

- Occurs in all racial and ethnic groups
- Slightly greater frequency in males than females
- Occurs in 1 in 650–1000 live births
- Associated with advanced parental age, particularly maternal age over 40
- 95% of cases are simple trisomy with three freestanding copies of chromosome 21
  - 4% translocation of chromosome 21 (2% de novo mutation and 2% balanced translocation)
  - 1% mosaic with some normal chromosome pairs
- Coexisting conditions include:
  - Thyroid disease in 40% of patients
  - 15-fold increased risk of leukemia
  - Increased incidence of autism spectrum disorders, diabetes mellitus, Alzheimer disease, and celiac disease
  - Almost all cases have significant morbidity from frequent upper and lower respiratory tract infections

PATIENT PRESENTATION

- Hypotonia and microcephaly
- Mild to moderate mental retardation
- Atlanto-axial instability
- Delay of almost all parameters of growth and development: physical growth, developmental milestones, cognition, and even tooth eruption
- Epicanthal folds, upward slanting palpebral fissures, glossal protrusion
- Stenotic ear canals and eustachian tubes
- Frequent upper and lower respiratory tract infections and gingival disease
- Congenital heart defects and VSD
- Congenital abdominal defects (duodenal atresia, tracheoesophageal fistula or atresia, pyloric stenosis, and Hirschsprung disease), which present as intestinal obstruction or aspiration
- Single palmar crease
- Separation of first and second toes

DIFFERENTIAL DX

- May be confused with Zellweger syndrome because of similar facial phenotype
- Other chromosome abnormalities (including Smith-Magenis)

DIAGNOSTIC EVALUATION

- Prenatal screening:
  - Maternal serum screen may reveal low α-fetoprotein, low unconjugated estriol, and elevated human chorionic gonadotropin
  - Prenatal ultrasound may show characteristic findings such as increased nuchal fold
  - Definitive prenatal diagnosis by chorionic villous sampling, amniocentesis, percutaneous umbilical blood sampling, and sometimes extraction of fetal cells from maternal circulation
  - For in vitro fertilization, pre-implantation genetic testing is performed before selecting the embryo to be implanted
- After birth, infants may often be suspected of having Down syndrome via recognition by phenotypic characteristics
- Karyotype analysis
- If the patient has a translocation defect, karyotyping of both parents is indicated to complete genetic counseling
- FISH (fluorescent in situ hybridization) may be used with both prenatal and postnatal specimens
- Other laboratory testing includes thyroid function studies to assess for hypothyroidism and quantitative immunoglobins with subclasses (because inadequate IgA is associated and may cause frequent respiratory and gingival infections)

TREATMENT & MANAGEMENT

- Early involvement in developmental support services to optimize cognitive and social progress
- Feeding and nutritional consults to support suboptimal feeding during the newborn period and prevent obesity in childhood and adolescence
- Growth and development expectations via Down-specific growth charts
- Cardiology evaluation:
  - Fetal echocardiogram is indicated when Down syndrome is known or suspected
  - Neonatal echocardiogram should be obtained expeditiously when features of Down syndrome are noted after birth, whether or not there is an audible murmur
- Audiology and ophthalmology evaluations in the newborn period and annually
- Meticulous dental care
- Screening for atlantoaxial instability by age 3
- Pneumococcal, respiratory syncytial virus, and influenza vaccines for children with chronic respiratory or cardiac disease
- Genetic counseling
- Screening for celiac disease by age 3

PROGNOSIS & COMPLICATIONS

- A majority of fetuses with Down syndrome undergo intrauterine fetal demise
- Life expectancy is reduced; among patients who survive infancy, many live to their 50s or 60s
- Physical prognosis is determined by the presence of major cardiac or gastrointestinal anomalies; outcome depends on the degree of developmental intervention and quality of medical care
- May develop early CHF and valvular disease due to high pulmonary vascular resistance
- Neurologic sequelae of atlantoaxial instability (spinal cord compression) include torticollis, gait abnormalities, loss of strength, and impaired bowel/bladder function

Klinefelter Syndrome

INTRODUCTION

- Klinefelter syndrome is the name for the genetic disorder created by one or more extra X chromosomes and sometimes one or more extra Y chromosomes
- The disorder is associated with hypogonadism and small testes, azoospermia or oligospermia, and infertility, as well as gynecomastia and reduced face and body hair; developmental, cardiac, and orthopedic aberrations may also be present
- The testicular failure of Klinefelter syndrome results in androgen deficiency, which leads to most of the typical phenotypic characteristics
- Mental retardation may be present, but the average IQ in classic Klinefelter syndrome is only slightly decreased (approximately 90) from the general population

ETIOLOGY, EPIDEMIOLOGY, & RISK FACTORS

- Associated with advanced parental age, which leads to chromosome nondisjunction
- Occurs only in males
- X chromosome aneuploidy may include 47,XXY (80%), 46,XX/47,XXY (10%), 48,XXXY, 48,XXYY, or 49,XXXXY
  - Increasing medical problems are associated with increased X chromosome aneuploidy
  - A decrease in IQ occurs with increased X chromosome aneuploidy; patients with 49,XXXXY function at a similar level as patients with Down syndrome
- Among fetuses with Klinefelter syndrome, over half undergo fetal demise
- Prevalence of 1 in 1000 male births
- There is increased incidence of autoimmune disorders in these patients

PATIENT PRESENTATION

- Few physical problems occur during childhood
- Testosterone-dependent effects include:
  - Altered body habitus with long arms and legs, slim build, and female type of fat distribution (eunuchoid)
  - Small testes: 1–2 cm (normal, 3.5–4.5 cm)
  - Sparse facial and body hair
  - Gynecomastia
  - Osteoporosis
- Neurodevelopmental problems include delays in speech and language; learning disabilities, such as memory deficits, ADHD, and dyslexia; and psychiatric disorders, such as anxiety and depression (sometimes secondary to the stress of societal unacceptance due to the phenotype)
- Cardiac manifestations include mitral valve prolapse and varicose veins, sometimes with recurrent DVTs or stasis ulcers

DIFFERENTIAL DX

- Similar body habitus seen in homocystinuria and Marfan syndrome
- Other causes of hypogonadism (eg, primary testicular failure, hypogonadotropic hypogonadism, panhypopituitarism, and Kallman syndrome)
- Transient gynecomastia may be a part of normal puertal development

DIAGNOSTIC EVALUATION

- May be an incidental finding during prenatal amniocentesis or chorionic villous sampling
- Clinical diagnosis is typically made during adolescence due to problems with pubertal development
- Laboratory testing includes peripheral blood chromosome analysis, low plasma testosterone levels in the presence of normal or high FSH, LH, and estrogen; and abnormal gonadotropin stimulation test (testosterone should normally increase when the patient is administered hCG)
- Echocardiography to assess for mitral valve prolapse
- Bone density studies

TREATMENT & MANAGEMENT

- Begin testosterone supplementation at the onset of puberty
  - Testosterone is given by periodic injections or patch
  - Appropriate virilization should normalize sexual desire, increase strength and muscle mass, and protect against osteoporosis
  - Testosterone supplementation may improve mood and prevent the psychosocial stress that often occurs due to inadequate male development
- Monitor for developmental and learning problems (testosterone supplementation does not protect against learning disorders)
- Surgical intervention may be warranted for severe gynecomastia
- Counseling for infertility

PROGNOSIS & COMPLICATIONS

- Sexual orientation is generally heterosexual, but there may be a decrease in libido
- Patients with 48XXXY and 49XXXXY have more marked symptoms, and mental retardation is common
- Life expectancy is not altered

Marfan Syndrome

INTRODUCTION

- Marfan syndrome is a genetic disorder of fibrillin, a building block of connective tissue
- Fibrillin is the main component of myofibrils, which are structural components of the aorta, lung, dura mater, and suspensory ligament of the lens of the eye
- The most striking external feature is the marfanoid body habitus: tall height and long arms, legs, fingers, and toes, none of which poses a medical threat
- The associated internal anomalies may be life-threatening:
  - Eyes: Dislocated lens (ectopia lentis)
  - Lungs: Spontaneous pneumothorax and apical blebs
  - Cardiovascular: Dilated aorta with or without aortic dissection and mitral valve prolapse

ETIOLOGY, EPIDEMIOLOGY, & RISK FACTORS

- Caused by a defect of the fibrillin-1 gene, leading to defects of the eyes, lungs, skeletal system, heart, and vasculature
- There are two genes for fibrillin; affected patients are usually heterozygous, with one gene coding for normal fibrillin and the other coding for defective fibrillin
- There are a number of types of mutations of the gene (FBN1 mutations)
- There is variable expression of the abnormal gene; patients with Marfan may exhibit isolated anomalies or any combination of associated features
- Incidence of 1–2 cases per 10,000 live births
- 75% of cases are familial autosomal dominant inheritance
- 25% of cases are new mutations (new mutations may result in the classic Marfan syndrome or a more severe neonatal form)

PATIENT PRESENTATION

- Marfanoid body habitus: reduced ratio of upper to lower body length, increased arm span, arachnodactyly (long fingers and toes), pectus deformity, scoliosis
- Developmental delay of gross motor skills secondary to decreased ligamentous integrity
- Cardiac manifestations: murmur of mitral valve prolapse and regurgitation, tricuspid regurgitation, and aortic dilatation and dissection, ranging from asymptomatic to sudden onset of chest pain progressing to sudden death
- Pulmonary: spontaneous pneumothorax is common; pectus deformities may impair lung function
- Ocular: ectopia lentis (dislocated lens of the eye)
- Skin stretch marks despite thin body habitus

DIFFERENTIAL DX

- Congenital contractural arachnodactyly (Beals syndrome)
- Ehlers-Danlos syndrome
- Shprintzen-Goldberg syndrome
- Trisomy 8
- Stickler syndrome
- Homocystinuria
- Klinefelter syndrome (in males)

DIAGNOSTIC EVALUATION

- The diagnosis is typically established by clinical criteria and family history
  - If there is a positive family history: Involvement of two or more organ systems suggests the diagnosis
  - If there is no family history: Diagnosis should only be made if there are typical skeletal findings plus involvement of two other organs with at least one major criterion (dislocated lens, aortic root dilatation, or dural ectasia)
  - In families with a known history of Marfan syndrome, linkage studies may also be used
  - In patients without a family history, homocysteine levels should be measured to rule out homocystinuria
  - The Ghent and Berlin criteria are systems of classifying marfanoid manifestations into major and minor criteria, with a formula for diagnosis
  - Major criteria include the presence of a genetic mutation known to cause Marfan in the general population or in a relative with Marfan syndrome and family history of a first-degree relative with Marfan syndrome
- Laboratory testing includes evaluation of microfibrils in cultured skin fibroblasts and DNA testing of the FBN1 gene
- Echocardiography to assess valvular function and aortic configuration
- MRI may show dural ectasia

TREATMENT & MANAGEMENT

- Monitor regularly for aortic changes with echocardiography and MRI
  - Once the aorta begins to dilate, β-blockers are used to slow progress
  - Surgical intervention becomes necessary when aorta dilates beyond 5 cm
- Valve replacement may be necessary; anticoagulation is necessary in patients who have undergone valve replacements
- Ocular involvement requires periodic visits with an ophthalmologist
  - Ectopia lentis and myopia may both be treated surgically
- Musculoskeletal involvement requires early intervention and occupational and/or physical therapy for gross motor delay
  - Scoliosis frequently requires surgery; bracing is not usually effective
  - Surgery for pectus may improve lung function, but relapses are common
  - Pain management (chronic pain often present due to joint problems)
  - Contact sports and physically rigorous activities should be avoided

PROGNOSIS & COMPLICATIONS

- With appropriate medical and surgical management, most patients have a nearly normal life expectancy
- Prior to prophylactic surgery for aortic pathology, life expectancy was 30–40 years
- The neonatal form of the disease frequently has more significant cardiac involvement that does not respond to treatment; significant mitral valve prolapse is more threatening in infancy
- Chronic skeletal pain may be debilitating
- Pregnancy in females with Marfan syndrome warrants careful screening for exacerbation of aortic pathology; risk of dissection is high during labor and post-delivery

Prader-Willi Syndrome

INTRODUCTION

- Prader-Willi syndrome is a distinct genetic syndrome characterized by hyperphagia and obesity, hypogonadism, characteristic physical features, and behavioral and cognitive manifestations
- Because the most important findings in infants are nonspecific (hypotonia and failure to thrive), the diagnosis is often made in childhood rather than in infancy
- Most of the findings in Prader-Willi have some relationship to hypothalamic function

ETIOLOGY, EPIDEMIOLOGY, & RISK FACTORS

- Due to a lack of expression of genes on chromosome 15
  - Deletion of material from the father's chromosome 15 occurs in 75% of cases
  - Inheritance of two maternally derived chromosomes 15 (uniparental disomy) and unbalanced translocations account for the remainder of cases
- Incidence of 1 in 10,000–15,000
- Both sexes are affected equally

PATIENT PRESENTATION

- Central hypotonia with poor sucking and failure to thrive during infancy
- Genital hypoplasia (clitoral, testicular)
- Characteristic facies: almond-shaped palpebral fissures, narrowed bitemporal diameter, and thin upper lip
- Small hands and feet
- Obesity begins in childhood as hypotonia improves and a voracious appetite ensues
- Developmental delays and mental retardation
- Short stature
- Generalized hypopigmentation

DIFFERENTIAL DX

- Spinal muscular atrophy
- Congenital myotonic dystrophy
- Other neuromuscular diseases
- Bardet-Biedl syndrome
- Albright hereditary osteodystrophy
- Cohen syndrome
- Familial obesity

DIAGNOSTIC EVALUATION

- May be discovered prenatally via amniocentesis or chorionic villous sampling
- Clinical findings include a constellation of obesity, characteristic facies, small hands and feet, and small gonads in males
  - A Prader-Willi rating scale exists to assess likelihood of the disease based on clinical findings
  - Bizarre food-seeking behaviors may be an important clue to the diagnosis
- Laboratory testing includes DNA-based methylation testing to detect abnormal parent-specific imprinting within the Prader-Willi control region on chromosome 15
- Other laboratory testing includes GnRH, FSH, LH, and sex steroid hormones in the evaluation of hypogonadotropic hypogonadism
  - Growth hormone deficiency may also be found
- Intelligence testing and testing for learning disabilities
- Psychiatric evaluation for behavior disturbances
- Sleep studies to evaluate for sleep apnea

TREATMENT & MANAGEMENT

- Early intervention in infancy to address feeding problems, hypotonia, and delayed gross motor skills
- Appropriate developmental support, including special education services as child approaches school age
- Short stature should be treated with growth hormone replacement
- When obesity develops, strict adherence to calorie-restricted diet and an exercise program
- Surveillance for ophthalmologic problems (eg, strabismus)
- Surveillance for osteoporosis (secondary to sex steroid insufficiency)
- Periodic screening for other endocrine problems, including diabetes and hypothyroidism
  - Growth hormone testing is not required; patients automatically qualify for growth hormone therapy for short stature

PROGNOSIS & COMPLICATIONS

- Morbid obesity and associated problems are the most serious complications (slipped capital femoral epiphysis, diabetes mellitus, cardiovascular disease, obstructive sleep apnea)
- A phenomenon of acute gastric distension and necrosis has been described after binge eating
- Most patients are mildly mentally retarded
- Behavioral and psychiatric problems present a significant challenge to the management of the adult patient with Prader-Willi
- Life expectancy can be improved by strict management of obesity

Turner Syndrome

INTRODUCTION

- Turner syndrome is a disorder of females consisting of an absent or incomplete X chromosome, previously referred to as 45,XO or 45,X
- Gonadal dysgenesis occurs secondary to X chromosome abnormalities
- It is typified by short stature and impairment of sexual development, including eventual infertility, as well as other morphologic findings and behavior and developmental problems
- When Turner syndrome is not recognized by the constellation of phenotypic characteristics, the diagnosis may be made during the investigation of short stature or infertility

ETIOLOGY, EPIDEMIOLOGY, & RISK FACTORS

- Affects only females
- No known racial or ethnic predilection
- Incidence is 1 in 2000–5000 live female births
- 50% have absence of an X chromosome (XO karyotype)
  - This occurs as a result of nondisjunction during meiosis
  - When one X chromosome is missing entirely, it is usually the paternal X chromosome
- Other patterns are possible, including mosaic 45,XX/46,XY
- 20% of spontaneously miscarried fetuses have Turner syndrome
- Only 1–2% of conceptions with Turner syndrome survive beyond 28 weeks of gestation
- Hypothyroidism is a common coexisting condition
- Diabetes and carbohydrate intolerance issues are common

PATIENT PRESENTATION

- Short stature, particularly after age 11–12, since pubertal growth spurt does not occur
- Low hairline, low-set ears, ptosis, and high-arch palate
- Webbed neck
- Shield (broad) chest with widely spaced nipples
- Cardiac complications include coarctation of the aorta, aortic dissection, bicuspid aortic valve, and hypertension
- Streak gonads, which present as delayed onset of estrogen-dependent features of puberty, amenorrhea, and renal anomalies
- Lymphedema of hands and feet
- Hip dislocation, cubitus valgus, scoliosis, hypoplastic nails
- Learning disabilities

DIFFERENTIAL DX

- Noonan syndrome (sometimes called "male Turner syndrome," although this is an unrelated disorder)
- Milroy disease
- Type E brachydactyly
- Multiple pterygium syndrome
- Leri-Weill dyschondrosteosis

DIAGNOSTIC EVALUATION

- Clinical evaluation:
  - One-third of patients are diagnosed at birth by the identification of a webbed neck and lymphedema of the dorsum of hands and feet
  - Another one-third are diagnosed in childhood during evaluation of short stature or other anomalies
  - The final one-third are diagnosed in the teenage years during the evaluation of abnormal pubertal development
- Suspicion may arise during prenatal ultrasound; definitive diagnosis can be made prenatally by amniocentesis or chorionic villous sampling
  - Prenatal findings consistent with Turner syndrome include hydrops fetalis and cystic hygroma
- Chromosome analysis with adequate cell counts to rule out mosaicism
- Fluorescent in situ hybridization (FISH) may be used
- Buccal smear to evaluate for Barr bodies was an earlier method of diagnosis; however, this method should not be used because there are many false-negative results in mosaic patients
- Echocardiogram to evaluate for cardiac anomalies
- Renal, abdominal, and/or pelvic ultrasound to look for genitourinary anomalies

TREATMENT & MANAGEMENT

- Surgical intervention for cardiac defects
- Growth hormone replacement beginning at 3–4 years of age
  - Growth hormone administration may worsen glucose intolerance; urine should be checked for glucose after administration
- Estrogen and progesterone replacement to establish secondary sexual characteristics in adolescence
- Appropriate educational interventions for patients with learning disabilities
- Monitor for other health problems:
  - Hypothyroidism: Thyroid function studies in neonates and periodically afterwards
  - Obesity and diabetes mellitus: Weight management, glucose tolerance testing or fasting blood glucose, lipid studies
  - Hypertension, secondary to cardiac disorders, obesity, or renal anomalies
  - Otic conditions: Hearing screens (canals may be stenotic; otitis media is frequent)
- In cases with a Y chromosome, surgical removal of the gonad is required to prevent gonadoblastoma

PROGNOSIS & COMPLICATIONS

- Mental retardation is uncommon, but learning disabilities with visual-spatial deficits are common
- Patients with mosaicism have fewer physical findings
- Cardiac concerns increase morbidity and mortality; if not coarctation or aortic dissection, then cardiovascular disease secondary to obesity is more frequent
- Pregnancy is possible with donor egg and assisted reproduction

Cleft Palate

INTRODUCTION

- Cleft palate describes a failure of midline fusion of the embryonic palatal processes and inadequate migration and fusion of the associated nasopharyngeal structures that normally occur during the first trimester
- May involve the hard palate, soft palate, or both; it may be submucosal or affect primarily the function of the associated structures
- Cleft palate may occur with or without an associated cleft lip
- Feeding, speech, maxillofacial growth, ears, nose, throat, and dentition are all affected, requiring substantial intervention, particularly in the first year of life

ETIOLOGY, EPIDEMIOLOGY, & RISK FACTORS

- Incidence of up to 1 case per 1000 births
- May be caused by chromosome disorders, single gene defects, or teratogenic exposures
  - Autosomal dominant, autosomal recessive, and X-linked patterns have been described
  - Known teratogens include agents of maternal smoking, phenytoin, retinoids, alcohol, and cocaine
- Other anomalies are found in 13–50% of patients; many have an identifiable genetic syndrome
- Among cleft lip/palate defects, 30% are isolated cleft palate, 20% are isolated cleft lip, and the rest are cleft palate with unilateral or bilateral cleft lip
- Cleft palate may occur in the following configurations:
  - True cleft palate (failure of midline fusion of the hard and soft palate)
  - Submucous cleft palate (midline fusion of mucosa but not underlying bony and soft tissue structures)
  - Velopharyngeal insufficiency (malfunction of the palatal and pharyngeal muscles)
  - Pierre-Robin sequence (micrognathia, U-shaped cleft palate, and glossoptosis, which is excessive tongue size relative to the size of mouth and may compromise the upper airway)

PATIENT PRESENTATION

- Isolated cleft palate is usually identified on newborn exam
- Feeding difficulties occur early:
  - Inability to generate adequate suction due to the oral cavity being open to the nasopharynx
  - Reflux of feeding into the nasal cavity, which may cause aspiration of feedings
  - Early fatigue during feeding due to the increased effort in sucking
- Ear infections and middle ear dysfunction
- Upper airway obstruction due to protrusion of the tongue into the inferior nasal cavity, especially when micrognathia is associated
- Articulation problems after infancy
- Associated anomalies include congenital heart defects, hypopituitarism, myopia, micrognathia (mandibular hypoplasia), and glossoptosis (excessive tongue size relative to size of mouth)

DIFFERENTIAL DX

- Cleft lip/cleft palate
- Isolated cleft palate
- Pierre-Robin sequence
- Associated syndromes include Spitzen, Vanderwoude, Stickler, and oral-facial-digital syndromes

DIAGNOSTIC EVALUATION

- Prenatal testing via second-trimester ultrasound may detect cleft palate
- Prenatal history to screen for teratogenic exposures, including alcohol and smoking
- The presence of cleft palate is documented by physical exam; however, submucous cleft palate may be missed if the examiner does not palpate the palate carefully
  - Bifid uvula is a clue to potential cleft palate
  - Velopharyngeal insufficiency and submucous cleft may be seen by indirect laryngoscopy
  - Detailed family history, with attention to other family members with cleft defects or other syndromic features, may assist in detecting a possible etiology
- Careful evaluation to rule out other anomalies and/or associated syndromes, such as Apert syndrome, Treacher-Collins syndrome, and Stickler syndrome
- Chromosome analysis with FISH (fluorescent in situ hybridization) probe to evaluate for deletion 22q11

TREATMENT & MANAGEMENT

- Referral to cleft palate team or cleft palate center for specialized management
- Oromaxillofacial surgeons provide the majority of the care
  - In the early newborn period, infants may be fitted with a palatal prosthesis to prevent flow of milk into the nasopharynx during feeding
  - Surgical correction is done within the first year of life; the repair may be in stages, depending on the degree of deformity and presence or absence of a cleft lip
- Cleft palate–specific nipples and feeding devices are available for both breastfed and formula-fed babies
  - Breastfeeding is more difficult but may be attempted
  - Fortified formulas help patients obtain enough calories
- Speech therapy may be able to assist patients with velopharyngeal insufficiency to learn more effective sucking and swallowing
- Otitis media may be chronic and severe and should be treated aggressively
- Early dental consultation because dental anomalies and caries are common

PROGNOSIS & COMPLICATIONS

- In isolated cases of cleft palate when a good surgical repair is achieved, there are no significant medical sequelae; however, psychosocial issues may be significant
- Hearing loss may occur if ear infections are not treated aggressively
- Genetic counseling is indicated for the patient and family
- Due to the broad needs of cleft palate patients, good outcomes depend on a cohesive, multidisciplinary approach utilizing nutrition, speech pathology, otolaryngology, dentistry, and oromaxillofacial surgery; cleft palate centers with coordinated services achieve good outcomes

Section 12

Metabolic Disorders

Metabolic Disorders, Part 1

Phenylketonuria

- A deficiency of phenylalanine hydroxylase, which converts phenylalanine to tyrosine; tyrosine is a precursor of catecholamines and fumarate, which enters the Krebs cycle
- Accumulation of the resulting metabolites (phenylpyruvate and phenylacetate) leads to mental retardation; since tyrosine cannot be synthesized, it becomes an essential amino acid
- It is the most common clinically encountered inborn error of amino acid metabolism
- Incidence is 1 in 10,000 live births; 1 in 50 are carriers
- Many mutations in the phenylalanine hydroxylase gene exist
- Presentation includes microcephaly, mental retardation, growth retardation, developmental delay, behavioral problems, seizures, and hypopigmentation
- Universal state screening in every newborn has led to early diagnosis
- High serum phenylalanine and low serum tyrosine confirm the diagnosis
- A variant of the disease is deficiency of the cofactor tetrahydrobiopterin (BH4), resulting in hyperphenylalaninemia; distinguish classic phenylketonuria from BH4 deficiency by measurement of biopterin and neopterin, which are byproducts of cofactor synthesis
- Treat with dietary restriction of phenylalanine (eg, aspartame), overall dietary protein restriction, and tyrosine supplementation; it was once thought that dietary restrictions were only necessary during childhood, but there is now a movement toward lifelong dietary compliance
- Without treatment, severe mental retardation occurs, which may be detected as early as 1 year of age; even with treatment, behavior problems are increased in this population
- Phenylalanine is teratogenic; thus, women attempting to become pregnant must maintain the dietary restrictions prior to conception and throughout the duration of pregnancy

Lesch-Nyhan Disease

- An inherited disorder of purine metabolism and salvage, leading to an accumulation of uric acid and a clinical syndrome of mental retardation, self-mutilation, movement disorder, and inability to walk
- Due to an X-linked recessive defect in the hypoxanthine-guanine phosphoribosyl transferase (HGPRT) enzyme, which catalyzes the reaction of hypoxanthine or guanine with phosphoribosyl pyrophosphate to form nucleotides
- Primarily a disease of males affecting 1 in 100,000 live births
- Normal development occurs until 6–8 months of age; the initial manifestation is orange crystals in the diaper, which may be accompanied by hematuria and renal stones
- Other symptoms include poor feeding and failure to thrive due to oral apraxia and behavioral vomiting; gross motor delay and regression of motor skills (head control, sitting); spastic cerebral palsy (scissoring of legs, flexion contractures, dislocated hips, hyperreflexia, positive Babinski sign); involuntary dystonic and choreoathetoid movements with opisthotonic spasms; incontinence; self-injurious behavior (eg, biting); and gouty arthritis
- Prenatal testing is available via chorionic villous sampling or amniocentesis
- Diagnosis via deficient activity of the HGPRT enzyme and elevated uric acid levels in the serum and urine
- Treat with allopurinol, an inhibitor of xanthine oxidase, which decreases the formation of uric acid from nucleotide degradation; however, treatment does not result in complete resolution of symptoms and prognosis is poor
- Patients are nonambulatory secondary to severe gross motor delay
- Dental extraction and physical restraint may be necessary to prevent self-injury, but measures to avoid self-injury may be difficult to maintain

Tay-Sachs Disease

- Caused by deficiency of hexosaminidase A, a lysosomal enzyme, which results in accumulation of G_{M2} ganglioside in lysosomes of various tissues
- Autosomal recessive transmission of the HEXA gene, located on chromosome 15

- Approximately 80% of affected children are of Jewish ancestry
- Signs of the disease appear during infancy:
  - The earliest symptoms are irritability and exaggerated reactions to routine stimuli
  - Hypotonia with delayed motor development occurs
  - Vision begins to deteriorate by 6 months of age; blindness occurs by 1 year
  - Seizure activity (often myoclonic) can begin as early as 6 months of age; a cherry-red spot on the macula occurs due to degeneration of the ganglion cells surrounding the fovea
  - Macrocephaly occurs later due to cerebral G_{M2} accumulation
- Primarily a clinical diagnosis; identifiable symptoms occur as early as 6 months of age
  - Prenatal screening via amniocentesis or chorionic villous sampling
  - Blood sampling of suspected children or carriers
  - Gene testing for known mutations
  - MRI shows an enlarged caudate nucleus, later progressing to cerebral atrophy
- Definitive therapy is not available; supportive care is important
  - Enzyme replacement is being studied
  - Bone marrow transplant is not effective
- The disease follows a relentless course over the initial few years of life; affected children usually die by 4 years of age

Niemann-Pick Disease

- An autosomal recessive deficiency of sphingomyelinase, resulting in sphingomyelin accumulation in lysosomes
- Niemann-Pick cells ("foam cells") are formed, which cause damage to multiple organ systems, including the reticuloendothelial system, brain, spinal cord, and lung
- More common in patients of Ashkenazi Jewish descent
- Feeding difficulties and failure to thrive are often the presenting symptoms
- Other symptoms include global developmental delay and deterioration, mental retardation, hypotonia, weakness, hearing and vision loss, and seizures
- Findings include growth delay, hepatosplenomegaly, and a cherry-red spot on the macula
- Prenatal diagnosis is available using chorionic villous sampling
- Diagnosis is made by measuring the sphingomyelinase activity in white blood cells (a blood test), in skin fibroblasts (via biopsy), in liver cells (via biopsy), or by DNA testing (which can also identify the carrier status)
- There is no definitive treatment; developmental therapy and nutrition support are used

Gaucher Disease (Glucocerebrosidosis)

- Caused by a deficiency of β-glucosidase, which results in accumulation and deposition of glucocerebrosidase (a lysosomal enzyme) in the reticuloendothelial system; Gaucher cells fill the liver, spleen, lymph nodes, bone, bone marrow, and lungs
- Autosomal recessive inheritance; very common in Ashkenazi Jews
- Diagnosed by enzyme analysis of white blood cells or fibroblasts and bone marrow biopsy
- Type 1 (chronic nonneuronopathic) is the most common sphingolipid storage disorder
  - Severely affected patients present in childhood with severe splenomegaly/pancytopenia; cirrhosis, liver failure, poor pulmonary function, and cor pulmonale occasionally occur
  - The distal femur has an expanded cortex (Erlenmeyer flask deformity)
  - The disease is progressive, but children will live into adult life
- Type 2 (acute neuronopathic) presents between birth and 18 months; death occurs by age 2
  - Patients have massive hepatosplenomegaly and rapidly progressing CNS deterioration
  - Trismus, strabismus, and retroflexion of the head are pathognomonic
  - Enzyme replacement will not prevent CNS deterioration
- Treat with enzyme replacement using glucocerebrosidase (either synthetic or derived from human placenta), which will improve splenomegaly and blood counts but not neurologic manifestations; bone marrow transplantation may improve neurologic symptoms as well as pulmonary and bone involvement

Metabolic Disorders, Part 2

Cystinuria
- Cystinuria is one of the most common inherited disorders (1 in 7000 live births) and is the most common genetic defect of amino acid transport; autosomal recessive inheritance
- Occurs due to mutations of a renal transport protein that normally reabsorbs four amino acids (cysteine, ornithine, arginine, and lysine) in the renal tubules; as a result, there are increased concentrations of amino acids (primarily cysteine) in the renal tubules, collecting ducts, ureters, and bladder, which then precipitate and form radiopaque urinary stones (cystine stones account for 1–2% of all cases of urolithiasis)
- May be asymptomatic, but most patients have renal symptoms (renal colic, calculi, frequent urinary tract infections, renal hypertension)
- Diagnostic workup is similar to other causes of urolithiasis, including urinalysis, urine pH, urine culture, and plain abdominal X-rays or spiral CT scan without contrast
- Consider the diagnosis in patients (especially males) with recurrent UTIs or urolithiasis
- Treat with hydration, pain control, D-penicillamine (reacts with cysteine to form a more soluble compound that can be eliminated in the urine), and appropriate antibiotics for associated urinary tract infections; surgical removal of obstructive stones may be necessary

Homocystinuria
- A deficiency of cystathionine β-synthase, which converts homocysteine to cystathionine, resulting in accumulation of homocysteine
- Results in developmental delay, mental retardation, failure to thrive, eye disease (lens dislocation or subluxation, which may result in severe myopia, astigmatism, glaucoma, cataracts, and retinal detachment), osteoporosis, seizures, and marfanoid appearance
- Psychiatric disorders occur in more than half of affected children
- Heterozygous carriers have an increased risk of thromboembolic disease
- Autosomal recessive inheritance; the gene is located on chromosome 21
- Diagnosis is based on elevated methionine and homocysteine in the serum and urine and is confirmed by elevated homocysteine levels in a tissue sample (eg, fibroblasts)
- Treat by restriction of dietary methionine (an essential amino acid) and supplementation of cysteine, folic acid, vitamin B_6, and betaine

Mitochondrial Cytopathies
- Mitochondria are present in nearly every cell, where they produce ATP for cellular energy; they contain their own DNA, which is maternally inherited; because the mutation rate is 10 times higher than that of nuclear DNA, mitochondrial disorders are fairly common
- Organs with high energy requirements are affected (brain, muscle, heart, liver, kidney)
- Various discrete syndromes have been described, including MERRF (myoclonus epilepsy and ragged red fibers) and MELAS (mitochondrial myopathy, encephalopathy, lactic acidosis, and stroke-like episodes)
- May present in infancy with profound lactic acidosis, failure to thrive, and seizures
- Other presentations include sensorineural hearing loss, optic atrophy with possible visual loss, myopathies, exercise intolerance, cardiomyopathy and conduction defects, and neurologic manifestations (eg, seizures, stroke-like episodes, neuropathy, ataxia)
- Have a high suspicion in patients with disease in three or more organ systems not attributable to routine pathologies
- Laboratory studies may reveal elevated lactate and pyruvate; lactic acidosis; and abnormal serum amino acids, urine amino acids, and urine organic acids
- Further testing includes mitochondrial DNA testing, Southern blot, and skin/muscle biopsy
- Treat with supplementation of mitochondrial cofactors (eg, carnitine, coenzyme Q, B vitamins, alpha-lipoic acid, antioxidants)

Urea Cycle Abnormalities
- Urea is the primary waste product of amino acid metabolism; any enzyme deficiency in the cycle creates a backup of urea and results in hyperammonemia; the urea cycle disorders include carbamoyl phosphate synthetase deficiency, ornithine transcarbamylase (OTC) deficiency, citrullinemia (arginosuccinate synthetase deficiency), arginosuccinic aciduria (arginosuccinate lyase deficiency), and argininemia (arginase deficiency)
- OTC deficiency is an X-linked defect; the rest are autosomal recessive
- Presentation may include lethargy, protein aversion or intolerance, anorexia, vomiting (especially recurrent or cyclic), hepatomegaly with abnormal liver function studies, blurred vision, neurologic symptoms (eg, seizures, dystonia, irritability, tremor, stroke), bizarre behavior, screaming episodes, mental retardation, and coma
- This condition should be considered in severely ill neonates; screening should include serum ammonia and lactate levels
- Definitive diagnosis via liver biopsy and enzyme assay; prenatal diagnosis is available
- Treat with hemodialysis for rapid removal of ammonia, sodium benzoate and phenylacetate to bypass urea production, mannitol to treat cerebral edema and increased intracranial pressure, avoidance of nitrogen intake via protein restriction, and dietary supplementation (arginine, folate, vitamin B_6)
- Few affected patients survive infancy; those who do have a poor prognosis

Organic Acidemias
- A group of inherited disorders (maple syrup urine disease, propionic acidemia, methylmalonic acidemia, isovaleric acidemia, and glutaric acidemia) that result in excess organic acids in the blood and increased excretion in the urine; pathology occurs due to accumulation of toxic metabolites and/or deficiency of end products
- Newborns do well for the first few days of life but then develop a toxic encephalopathy
- Presentations include vomiting, poor feeding, poor muscle tone, seizures, developmental delay, encephalopathy, lethargy, and coma
- Newborn screening is available but must be confirmed by more definitive testing
- The diagnosis should be considered in severely ill neonates; screening includes levels of glucose, lactate, ammonia, blood gas, serum amino acids, and urine organic acids
- Organic acids are generally measured in urine only (difficult to detect in serum) by mass spectroscopy; a serum amino acid profile may be helpful to determine the precise disorder
- Labs show metabolic acidosis, ketosis, hyperammonemia, elevated liver function tests, hypoglycemia, neutropenia, and thrombocytopenia
- Brain MRI reveals characteristic changes
- Treat with restriction of dietary precursor amino acids (special formulas are available), adjunctive treatments specific to each disorder (eg, vitamin B_{12} for methylmalonic acidemia), and supportive care during decompensations; liver transplant may be necessary

Galactosemia
- Deficiency of galactose-1-phosphate uridyl transferase, which is an important enzyme in the conversion of galactose to glucose; pathology arises from accumulation of the precursors (galactose-1-phosphate and galactitol) in the CNS, lens of eye, liver, kidney, and other organs
- The major dietary source of galactose is breast milk or cow's milk–based formula
- Infants become ill within a few days of milk intake (intractable vomiting, hepatomegaly, lethargy, poor growth); may be rapidly fatal if milk feedings continue
- Initial presentation includes hypoglycemia or neonatal sepsis
- Severe mental retardation occurs due to accumulation of precursors in the CNS
- Rapid diagnosis is essential to prevent/diminish mental retardation and other sequelae; universal neonatal screening can detect the enzyme deficiency early
- When consuming galactose, the urine contains reducing substances but not glucose
- Treat with strict dietary avoidance of galactose and lactose; infants use soy-based formula

Developmental Disorders

Attention Deficit Hyperactivity Disorder

INTRODUCTION

- Attention deficit hyperactivity disorder (ADHD) is a relatively prevalent childhood disorder that may have a profound effect on a child's global functioning
- In addition to impairing the child's learning, psychosocial development and self-concept may be negatively impacted; similarly, family, peer, and other relationships are subject to discord
- Thus, prompt recognition and effective treatment are essential for better immediate and long-term outcomes in children and adolescents with ADHD
- The American Academy of Pediatrics has an ADHD toolkit that is available on their website

ETIOLOGY, EPIDEMIOLOGY, & RISK FACTORS

- Characterized by inattentiveness, hyperactivity, and/or poor impulse control
- No specific etiology has been identified; probably multifactorial
  - Probable genetic contribution
  - Possible neurotransmitter abnormalities
  - CNS and neurologic disorders may serve as predisposing factors
- Prevalence of 3–8% of school-aged children
- Onset before age 4 in half of cases
- Although more boys than girls have this diagnosis, recent studies suggest that there may not be an actual male predominance
- Coexisting conditions are frequent and include learning disabilities, anxiety and depression, oppositional defiant disorder, and conduct disorder

PATIENT PRESENTATION

- Inattentiveness:
  - Difficulty sustaining attention in activity
  - Avoids tasks requiring sustained mental effort
  - Easily distracted, unable to finish tasks
  - Careless mistakes at school
  - Frequently misplaces items
  - Does not follow instructions
  - Forgetful and disorganized
- Hyperactivity:
  - Squirming and fidgeting
  - Cannot sit still or stay seated
  - Cannot play or work quietly
  - Excessive running/climbing
  - Restlessness, "on the go," "motor-driven"
  - Talks excessively
- Poor impulse control:
  - Interrupts; cannot take turns
  - Risky acts without considering consequences

DIFFERENTIAL DX

- Sensory impairments (hearing, vision)
- Depression or bipolar disorder
- Adjustment disorder
- Anxiety disorder
- Mental retardation
- Developmental delay
- Autism spectrum disorder
- Substance abuse
- Hyperthyroidism
- Seizure disorder
- Sleep disorder (eg, sleep apnea)
- Lead poisoning

DIAGNOSTIC EVALUATION

- Three types of ADHD have been recognized: attention deficits only (inattentive type), hyperactivity/impulsivity, and combined inattentiveness and hyperactivity
- Diagnostic and Statistical Manual of Mental Disorders (DSM) IV criteria require six symptoms from either the inattentive category or the hyperactivity/impulsivity category, or a combination totaling six
  - Symptoms should be present in two or more settings (eg, school and home)
  - Symptoms of maladaptive behavior inconsistent with developmental level persisting for 6 months
  - Signs of ADHD must be present before 7 years of age
- The ADHD rating scale, the Vanderbilt scale, and the Connors scale are behavioral rating scales that formalize input from parents and teachers to assist in diagnosis
- Thorough evaluation to rule out underlying medical causes
- Psychological and cognitive testing to differentiate learning disabilities and mental retardation

TREATMENT & MANAGEMENT

- Behavior modification, including a structured, calm environment; clear, simple rules and consequences; and a reward system for improved behaviors
- Stimulants are the mainstay of pharmacologic therapy (eg, methylphenidate, dextroamphetamine, amphetamine combinations) and block dopamine and norepinephrine reuptake into the presynaptic area
  - Side effects include appetite suppression, weight loss, irritability, and sleep problems
  - When used to treat ADHD, stimulants are not extremely likely to be substances of abuse, although there are cases of people (patients, parents, and others) crushing and snorting stimulants; more likely, adverse effects are related to misuse of the mediations (eg, a teenager who is not very prompt or compliant with medications and ends up with extra tablets that he or she later uses to pull an "all-nighter" or shares with a friend who is dieting)
- Antidepressant medications (eg, bupropion, tricyclic antidepressants) may be useful in some children by inhibiting dopamine or norepinephrine reuptake
- Nonstimulant medications (eg, Strattera) inhibit norepinephrine reuptake
- Alpha-agonists (eg, clonidine) decrease catecholamine production and are primarily used in children with comorbidities (eg, anxiety disorders) or children who need stimulants but cannot tolerate the side effects
- Treat coexisting conditions as necessary

PROGNOSIS & COMPLICATIONS

- ADHD should be viewed as a chronic illness; therefore, treatment should follow a chronic illness model with an initial treatment method and ongoing management strategy
- During treatment with stimulants, patients must be monitored for weight loss, growth failure, sleep disturbance, hypertension, and exacerbation of tic disorder
- Many patients take a "drug holiday" on weekends and during the summer
- Patients who receive appropriate treatment and follow-up learn compensatory mechanisms and live productive lives
- May persist into adolescence and adulthood (contrary to earlier reports)
- Later psychopathology may be related to anxiety, depression, or aggressiveness in childhood

Autism Spectrum Disorders

INTRODUCTION

- A spectrum of developmental disorders characterized by abnormalities in social interaction, communication, and patterns of behavior, activities, and interests
- Also referred to as pervasive developmental disorders
- The most common disorders include autism, Rett disorder, Asperger disorder, and childhood disintegrative disorder (CDD)
- Early detection and intervention are crucial because the eventual severity of the diagnosis may be significantly impacted by intensive therapy during early childhood

ETIOLOGY, EPIDEMIOLOGY, & RISK FACTORS

- The etiology is unknown; infectious, traumatic, and neurochemical factors have been implicated
- A genetic contribution is suggested by high twin concordance rates
- Not caused by parenting style, as was previously postulated
- Not caused by the MMR or any other vaccines, a theory that has unfortunately received widespread media attention
- The general presence of these disorders is 1–2 cases per 10,000
- Male predominance
- Typical onset in infancy or early childhood

PATIENT PRESENTATION

- Onset generally occurs between ages 15 and 30 months
- Personal/social abnormalities (eg, lack of empathy, failure to seek comfort from caregivers)
- Language abnormalities (eg, lack of conversational reciprocity, echolalia, abnormal verbal sequencing)
- Self-stimulatory motor behaviors (eg, rocking, spinning, and hand-flapping; mouthing of objects; self-injurious behaviors)
- Stereotyped body movements
- Ritualistic behavior and need to follow strict routine
- Preoccupation with insignificant details
- Restricted interests, including numbers and counting, hyperlexia (letters and words), preoccupation with parts of things, lining things up and categorizing things

DIFFERENTIAL DX

- Mental retardation
- Language delay
- Hearing or vision impairments
- Degenerative neurologic disorders
- Reactive attachment disorder of infancy
- Schizophrenia
- Fragile X syndrome
- Trisomy 21
- Epilepsy
- Neurocutaneous disorders
- Phenylketonuria
- Mucopolysaccharidoses
- Mitochondrial disorders
- HIV

DIAGNOSTIC EVALUATION

- There is no biologic marker; screening depends on history and developmental assessment
- Diagnosis is made based on DSM-IV criteria; specific evaluation tools are available
- Autism is characterized by impairments in social interaction (lack of social reciprocity, lack of empathy, difficulties in forming attachments, inability to employ and understand nonverbal cues and facial expressions), impairments in communication (limited spoken language, lack of conversational reciprocity, echolalia, stereotyped language), stereotyped motor movements, and restricted or repetitive interests and patterns of behavior
- Asperger is characterized by normal language development but social maldevelopment (inadequate emotional reciprocity, inability to form peer relationships, inability to use nonverbal cues or facial expressions), as well as restricted patterns of interest and behavior
- CDD: normal development through first 2 years of life, followed by loss of developmental milestones in language, social and self-help skills, play and imagination, and motor skills; restricted and repetitive interests and behavior with stereotyped motor patterns are often present
- Rett disorder is characterized by a normal physical and developmental infantile course through the age of 5 months, followed by deceleration of head growth, loss of social engagement, limited development of gross motor and language skills, and altered fine motor skills (patients have stereotyped hand movements rather than advancing fine motor skills)
- Be sure to rule out sensory deficits (eg, deafness) that affect normal interaction
- Assess for metabolic/degenerative disorders characterized by developmental delay or regression (eg, phenylketonuria, mucopolysaccharidoses, mitochondrial disorders, HIV)

TREATMENT & MANAGEMENT

- Treatment is more successful when individually designed
- The mainstay of treatment is behavioral and educational therapies
- Behavioral techniques that families can use are a well-adhered to schedule, a system of warning before making transitions in activities, a calm environment, and visual communication aids (eg, picture cards for children who cannot use language to express themselves)
- Antidepressants and antipsychotics have been used to reduce global symptoms
- Specialized therapeutic educational programs use all of the above measures and usually involve an individual therapist who can buffer the effects of a mainstream class while working on attachment, basic social engagement, and conversational reciprocity; music and art therapy are sometimes used

PROGNOSIS & COMPLICATIONS

- Complete resolution of symptoms rarely occurs
- Successful symptom reduction may occur with behavior modification, environmental adaptations, and pharmacotherapy
- Level of function dictates ability to be self-sufficient in the community versus long-term monitored living arrangements
- Better prognosis in patients with higher intelligence
- Risk of seizures increases with age

Developmental Delay

INTRODUCTION

- Developmental evaluation is one of the most important elements of well child care
- Assessment of developmental progression should occur at all preventive health visits, as well as at any point that a concern is raised by a clinician or caregiver
- Developmental acquisition may be divided into five categories: fine motor, gross motor, speech, self-help, and personal/social
- Developmental delay may occur in one or more of these categories; when there are delayed milestones in all of them, it is referred to as global developmental delay
- A formal screening tool helps to standardize assessment and improve accuracy; it should be based on observation as well as parental report

ETIOLOGY, EPIDEMIOLOGY, & RISK FACTORS

- "Developmental delay" is a basket term that refers to late or absent acquisition of expected developmental milestones for any reason
- May include permanent global deficits (commonly referred to as mental retardation) or isolated deficits in one or more developmental skills or categories
- May be due to:
  - Genetic defects (eg, fragile X syndrome, neurofibromatosis)
  - Environmental factors (eg, neglect, lead poisoning)
  - Prenatal/perinatal factors (eg, prematurity, prenatal drug exposure)
  - CNS disease or injury (eg, hypoxic-ischemic or infectious encephalopathy)
  - Idiopathic
- One of the most common chronic diseases in children
- Accounts for considerable portion of health care and education spending

PATIENT PRESENTATION

- Delayed developmental skills:
  - Gross motor skills (eg, head control, rolling, sitting, walking)
  - Fine motor skills (eg, pincer grasp, using a writing instrument)
  - Personal/social skills (eg, social smile, waving, sharing)
  - Self-help/adaptive skills (eg, feeding self, dressing self)
  - Language skills (eg, word acquisition and syntax learning)
- Focal neurologic deficits
- Dysmorphic features
- Nonspecific (eg, microcephaly) or specific (eg, neurocutaneous lesions) exam findings

DIFFERENTIAL DX

- Static global delay/mental retardation: cerebral palsy, perinatal asphyxia
- Progressive global delay: progressive neurologic or metabolic disorders
- Gross motor delay: benign hypotonia of infancy
- Sensory deficits: hearing impairment (will lead to speech delay), visual deficits (will impair global functioning)
- Language disorders: autism spectrum disorders, selective mutism
- Learning disabilities

DIAGNOSTIC EVALUATION

- History should pay attention to birth history (eg, trauma, perinatal depression or asphyxia, maternal substance abuse, prematurity), medical history (eg, significant illnesses, injuries, or infections, including neonatal sepsis or meningitis at any age), and developmental milestones, both current and previous (eg, at what age did the child sit, walk, say "mama")
- Physical examination should include all growth parameters (height, weight, and head circumference) and evaluate for dysmorphic characteristics, cardiac murmurs, or orthopedic anomalies that may suggest a genetic syndrome; a thorough neurologic examination is necessary
- Distinctions are drawn among *surveillance* (assessment of whether or not developmental delay may be present), *screening* (the use of standardized tools to identify and describe delay or deficits), and *evaluation* (the potentially complex process of identifying the developmental disorders or medical condition causing the developmental delay)
- Use the available developmental testing protocols: The Denver Developmental Assessment, the Ireton Child Development Scale, and the Early Childhood Language Scale are screening tools that integrate items of parental report with milestones that are readily demonstrable in an office setting; they are used widely for developmental assessments in children up to 6 years old

TREATMENT & MANAGEMENT

- The treatment plan should be individually constructed and periodically adjusted based on the patient's needs and progress
- Specific treatment for individual needs may include occupational therapy, physical therapy, adaptive skills learning, and cognitive therapy
- Treat associated medical conditions
- Some disorders have specific therapeutic protocols (eg, Down syndrome)
- Through age 3, developmental services are usually provided in regional early intervention programs
- After age 3, provision of developmental services is usually the responsibility of the school district, even prior to entering kindergarten
- Much developmental support takes place within the school system in the form of special education, which may be supplied as instructional support, emotional support, or general assistance with routine activities, and which may occur in a mainstreamed classroom or in a special education setting

PROGNOSIS & COMPLICATIONS

- The prognosis is highly variable depending on the etiology and severity; those with genetic syndromes and neurologic disorders have the worst prognosis
- Children with developmental delay due to prematurity alone should be "caught up" before age 2 and usually have a good prognosis unless there is a history of significant hypoxia or intracranial hemorrhage
- There is an improved prognosis in patients with well-developed, comprehensive management plans, as well as in patients who receive the earliest possible referral to interventional services
- Developmental delay creates a significant impact on individual and family quality of life

Fetal Alcohol Syndrome

INTRODUCTION

- Alcohol is teratogenic; infants of mothers who consumed alcohol during pregnancy may experience a syndrome of dysmorphology, growth abnormalities, and intellectual impairment
- Birth defects may appear along a spectrum that is related to the dose of alcohol intake; fetal alcohol syndrome is the term for the most severe damage, whereas fetal alcohol effects refer to less severe or fewer findings
- The type of fetal alcohol effects varies with gestational age and duration of alcohol consumption; alcohol use during organogenesis in the first trimester contributes to structural maldevelopment, whereas third-trimester effects are primarily neurologic

ETIOLOGY, EPIDEMIOLOGY, & RISK FACTORS

- Severity is proportional to the amount of alcohol intake; no safe dose of alcohol during pregnancy has been established
- There is a high incidence in women who drink more than three alcoholic beverages a day
- Fetal alcohol syndrome appears in 10% of cases of alcoholic mothers; substantially more cases will have some degree of fetal alcohol effects
- Fetal alcohol syndrome is one of the most common causes of mental retardation; it is the most preventable cause of mental retardation
- Incidence of 1 in 1000 in the general population
- Exacerbating factors include Native-American race, poor maternal nutrition (inadequate folate, magnesium, and zinc compound the problem), parity (worse effects in multiparas), and maternal liver dysfunction (whether due to alcohol or other reasons) because alcohol clearance is reduced

PATIENT PRESENTATION

- Facial dysmorphism: short palpebral fissures, microphthalmia, long flat philtrum, thin upper lip, midface hypoplasia, wide nasal bridge, micrognathia
- CNS manifestations: microcephaly, mental retardation, hypotonia
- Behavioral problems (eg, ADHD, learning disabilities)
- Intrauterine growth retardation and/or postnatal growth restriction
- Failure to thrive in infancy
- Cardiac anomalies, especially atrial septal defects
- Urogenital anomalies

DIFFERENTIAL DX

- Other causes of microcephaly, intrauterine growth retardation, and facial dysmorphism:
- Fetal hydantoin syndrome
- Maternal phenylketonuria
- Cornelia de Lange syndrome
- Noonan syndrome

DIAGNOSTIC EVALUATION

- History and physical examination
  - The diagnosis is suggested by a maternal history of alcohol abuse, intrauterine growth retardation, and low birth weight
  - History of developmental delay, hypersensitivity to routine stimuli, learning difficulties, and social difficulties are common
  - Record and compare height, weight, and head circumference with historical growth charts
  - Facial examination for dysmorphic characteristics
  - Head and neck findings of strabismus, chronic otitis media, hearing impairments, and cleft palate are supportive
- Delayed bone growth is characteristic; radioulnar synostosis is a less common finding
- There is no specific test to diagnose fetal alcohol syndrome or its effects; it is a clinical diagnosis based on anatomic stigmata
- Must have all three components (dysmorphology, evidence of CNS dysfunction, and history of growth restriction) to qualify for diagnosis
- Cardiac evaluation
- Urogenital anomalies, particularly hypospadias

TREATMENT & MANAGEMENT

- Therapy depends on individual characteristics and medical needs
- Appropriate developmental and educational support is of paramount importance
  - Sensory integration therapy to minimize the impact of hyperreactivity
  - Social skills training to improve peer relationships or prevent social isolation
  - Treatment of attention deficit hyperactivity symptoms, particularly by nonpharmacologic methods
  - Special education, because poor school performance is typical, especially in math
  - A stable, structured environment will help with impulse control, adapting to transitions, and mastering activities of daily living
- Nutritional support to maximize growth potential
- Referral to subspecialists for cardiac, renal, or orthopedic anomalies
- Social services or family therapy to engage the family in the necessary measures to understand the disorder, deal with parental guilt, and construct methods to meet the developmental needs
- Surveillance and referral for ongoing alcohol or other substance abuse

PROGNOSIS & COMPLICATIONS

- Prognosis is variable depending on the degree of severity
- The degree of mental retardation dictates eventual outcome; some patients with fetal alcohol effects have an IQ in the normal range, while a few are severely retarded
- Children who remain in special education or who receive long-term supportive services are more likely to achieve their developmental potential
- Psychiatric problems, criminal behavior, unemployment, and incomplete education are common adverse outcomes
- The worst outcomes are in patients who have families with ongoing substance abuse

Allergy/Immunology

Allergic Rhinitis

INTRODUCTION

- Allergic rhinitis is a common disorder that affects patients of all ages and manifests as a variety of mild to moderately severe upper and lower respiratory symptoms
- It is caused by interaction of the nasal mucosa with airborne allergens
- Results in formation of antigen-specific IgE antibodies that lead to mast cell degranulation and release of inflammatory mediators (histamine, leukotrienes, and prostaglandins)
- There is an immediate-phase reaction, with acute local symptoms after exposure to the allergen, and a late-phase reaction, when the release of inflammatory mediators continues the inflammatory response, sometimes affecting the lower respiratory tract; it may complicate asthma or trigger an asthma exacerbation
- As an atopic process, there is considerable overlap between allergic rhinitis, asthma, and atopic dermatitis

ETIOLOGY, EPIDEMIOLOGY, & RISK FACTORS

- Up to 20% of the population have symptoms of allergic rhinitis
- There is a genetic predilection: Patients with a family history of allergic rhinitis on one side have a 30% chance of developing symptoms; patients with a family history on both sides have a >70% chance of developing symptoms
- Pollen and molds are the most common outdoor triggers
- Dust mites, cockroaches, and pet dander are the most common indoor allergens
- Depending on the causative allergen and the frequency of exposure, symptoms may be intermittent, seasonal, or perennial
- First episodes almost always occur in childhood, usually by the second decade, with the average age of presentation at 8–10 years of age
- Perennial allergic rhinitis may be seen in infants because some indoor allergens are potent sensitizers with a greater impact on the immune system and because the exposure is more constant
- Seasonal allergic rhinitis is not usually seen until after age 3 because the immune response to the allergen becomes cumulative over two or more seasons

PATIENT PRESENTATION

- Nasal congestion, itching, and sneezing
- Nose rubbing ("allergic salute")
- Clear nasal discharge, sniffling
- Epistaxis
- Frequent cough with throat clearing
- Mouth breathing; snoring
- Watery, red, itchy eyes
- Suborbital venous congestion ("allergic shiners")
- Creases beneath the lower eyelids ("Dennie lines")
- Pale, swollen nasal turbinates; transverse nasal crease
- "Cobblestoning" in posterior pharynx secondary to drainage
- Sinus pressure and tenderness
- Headache

DIFFERENTIAL DX

- Recurrent upper respiratory illnesses
- Recurrent sinusitis
- Adenoidal hypertrophy (causing chronic nasal congestion)
- Nasal polyps
- Vasomotor rhinitis
- Rhinitis medicamentosa due to overuse of over-the-counter nasal sprays

DIAGNOSTIC EVALUATION

- History
  - Note timing, duration, and intensity of symptoms
  - Note seasonality of symptoms, with special focus on the environment
  - Note exposure to smokers, pets, dust mites (eg, stuffed toys, carpet), or cockroaches
  - Note the effect of over-the-counter medications or antibiotics on symptoms
  - Consider the environment in places other than the patient's home, such as relatives' homes, sitters' homes, daycare, school, and work
- Physical findings consistent with allergic rhinitis include allergic shiners, Dennie lines, transverse nasal crease, edematous or pale nasal mucosa, high-arched palate or poor dentition from chronic mouth breathing, and pharyngeal cobblestoning
- Testing may include skin tests or blood tests
  - Allergy skin testing with specific antigens; positive response is a wheal-and-flare reaction
  - Specific serum IgE measurements (previously called RAST testing)
  - Eosinophilia may be present in nasal discharge

TREATMENT & MANAGEMENT

- Avoid allergens, if possible
  - Use dust covers on bedding, wash linens weekly in high heat, and avoid stuffed toys
  - Avoid carpets and curtains in bedrooms
  - Decrease exposure to pets, and avoid pets in bedrooms
- Symptomatic treatment is effective in most patients
  - Oral antihistamines (eg, cetirizine, fexofenadine, loratadine)
  - Intranasal antihistamines (eg, azelastine)
  - Intranasal steroids (eg, fluticasone, flunisolide, mometasone, beclomethasone, budesonide)
  - Antileukotrienes (eg, montelukast), either alone or with antihistamines
  - Mast cell stabilizers (eg, cromolyn)
  - Decongestants are of limited use due to side effects and rebound symptoms
- For severely affected patients, consider allergen-specific immunotherapy ("allergy shots")
  - Series of weekly injections of antigen based on the patient's profile of allergenic triggers; begins with a low dose and increases monthly to a maintenance dose
  - Patients begin to make antigen-specific IgG that bind to IgE, thereby stabilizing mast cells
  - Results may be seen within 6 months and may be long lasting; length of treatment is usually 3 to 5 years

PROGNOSIS & COMPLICATIONS

- Allergic rhinitis amounts to a notable number of missed work and school days and health care spending, especially when the affect on asthma is considered
- Out-of-pocket expenses for much of the treatment may be substantial
- Environmental control and pharmacotherapy usually provide adequate relief
- Patients can expect to need treatment on an ongoing or intermittent basis
- Patients sometimes have difficulty maintaining compliance with ongoing medical treatment, especially intranasal medications and allergy shots

Drug Allergy

INTRODUCTION

- There are many types of adverse reactions to drugs; drug allergy differs from other reactions, such as routine side effects, drug interactions, drug fevers, overdose, and some cutaneous reactions
- Drug allergy may include a spectrum of allergic responses, ranging from simple cutaneous eruptions to hematologic, renal, vasculitis, and life-threatening anaphylactic reactions
- Well-described syndromes with cutaneous findings include serum sickness, Stevens-Johnson syndrome, and toxic epidermal necrolysis
- 5% of adults have a true drug allergy, and 5–10% of adverse drug reactions are true allergic reactions; up to 15% of adults mistakenly believe they have a drug allergy

ETIOLOGY, EPIDEMIOLOGY, & RISK FACTORS

- Antibiotics and pain medications are the most frequent cause of allergic drug reactions
- Immediate generalized reactions occur due to release of vasoactive and inflammatory mediators from mast cells and basophils, causing multisystem dysfunction
- Children have a lower incidence of drug allergy compared with adults
- Allergic reactions are more common in hospitalized patients
- Gell and Coombs classification of allergic reactions:
  - Type I: IgE mediated (eg, anaphylaxis from a β-lactam drug)
  - Type II: Cytotoxic antibody mediated (eg, hemolytic anemia from penicillin)
  - Type III: Mediated by immune complex formation (eg, serum sickness from a cephalosporin)
  - Type IV: Cell mediated (eg, contact dermatitis from topical neomycin)
- Reactions may also be classified according to time of onset: immediate (<1 hour after administration, resulting in anaphylaxis, hives, and wheezing), intermediate (within the first 3 days, resulting in hives, laryngeal edema, and wheezing), and late (after 3 days, resulting in the above presentations plus cutaneous eruptions, hematologic aberrations, vasculitis, serum sickness, or Stevens-Johnson syndrome)

PATIENT PRESENTATION

- Rashes are the most common manifestation of drug allergy in children
  - Urticaria, angioedema
  - Morbilliform rashes
  - Photoreaction
  - Erythema multiforme, Stevens-Johnson syndrome, and toxic epidermal necrolysis are a range of severe dermatologic reactions with circular or target mucocutaneous lesions that may progress to severe blistering and sloughing of skin
- Respiratory symptoms may include hoarseness or wheezing
- Edema may occur due to angioedema, nephritis or nephrotic syndrome, or serum sickness
- Hypotension
- Anemia, neutropenia, or thrombocytopenia may occur due to destruction of peripheral cells

DIFFERENTIAL DX

- Mild skin exanthems
  - Viral illness
  - Atopic dermatitis
  - Urticaria from other causes
  - Contact dermatitis
- Anaphylaxis
  - Food allergy
  - Stinging insect (venom) allergy

DIAGNOSTIC EVALUATION

- A thorough history is the most important diagnostic factor
  - Note medications the patient is taking or has recently taken, as well as the time of intro-duction, route, dose, and duration
  - Medications used frequently or chronically have lower chance of causing reactions than ones that were recently introduced
  - A history of other drug allergies raises the likelihood of drug allergy
- Serum-specific IgE testing for a specific allergen (previously called RAST testing) is not helpful because many drugs are allergenic only when bound to a carrier protein in vivo
- Skin testing for penicillin may be helpful
  - A scratch or pinprick test is safer but less definitive than an intradermal skin test
  - If positive, drug should be avoided
  - If negative, there is still a risk of allergy; however, more than half of patients with a negative skin test can safely take penicillin
- A provocative drug challenge (administration of the suspected agent under controlled circumstances) is rarely performed
- Skin testing and provocative drug challenge are contraindicated in patients who have had Stevens-Johnson syndrome, toxic epidermal necrolysis, or anaphylaxis

TREATMENT & MANAGEMENT

- Discontinue the drug and avoid future exposure to the same drug, as well as drugs in the same category
- In cases of anaphylaxis, emergent treatment is necessary with epinephrine, antihistamines, and corticosteroids
- If a drug is needed despite a severe, IgE-mediated allergy, desensitization may be performed
  - Desensitization consists of administering small, incrementally increased doses of the medication under a controlled, inpatient environment
  - Desensitization must be repeated each time the medication is used
- In cases of a needed medication or treatment with a history of questionable allergy, pretreatment with diphenhydramine may allow safe administration
- Exanthematous or morbilliform rashes resolve within 2–3 days after removal of the offending agent; antihistamines may be used for pruritus
- Topical steroids may improve localized cutaneous eruptions

PROGNOSIS & COMPLICATIONS

- Children with a history of allergic rhinitis, asthma, or atopic dermatitis do not appear to have an increased risk of developing drug hypersensitivities
- Children whose parents have had an allergic reaction to an antibiotic may be at increased risk of developing an allergic reaction to an antibiotic
- Some children with chronic illness, such as cystic fibrosis and HIV, are more prone to drug allergies that cannot be explained by multiple medication exposures alone

Food Allergy

INTRODUCTION

- Food allergy is separate from other adverse reactions to foods, including intolerance (such as lactose intolerance or sucrase-isomaltase deficiency), other enzyme deficiencies (such as galactosemia), and food poisoning
- Food allergy may present in a variety of ways:
  - Cutaneous: atopic dermatitis, urticaria, diaper rash
  - Oral allergy syndrome: local symptoms due to food and pollen cross-reactivity
  - Respiratory: rhinorrhea, nasal congestion, cough, wheezing
  - Gastrointestinal: milk-protein allergy (non-IgE), eosinophilic enteritis (IgE)
  - Anaphylactic: angioedema, hypotension, bronchospasm

ETIOLOGY, EPIDEMIOLOGY, & RISK FACTORS

- Foods are one of the most common causes of anaphylaxis
- Patients with asthma are more likely to have food allergies and more likely to have a severe reaction
- Up to 6% of young children have food allergies; the most common allergenic foods in children are milk, egg, peanuts, wheat, and soy
- Less than 1% of adults have food allergy; the most common allergenic foods in adults are peanuts, tree nuts, fish, and shellfish
- Food hypersensitivity is often an IgE-mediated process:
  - Mast cell–bound IgE cross-links with a food allergen, causing release of inflammatory mediators (histamine, leukotrienes, prostaglandins)
  - IgE-mediated food allergy typically manifests acutely within minutes to hours of eating the allergenic food with symptoms of mouth discomfort, itching, swelling, hives, and wheezing
- Non–IgE-mediated food allergy has a more insidious course:
  - Evolves over hours and typically follows a chronic course
  - Eosinophilic infiltration of the gut results in inflammation with ensuing diarrhea, vomiting, abdominal pain, and failure to thrive in infants

PATIENT PRESENTATION

- Cutaneous manifestations: atopic dermatitis, urticaria
- Gastrointestinal manifestations: nausea, vomiting, abdominal pain, diarrhea, failure to thrive
  - Anemia may occur due to microscopic blood loss from the inflamed gut
- Respiratory manifestations: sneezing, rhinorrhea, coughing, wheezing
- Anaphylaxis (eg, hypotension, tachycardia)

DIFFERENTIAL DX

- Food intolerance (eg, lactase deficiency)
- Food-induced colitis syndrome (eg, infant "milk protein allergy")
- Food poisoning
- Gastroesophageal reflux disease
- Celiac disease
- Inflammatory bowel disease
- Drug allergy
- Idiopathic urticaria

DIAGNOSTIC EVALUATION

- A detailed history is the mainstay of diagnosis
  - Note ingestions of suspected foods and timing of symptoms related to ingestion; keeping a "diet diary" is often helpful
  - Note type, severity, and reproducibility of symptoms
  - Note family history of food allergies
  - Distinguish food allergy from food intolerance
- Skin testing:
  - A negative puncture skin test essentially rules out IgE-mediated food allergy
  - A positive puncture skin test, especially without a significant history, may be a false-positive result
  - Skin testing alone can provoke anaphylaxis in extremely sensitive individuals
- Elevated eosinophils on CBC or elevated total IgE are supportive but not diagnostic findings
- Serum measurement of specific IgE antibodies using RAST testing
- Fluorescent enzyme immunoassay is becoming more available
- A double-blind, placebo-controlled food challenge is the gold standard for diagnosing food allergy but is difficult to perform and has a questionable safety profile; other food challenges are sometimes undertaken to aid the diagnosis
  - Any food challenge should take place in a medical setting

TREATMENT & MANAGEMENT

- For children with a history of anaphylaxis from a food allergy, strict avoidance of the food is necessary
  - Epinephrine should be available at all times
  - Patient and parent education, including label reading and food preparation
- For children with a history of atopic dermatitis and food allergy, an elimination diet may be helpful
  - Remove all skin test- or blood test-positive foods for 2 weeks
  - If skin improves, slowly reintroduce each food, one at a time, and observe any skin changes to determine which foods are allergenic
  - If there is no skin improvement after 2 weeks of a strict elimination diet, it is less likely that food is contributing to the atopic dermatitis
- For patients with asthma, initiate bronchodilator therapy, begin or increase inhaled steroids, and consider systemic steroids if the reaction is significant
- Consider nutrition consultation if diet is restrictive
- Antihistamines are generally useful and well tolerated

PROGNOSIS & COMPLICATIONS

- Food allergies to milk, egg, wheat, and soy are usually outgrown by age 3 years
- Allergies to peanuts, tree nuts, fish, and shellfish tend to be lifelong
- Constant vigilance is required when eating in restaurants or other places where prepared food is served
- Schools should be informed when a child is diagnosed with food allergy
- Epinephrine must remain immediately available in case of accidental ingestions; parents, schoolteachers, and other caregivers must know how to use the epinephrine autoinjector

Primary Immunodeficiencies

INTRODUCTION

- More than 150 different primary immunodeficiencies have been identified
- Primary immunodeficiencies cause increased susceptibility to infections and may present as repeated minor infections, one or more severe infections, infections with unusual or opportunistic pathogens, or quick relapse after treatment of an infection
- Primary immunodeficiencies are the result of a defect in any arm of the immune system or immune cell type within the body's defense systems, including innate defenses (neutrophils, macrophages/phagocytic cells, natural killer cells, complement function) or adaptive defenses (antigen-presenting cells, B-cell, T-cell, combined B- and T-cell actions)

ETIOLOGY, EPIDEMIOLOGY, & RISK FACTORS

- Overall incidence of 1 per 10,000 births
  - Incidence is as high as 1 in 333 for selective IgA deficiency and as low as 1 in 200,000 for chronic granulomatous disease (CGD)
  - The most commonly diagnosed disorder is common variable immunodeficiency
  - Most cases present in infancy or childhood, but milder forms may be diagnosed later in adolescence or adulthood
- The most common or significant diagnoses include:
  - B-cell: X-linked agammaglobulinemia, selective IgA deficiency
  - T-cell: DiGeorge syndrome, chronic mucocutaneous candidiasis
  - Combined B- and T-cell: Wiskott-Aldrich syndrome, hyper-IgM syndrome, severe combined immunodeficiency (SCID)
  - Phagocyte: CGD, leukocyte adhesion defect
  - Complement: C5 deficiency, C2 deficiency
- These disorders have genetic inheritances:
  - X-linked: SCID, hyper-IgM, CGD, Wiskott-Aldrich
  - Autosomal recessive: Ataxia-telangiectasia, many complement deficiencies
  - Autosomal dominant: DiGeorge syndrome

PATIENT PRESENTATION

- B-cell defects: sinus and respiratory diseases, chronic otitis media (infection with encapsulated organisms), thick purulent nasal secretions, abnormal lung exam consistent with pneumonia
- T-cell defects: opportunistic infections with viruses and fungi, growth failure, candidiasis, dysmorphic features, tonsils may be absent
- Phagocyte defects: recurrent infections with catalase-positive bacterial organisms and fungi, abscesses, lymphoid hyperplasia
- Complement defects: high incidence of severe infections with *Neisseria* organisms, arthritis/arthralgias

DIFFERENTIAL DX

- Normal patient with frequent infections
- Cystic fibrosis
- HIV
- Failure to thrive for other reasons
- Nephrotic syndrome
- Leukemia
- Lymphoma

DIAGNOSTIC EVALUATION

- Detailed infection history, including age of onset
  - B-cell defects usually present around 6 months of age
  - T-cell defects usually present shortly after birth
  - Variable presentations with phagocyte and complement defects
  - Factors and findings suggestive of primary immunodeficiency include eight or more ear infections, two or more cases of pneumonia, or two or more deep infections in 1 year; any history of unusual or opportunistic infections; recurrent skin abscesses; or a family history of an immune disorder
- Physical exam may reveal poor weight gain, failure to thrive, absent lymph nodes or tonsils, and skin findings (eg, eczematous lesions, cutaneous infections including *Candida*)
- Laboratory testing:
  - Complete blood count with visual differential cell count
  - B-cell testing: Quantitative serum immunoglobulins, IgG subclasses, and specific antibody testing (eg, pneumococci, tetanus)
  - T-cell testing: Absolute lymphocyte count and lymphocyte subset counts (CD4, CD8), lymphocyte proliferation response to mitogens, delayed-type hypersensitivity reactions
  - Phagocyte testing: Absolute neutrophil count, neutrophil oxidative burst assay
  - Complement testing: CH_{50} assay as a screen of complement activity; if abnormal, test for specific complement levels

TREATMENT & MANAGEMENT

- Treatment varies depending on the type of immunodeficiency
- Aggressive management of infections, with culture and sensitivities when obtainable and early empiric therapy
- Prophylactic antibiotics for patients prone to opportunistic infections (eg, trimethoprim-sulfamethoxazole for *Pneumocystis carinii* prophylaxis in patients with CGD)
- Immunoglobulin is useful for X-linked agammaglobulinemia, common variable immunodeficiency, X-linked hyper-IgM, SCID, Wiskott-Aldrich syndrome, and selective IgG class deficiency
- Bone marrow transplantation from HLA-identical donors may be curative and is used in patients with cellular immune deficiencies, such as SCID, Wiskott-Aldrich syndrome, DiGeorge syndrome, and CGD
- Live vaccines should not be given to immunodeficient patients or their close contacts
- If a transfusion is given to a patient with a primary immunodeficiency, it should be irradiated to prevent graft-versus-host disease

PROGNOSIS & COMPLICATIONS

- Prognosis and clinical course vary from asymptomatic (eg, in some cases of IgA deficiency) to severe disease and death in early childhood (eg, in cases of SCID that do not receive a bone marrow transplantation)
- Prevention and management of infections require meticulous health and hygiene habits, as well as prompt medical attention and good compliance to optimize outcomes

DiGeorge Syndrome

INTRODUCTION

- DiGeorge syndrome is a disorder comprised of immune deficiency, dysmorphism, abnormal calcium metabolism, and cardiac defects
- Occurs when there is defective embryonic development of the fourth branchial arch and third and fourth pharyngeal pouches, resulting in hypoplasia of the thymus and parathyroid glands, conotruncal heart defects, facial anomalies, and neuropsychiatric disorders
- It is one of a related group of anomalies involving neural crest migration and pharyngeal pouches and arches, alongside velocardiofacial syndrome and CHARGE syndrome (coloboma, heart defects, choanal atresia, mental retardation, genital anomalies, and ear anomalies)

ETIOLOGY, EPIDEMIOLOGY, & RISK FACTORS

- Affects 1 in 4000 live births
- Most often the result of a genetic defect of chromosome 22q11, usually due to a spontaneous mutation
- If the parent carries a deletion, the defect is passed in an autosomal dominant pattern, although autosomal recessive and X-linked cases have also been identified
- The hypoplastic thymus leads to failure of T-cell maturation, which predisposes to early and severe infections
- The missing parathyroid tissue leads to hypocalcemia, potentially causing severe seizures tetany, especially in the neonatal period
- Cardiac anomalies and their complications are the most frequent causes of death

PATIENT PRESENTATION

- Congenital heart disease, especially aortic arch anomalies (right aortic arch, interrupted aortic arch, truncus arteriosus, tetralogy of Fallot)
- Hypocalcemia, resulting in seizures and tetany
- Recurrent infections, especially viral
- Abnormal facies:
  - Hypertelorism
  - Down-slanting palpebral fissures
  - Prominent ears, sometimes low set
  - Micrognathia
- Mild cognitive impairment

DIFFERENTIAL DX

- Velocardiofacial syndrome
- Conotruncal anomaly face syndrome
- Congenital heart disease with aortic arch anomalies
- Other causes of hypocalcemia, tetany, and seizures
- Other T-cell immunodeficiencies that result in recurrent viral and fungal infections and opportunistic infections, such as *Pneumocystis carinii* pneumonia

DIAGNOSTIC EVALUATION

- History and physical examination
  - The characteristic phenotype varies from subtle facial findings and mild learning problems to profound cardiac, immunologic, and endocrine abnormalities
  - Characteristic facial dysmorphism
  - Hypocalcemic seizures or tetany
  - Frequent infections
  - Associated congenital heart defects
- Laboratory testing:
  - FISH (fluorescence in situ hybridization) analysis for 22q11.2 followed by cytogenetic analysis
  - Low CD3 T-cell count
  - "Complete" DiGeorge syndrome is characterized by markedly low T-cell counts with impaired responses to mitogens on flow cytometry
  - "Partial" DiGeorge syndrome is characterized by normal or near-normal T-cell counts with normal or near-normal responses to mitogens on flow cytometry
  - Hypocalcemia occurs secondary to hypoparathyroidism; indeterminate parathyroid hormone function can be evaluated by a disodium edentate challenge
- Chest X-ray reveals an absent thymic shadow in a newborn or young infant
- Echocardiography is necessary to assess for congenital heart defects

TREATMENT & MANAGEMENT

- Neonates suspected to have DiGeorge syndrome based on the typical facies, associated congenital heart defect, abnormal thymic shadow, or family history should be monitored carefully for hypocalcemia and treated as necessary; an echocardiogram should be obtained as early as possible, even if patient is cardiovascularly stable
- Bone marrow or thymic tissue transplantation is indicated in cases of "complete" DiGeorge syndrome but is not necessary for "partial" DiGeorge cases
- Antibiotic treatment or prophylaxis for opportunistic infections
- Serum calcium regulation using calcium and vitamin D supplementation
- Correction of congenital heart defects, when present
- Any blood transfusions must be confirmed negative for cytomegalovirus and irradiated to prevent graft-versus-host disease
- Early intervention to maximize developmental outcome

PROGNOSIS & COMPLICATIONS

- The extent and severity of associated cardiac defects are the major determinants of prognosis
- The majority of children have mild and transient immune problems
- Increased risk for autoimmune diseases
- Genetic counseling is indicated

Serum Sickness

- Serum sickness is a type III hypersensitivity reaction that occurs as a result of exposure to a foreign substance
- Historically, serum sickness occurred when a patient was given a heterologous antigenic protein in the form of an antitoxin, such as rabies or tetanus from horse serum; because these are less frequently used, serum sickness and serum sickness–like reactions are now most likely to occur after administration of drugs, blood products, hormones, and vaccines
- Results in vasculitis manifested as fever, arthralgias, arthritis, lymphadenopathy, and rash, along with a broad range of other clinical findings

ETIOLOGY, EPIDEMIOLOGY, & RISK FACTORS

- A classic example of a type III hypersensitivity reaction
- Following administration of a foreign antigenic substance, antibody-antigen complexes are formed and become trapped in small vessels, resulting in complement activation
- The presence of immune complexes in the vessels causes an inflammatory response, resulting in vasculitis and tissue damage
- In pediatrics, the most commonly implicated drugs are penicillins, cephalosporins (especially cefaclor), and sulfonamides, but a number of other drugs in various categories are also causes
- Other iatrogenic etiologies of serum sickness include blood products, allergen extracts (for allergy shots), exogenous hormones, vaccines, and snake and spider bite antidotes
- Serum sickness also sporadically occurs following viral or bacterial infections

PATIENT PRESENTATION

- Symptoms usually occur 1–3 weeks after exposure (sooner if the child is already sensitized to the antigen)
- A local reaction at an injection site may precede systemic symptoms
- Fever, usually high grade
- Malaise, which may present as fussiness or irritability in young children
- Skin findings may include urticaria, scarlatiniform or polymorphous rash, and pruritic eruptions
- Arthritis and arthralgias, usually of the hips, knees, and elbows; may also involve the spine or small joints
- Less common presentations include hematuria, nephritis, neuropathy, and myocarditis or pericarditis

DIFFERENTIAL DX

- Other diseases that involve circulating immune complexes (eg, vasculitis, SLE, and glomerulonephritis)
- Mononucleosis
- Rocky Mountain spotted fever

DIAGNOSTIC EVALUATION

- Clinical history and physical examination with special attention to recent medications, vaccines, other medical treatments, and recent illness
- Laboratory testing includes:
  - Decreased complement levels (C3 and C4) occur early and resolve quickly
  - Erythrocyte sedimentation rate (ESR) may be elevated
  - Urinalysis may show proteinuria and/or hematuria
  - Testing of serum for immune complexes is generally not helpful because it is not readily available and many false-positive results occur
- Biopsy of skin lesions shows direct immunofluorescence of IgM, IgA, IgE, and C3 complexes deposited in capillary walls

TREATMENT & MANAGEMENT

- Supportive care
- Remove offending agents
- Further administration of a potential causative agent is relatively contraindicated
- The goal of treatment is to decrease inflammation and tissue damage
- NSAIDs are useful for fever and general reduction of inflammation
- Antihistamines can blunt the effects of the inflammatory response
- Topical corticosteroids for localized skin eruptions
- Systemic corticosteroids may be needed in more severe cases to address the joint symptoms; they are also indicated when there is renal, cardiac, or neurologic involvement

PROGNOSIS & COMPLICATIONS

- Usually self-limited
- Symptoms often resolve within a few days to a few weeks; ongoing complications or sequelae do not usually occur
- Re-exposure results in further episodes, and subsequent episodes may be more severe
- If an antigenic drug is necessary (eg, penicillin), desensitization can be performed to prevent anaphylaxis; however, desensitization will not prevent serum sickness

Orthopedics

Developmental Dysplasia of the Hip

INTRODUCTION

- Developmental dysplasia of the hip refers to a spectrum of hip disorders with varying degrees of involvement and different ages of presentation
- Early diagnosis and treatment are important for successful remodeling of dysplastic hips
- Neonatal screening showing hip instability is a crucial aspect of diagnosis

ETIOLOGY, EPIDEMIOLOGY, & RISK FACTORS

- A congenital or acquired abnormality of hip development
- May be due to capsular laxity or mechanical factors (eg, abnormal intrauterine positioning)
- Occurs in the left hip more often than the right hip
- Risk factors include positive family history (20% of cases), female sex (85% of cases), breech position (nearly 50% of cases), multiple gestations, and oligohydramnios
- There is a higher incidence in Native-Americans and whites and lower incidence in blacks and Asians

PATIENT PRESENTATION

- Usually asymptomatic at birth
  - Hip click upon hip movement (Ortolani and Barlow maneuvers) is often the initial presentation
- Older infants may have decreased hip abduction or shortening of the affected leg
- Diagnosis may be delayed until the patient becomes ambulatory
  - Shortening of the affected leg and altered gait suggest the diagnosis
- If the diagnosis has not been made until older childhood, adolescence, or adulthood, affected patients may present with hip pain, limping, or early arthritis

DIFFERENTIAL DX

- Proximal femoral focal deficiency
- Benign labral hip click

DIAGNOSTIC EVALUATION

- Routine newborn screening by examination for a hip click is necessary
  - Barlow test: Adduction and depression of the femur dislocates the hip
  - Ortolani test: Elevation and abduction of the femur relocates the dislocated hip
- Patients with a hip click or significant risk factors should be evaluated by ultrasound
- Physical exam in older children may reveal decreased hip abduction of the affected hip or Galeazzi sign (shortened femur on the affected side)
- X-ray in older infants (>3 months) may reveal an increased acetabular index or delayed ossification of the femoral head
  - Perkins and Shenton line are radiographic parameters that are useful in identifying or tracking the progression of hip dysplasia
- Dynamic ultrasonography may be useful in younger children

TREATMENT & MANAGEMENT

- Early diagnosis allows for nonsurgical treatments because the anatomic changes are initially reversible
  - In patients with undiagnosed hip dysplasia, the acetabulum (hip socket) becomes shallow with irreversible soft tissue and bony changes, making surgery necessary to improve the articulation of the femoral head and acetabulum
- Early treatment aims at reducing the femoral head to apply a force to deepen the acetabulum during the neonatal period
- Infants (<6 months) may be treated with a Pavlik harness to reduce the hip in 100 degrees of flexion and mild abduction
  - Educate the family to appropriately apply and maintain the Pavlik harness; otherwise, the harness can be adjusted in the clinic on a weekly basis
- In patients aged 6–18 months or those who have failed the Pavlik harness, treat with closed surgical reduction and hip spica cast for 4 months
- Patients aged 12–18 months require open reduction if failed closed reduction, obstructive limbus, or unstable "safe zone" in Pavlik harness
- Patients presenting in adolescence often require more extensive surgery to reduce and reorient the acetabulum; this often requires acetabular osteotomies to achieve femoral head coverage

PROGNOSIS & COMPLICATIONS

- Excellent prognosis when diagnosed and treated early
- Risks of failed treatment include repeated dislocation, avascular necrosis of the femoral head, and early degenerative arthritis
  - Avascular necrosis is generally diagnosed when the femoral head fails to ossify or fails to grow within 1 year following hip reduction
  - Avascular necrosis may be prevented by avoiding abnormal hip positioning in the cast or Pavlik harness
  - Femoral shortening osteotomy may be required when the hip capsule is too tight following reduction

Slipped Capital Femoral Epiphysis

INTRODUCTION

- Slipped capital femoral epiphysis (SCFE) is the most common adolescent hip disorder
- Usually occurs during adolescence when rapid growth causes weakening of the proximal femoral physis, leading to displacement of the femoral head from its normal anatomic position
- The femoral head is displaced on the femoral neck, creating an abnormal angulation
- The slip may occur gradually with few symptoms or acutely following an extended period of milder symptoms
- When bilateral SCFE is diagnosed, an underlying endocrine disorder should be considered

ETIOLOGY, EPIDEMIOLOGY, & RISK FACTORS

- Mean age of onset is 11 years in girls and 13 years in boys
- SCFE may be related to hormonal changes in young children (eg, hypothyroidism and other endocrine abnormalities, renal disease), nutritional deficiencies, or trauma
- Risk factors include obesity, male sex, adolescent age, and family history
- Estimated incidence is approximately 2 cases per 100,000 with higher incidence in black males and in adolescents living in the eastern U.S.
- Occurs bilaterally in up to 25% of cases
- Chondrolysis (death of femoral joint cartilage) may occur (see Prognosis & Complications section)
  - Chondrolysis is a separate entity from avascular necrosis of the femoral head

PATIENT PRESENTATION

- Symptoms vary depending on whether the slip is acute, acute-on-chronic, or chronic
- Symptoms depend on the stability of slip
- Hip, groin, thigh, or knee pain
  - Patients may present with a dull, vague, achy pain that may be intermittent or constant and may be exacerbated by activity
  - Knee pain in adolescents is often caused by a slipped epiphysis, but the diagnosis is delayed or missed
  - Missed diagnoses often lead to more severe slips and a worse prognosis
- Limited internal rotation of the hip
- Coxalgic, externally rotated gait
- Thigh atrophy
- Limb shortening

DIFFERENTIAL DX

- Femoral cutaneous nerve entrapment
- Legg-Calvé-Perthes disease
- Osteochondral avulsion fracture
- Infection
  - Usually presents with fever, malaise, and pain due to hip capsule swelling
  - Infection may present as a psoas abscess or sacroiliac joint infection, which may be difficult to localize without other imaging studies such as CT scan or MRI

DIAGNOSTIC EVALUATION

- Clinical examination is the key to diagnosis
  - Antalgic gait with a limp on the affected side is often noted
  - The affected leg may be held in external rotation
  - Shortening of the affected leg and thigh atrophy may be present
  - Note body habitus and other signs of endocrine abnormalities; most patients will have a normal body habitus, but the stereotypical patient is an obese, hypogonadal male
  - A flexion contracture of the hip may suggest chondrolysis
- Anterior/posterior and lateral X-rays
  - The earliest radiologic sign is a widened and irregular proximal femoral physis
  - Mild slips may result in a slight posterior displacement of the femoral head
  - Klein line: On the AP view, a line drawn parallel to the superior femoral neck should intersect the lateral portion of the femoral head; in mild slips, this line does not intersect the capital epiphysis
- CT scan or bone scan may afford earlier diagnosis
  - CT scan may be more accurate in measuring the true head-neck angle, although it is generally not necessary for diagnosis
- Endocrine workup in preadolescent children may be indicated

TREATMENT & MANAGEMENT

- Triage and initial management include avoidance of weight bearing to avoid acute slip and displacement of the femoral head
  - A wheelchair transfer to radiology for X-ray evaluation is best
  - If the abnormality is unilateral, crutches may be used
- Surgical treatment is often indicated
  - Initially, surgical percutaneous pinning is done to stabilize the femoral head on the femoral neck, so that further displacement cannot occur
  - Further options for surgical intervention depend on the type and severity of the slip
  - Prophylactic pinning of the contralateral hip is recommended for patients with endocrinopathies
  - A primary goal of surgery is to prevent progression of the slip

PROGNOSIS & COMPLICATIONS

- Complications may include joint space narrowing (chondrolysis), avascular necrosis, osteonecrosis, pain, decreased range of motion, and early degenerative arthritis
- Chondrolysis is the death of femoral joint cartilage; this differs from avascular necrosis of the femoral head
  - The joint space narrows, and there is pain with worsening hip contracture
  - May be noted at presentation or postoperatively; postoperative chondrolysis is often related to metal penetration into the hip joint
- Avascular necrosis of the femoral head is the most severe complication; it occurs when the blood supply to the femoral head is compromised

Septic Arthritis

INTRODUCTION

- Bacterial infection of a joint space, usually from a hematogenous source
- Delayed diagnosis may lead to chondrolysis, avascular necrosis, joint destruction, or osteomyelitis
- A high index of suspicion is necessary in infants and toddlers because they may have a nonfocal clinical presentation
- Septic arthritis of the hip is a surgical emergency
- Before the introduction of antibiotics, mortality reached as high as 50%; however, improved detection and antibiotic treatments have significantly decreased the morbidity and mortality associated with joint sepsis

ETIOLOGY, EPIDEMIOLOGY, & RISK FACTORS

- Defined as acute infection of the synovial space
- Most commonly due to hematogenous spread but may also occur due to direct extension of osteomyelitis into the joint
- *Staphylococcus aureus* infection is the overall most common cause
- Group B streptococci are the most common cause in infants
- *Neisseria gonorrhoeae* is the most common cause in sexually active adolescents
- Vaccination has decreased the incidence of *Haemophilus influenzae* infection
- Most cases of septic hip arthritis occur in infants and children
- Some studies reveal an increased male predominance

PATIENT PRESENTATION

- Severe pain
- Fever
- Malaise
- Decreased range of motion or increased pain with motion of a joint
- Warmth, redness, and tenderness
- Failure to move or use the affected joint
- Pain with passive motion
- A history of minor trauma often precedes the presentation, which may confuse and delay the diagnosis of acute joint sepsis

DIFFERENTIAL DX

- Osteomyelitis
- Cellulitis
- Juvenile rheumatoid arthritis
- Fracture
- Avascular necrosis
- Transient synovitis
- Rheumatic fever
- Lyme disease
- Acute leukemia
- Diskitis

DIAGNOSTIC EVALUATION

- History and physical examination
  - In the case of a septic hip, the patient may hold the hip in a flexed, externally rotated and abducted position (this position allows for maximum volume expansion of the hip capsule)
- Laboratory testing includes complete blood count with differential, ESR, C-reactive protein, and blood cultures
- AP and lateral X-rays of the affected joint may show widened joint space or demonstrate concomitant osteomyelitis; however, the bone and joint often appear normal, and soft tissue swelling may be the only finding
- CT scan has limited efficacy in diagnosing an early septic arthritis but may be useful if there is suspicion of soft tissue abscess in the spine and pelvis region
- Ultrasound may demonstrate joint effusion
- Joint aspiration and synovial fluid cultures are diagnostic
  - White blood cell count >50,000 is common, but *N. gonorrhoeae* infection usually does not raise white blood cell count this high
  - Increased polymorphonuclear neutrophils >90%
  - Increased protein

TREATMENT & MANAGEMENT

- Septic arthritis is an acute surgical emergency
  - Aspirate the joint to confirm the diagnosis and send fluid for culture
  - Most studies support prompt surgical drainage of hip sepsis because of the limited success in effectively treating hip infection with medical management alone
  - Surgery of other joints is less well defined, although prompt aspiration, irrigation, and IV antibiotics in acute settings are appropriate
  - Patients who fail to improve require surgical arthrotomy and drainage
- Empiric IV antibiotics should be initiated immediately and continued for 3–6 weeks or until resolution of infection
  - Newborn (<3 months): Treat for *S. aureus* and group B streptococci
  - Children (3 months to 12–14 years): Treat for *S. aureus, Streptococcus pneumoniae, Streptococcus pyogenes*, Gram-negative bacilli, and *Haemophilus influenzae*
  - Adolescents and adults: Treat for *N. gonorrhoeae, S. aureus,* and streptococci

PROGNOSIS & COMPLICATIONS

- Good prognosis with early treatment
- Septic arthritis destroys the joint surface and may result in contractures, arthritis, chronic pain, recurrent infections, capsular scarring, joint malformation and osteonecrosis resulting in impaired and limited joint function

Legg-Calvé-Perthes Disease

INTRODUCTION

- Legg-Calvé-Perthes is a disease of the hip joint characterized by a vascular insult and growth disturbance of the femoral epiphysis
- Presents with variable severity; bilateral in 10% of cases

ETIOLOGY, EPIDEMIOLOGY, & RISK FACTORS

- Avascular necrosis of the femoral head (proximal femoral epiphysis) occurs, leading to osteonecrosis; the bone is then resorbed and replaced, but the replaced bone tends to be flattened and enlarged
- Most common in males aged 4–8 years
- Especially common in children with delayed skeletal maturity
- Other risk factors include family history, low birth weight, and abnormal birth presentation
- Medical conditions associated with Legg-Calvé-Perthes include coagulation abnormalities, protein C and S deficiencies, hemoglobinopathies (eg, sickle cell anemia, thalassemia), and leukemia and lymphoma

PATIENT PRESENTATION

- The deformity is variable in severity and depends on the age of presentation
- Painless limp, which may be exacerbated by activity and improved with rest
- Hip or knee pain
- Trendelenburg test: normally the pelvis is maintained in a horizontal position when standing on one leg; a positive test occurs when the pelvis drops on the contralateral side due to weakness of the hip abductor muscles
- Decreased range of motion of the hip with loss of abduction and internal rotation
- Antalgic gait

DIFFERENTIAL DX

- Septic arthritis
- Fracture
- Blood dyscrasias (eg, sickle cell disease)
- Hypothyroidism
- Epiphyseal dysplasias, including multiple epiphyseal dysplasia, spondyloepiphyseal dysplasia, and Morquio disease
  - In contrast to Legg-Calvé-Perthes disease, children with epiphyseal dysplasia generally have bilateral involvement, short stature, and distal femoral epiphyseal involvement

DIAGNOSTIC EVALUATION

- Clinical examination reveals abnormal gait and decreased hip range of motion (limited abduction and internal rotation)
- Radiology testing generally only includes AP and lateral pelvis X-rays
  - MRI, CT scan, ultrasound, and bone scan may be used but are not usually necessary
  - MRI is the most accurate imaging modality for early diagnosis
- Radiographic staging is based on the Waldenström classification, which includes four stages (initial, fragmentation, reossification, and residual)
  - Initial stage: Slightly smaller and lateralized femoral head ossific nucleus; frog-leg lateral view may show subchondral linear fracture (Waldenström sign)
  - Fragmentation stage: Lucencies develop in the ossific nucleus
  - Reossification stage: Healing stage with new bone formation in the subchondral part of the femoral head; improvement and rounding of the femoral head generally occur during this stage
  - Residual stage: No further healing occurs, but the shape of the femoral head may continue to remodel until skeletal maturity

TREATMENT & MANAGEMENT

- Rest
- Immobilization and traction may be necessary
- Symptomatic relief with anti-inflammatory medications
- Bracing to prevent further flattening of the femoral head
  - The rationale is to nonsurgically contain the femoral head
  - Many different braces have been developed with varying complexity in application and protocols
  - The type and duration of bracing are tailored to each patient; average length of treatment is 9–12 months
- Surgical intervention may be necessary for older children
  - Femoral varus derotational osteotomy may be indicated for late onset of disease (after 6 years old) or worsening radiographic signs
  - Innominate osteotomy and combined innominate and femoral osteotomy may be performed depending on severity

PROGNOSIS & COMPLICATIONS

- Most patients have moderate symptoms that last 12–18 months
- After this period, the symptoms subside and may completely resolve, allowing the child to resume normal activities; however, the severity of disease varies from patient to patient
- Prognosis depends on the age of onset and severity of femoral head involvement
  - A spherical-shaped femoral head improves the likeliness of a good outcome
  - Some studies suggest that up to 50% of cases may ultimately require hip replacement due to degenerative hip joint
- Younger patients have a better prognosis: Patients presenting at younger than 6 years old usually have a mild course; those presenting after 8 years usually have worse outcomes

Osgood-Schlatter Disease

INTRODUCTION

- Osgood-Schlatter disease is localized pain and swelling over the tibial tubercle in a growing, active child; it is likely due to traction-induced inflammation of the tibial tubercle apophysis
- The enlargement of the tibial tubercle and associated pain may cause concern that a tumor is growing
- The disorder is generally self-limiting for most patients; pain usually resolves at skeletal maturity
- Treatment includes education, reassurance, activity modification, and symptomatic therapy for pain

ETIOLOGY, EPIDEMIOLOGY, & RISK FACTORS

- Pain at the tibial tubercle occurs due to repetitive stress at the insertion of the patellar tendon into the tibial tuberosity
- Greater incidence in active children who are involved in athletic activities
- Pain may worsen in individuals involved in athletic activities but may persist despite activity modification
- Greater incidence in males
- Average age of onset is 14–15 years
- Bilateral in 25% of cases

PATIENT PRESENTATION

- Pain below the knee
  - Pain may be exacerbated by running, jumping, or kneeling exercises
  - Pain may occur while sitting with knees flexed, or shortly afterwards
- Exam usually elicits point tenderness over the tibial tubercle and swelling over the distal patellar tendon
- Symptoms may persist for months or even years during adolescence, but pain usually gradually diminishes with time

DIFFERENTIAL DX

- Infection (eg, osteomyelitis)
- Neoplasm (eg, osteosarcoma)
- Sinding-Larsen-Johansson lesion (pain and tenderness around the distal pole of the patella)

DIAGNOSTIC EVALUATION

- Clinical exam typically reveals pain, tenderness, and swelling at the insertion of the patellar tendon
- X-rays of the proximal tibia may demonstrate fragmentation of the tibial tubercle or ossicle formation in the patellar tendon
  - Carefully assess the soft tissue areas, especially if neoplasm is suspected; critical analysis of plain X-rays may lead to detection of malignant tumor, but subtle changes may be missed in the early stages
- MRI is generally not indicated

TREATMENT & MANAGEMENT

- Treatment usually consists of parent and patient education and reassurance that the disorder is self-limited and will improve in time
- Rest, ice, stretching, and NSAIDs
- Protective knee pads may be used
- Severe symptoms may require immobilization to permit healing of microscopic avulsion fractures
- Patellar tendon ossicles may require surgical excision, especially if disabling symptoms persist beyond adolescence and the ossicles are clearly evident on X-rays

PROGNOSIS & COMPLICATIONS

- The prognosis is generally excellent
- Although most patients improve in time with activity modification and skeletal maturity, there are reports of early proximal tibia tubercle physeal closure and progressive genu recurvatum

Leg and Foot Deformities

INTRODUCTION

- Rotational deformities involving the lower extremities, including intoeing and metatarsus adductus, are usually asymptomatic
- Often parental concerns prompt an orthopedic evaluation
- Many cases are minor and self-limited
- Education and reassurance are the mainstay of treatment in the many cases that will naturally resolve without intervention

ETIOLOGY, EPIDEMIOLOGY, & RISK FACTORS

- Intoeing, or "pigeon toes," is a condition in which the foot turns inward more than expected while walking or running
  - May occur secondary to deformities of the foot, inward rotation of the tibia or femur, or a combination of both
  - Tibial torsion is the most common cause of intoeing up to ages 3–4
  - Children begin walking with the foot about 10 degrees out from the line of progression
  - Parents may observe that the child's foot turns inward while walking or the child may stumble as his or her toes catch the back of the trailing leg
- Metatarsus adductus is a common neonatal problem that is often overlooked
  - It is a foot deformity in which the forefoot is deviated inward relative to the hindfoot
  - Presumed to be associated with intrauterine positioning; however, this has never been proven
  - The true incidence is difficult to determine because mild forms often spontaneously improve

PATIENT PRESENTATION

- Patients present without pain
- Referral often occurs because parents are concerned about their children's abnormal lower extremity alignment
- Normal hip, knee, and ankle motion

DIFFERENTIAL DX

- Tibial torsion
- Femoral anteversion
- Neuromuscular disorders
- Metatarsus adductus
- Serpentine foot
- Cavus foot
- Clubfoot
- Hyperactive abductor hallucis

DIAGNOSTIC EVALUATION

- Gait evaluation: Estimate the angle of the foot relative to the line of progression
  - If the patella faces inward, the femur may be anteverted
  - If the patella is pointing straight, deviation is due to the tibia or foot
- Femoral anteversion: Measure internal and external rotation of the hip while prone
  - The average child has 30–60 degrees of internal rotation and 20–60 degrees of external rotation
  - Increased internal rotation (>70 degrees) or limited external rotation (<20 degrees) indicates femoral anteversion
- Tibial torsion: Measure the thigh-foot angle, the axis of the neutral foot relative to the axis of the thigh with the knee flexed to 90 degrees
  - An angle less than 10 degrees indicates tibial torsion
  - Metatarsus adductus: Grading based on heel bisector line; in normal patients, a line bisecting the heel crosses the forefoot between the second and third toes
  - Mild deformity: Heel bisector line crosses the third toe
  - Moderate deformity: Heel bisector crosses between the third and forth toes
  - Severe deformity: Heel bisector crosses between the fourth and fifth toes

TREATMENT & MANAGEMENT

- Rotational variations will gradually normalize
  - Nonsurgical methods (eg, orthotics, shoe modifications, exercises) are ineffective
  - Femoral anteversion may spontaneously correct by age 10
  - Tibial torsion often spontaneously resolves by age 4–6
  - Surgical correction is reserved for children with severe gait deformity that persists into adolescence who find their gait appearance unacceptable
- Metatarsus adductus
  - Surveillance: Most cases (85%) resolve spontaneously
  - Physical therapy: If foot can be corrected to neutral alignment passively or by peroneal muscle stimulation, the deformity should respond to stretching exercises
  - If foot cannot be corrected to neutral alignment passively, then patient may need special orthotics or serial casting
  - Surgery is indicated in severe or refractory cases or if diagnosis occurs beyond infancy

PROGNOSIS & COMPLICATIONS

- Most cases of rotational variations will gradually improve; parents/families should be clearly educated on the natural progression
- Internal rotation variations have not been associated with premature degenerative joint disease
- Risk and complications of rotational deformities are related to the surgical treatment, not the rotational disturbance
- Treatment of metatarsus adductus with serial casting at younger ages generally has good results; older patients (>3 years) who present with fixed adductus with significant deformity have mixed results with casting alone

Torsional Deformities

INTRODUCTION

- Most children walk with their foot placed about 10 degrees out from the line of progression, which is an imaginary line drawn in the direction in which one is walking
- Intoeing, or "pigeon toes," is a condition in which the foot turns inward more than expected during walking or running
- Outtoeing is a condition in which the foot turns outward more than expected
- Often, parental concerns prompt an orthopedic evaluation; however, most cases are asymptomatic, minor, and self-limiting

ETIOLOGY, EPIDEMIOLOGY, & RISK FACTORS

- The true incidence is difficult to determine because mild forms are overlooked or spontaneously improve
- Tibial torsion is most common; it may be internal, causing intoeing ("pigeon toes") or external, causing outtoeing
- Intoeing may occur secondary to deformities of the foot (such as metatarsus adductus), inward rotation of the tibia or femur, or a combination of these
  - Tibial torsion is the most common cause of intoeing up to age 3–4 years
  - Internal femoral torsion (femoral anteversion) is more common in girls than in boys, may be related to intrauterine positioning, and is associated with sitting in the "W" position
- Outtoeing usually occurs due to external tibial torsion, which is another consequence of intrauterine positioning
  - External femoral torsion (femoral retroversion) is a less common condition and is less likely to be benign
  - Outtoeing is more likely to be idiopathic when it occurs bilaterally
  - When associated with pain or obesity, it may be due to slipped capital femoral epiphysis

PATIENT PRESENTATION

- Most cases are asymptomatic; usually, the child presents to a physician because the parent is concerned about abnormal lower extremity alignment
- With intoeing, parents may observe that the child's foot turns inward while walking or the child may stumble as the toes catch the back of the trailing leg
- Note several concerning signs:
  - Rotational deformities should only decrease with time; an increase in symptoms or apparent worsening should prompt an evaluation
  - Pain should not be attributed to torsional deformities

DIFFERENTIAL DX

- Tibial torsion
- Femoral anteversion
- Neuromuscular disorders
- Metatarsus adductus
- Serpentine foot
- Cavus foot
- Clubfoot
- Hyperactive abductor hallucis

DIAGNOSTIC EVALUATION

- Perform a gait evaluation to estimate the angle of the foot relative to the line of progression
  - If the patella faces inward, the femur may be anteverted
  - If the patella is pointing straight, the deviation is due to the tibia or foot
- To test for femoral anteversion, measure hip internal and external rotation while prone
  - Average children older than 2 years have 30–60 degrees of internal rotation and 20–60 degrees of external rotation
  - Increased internal rotation (>70 degrees) or limited external rotation (<20 degrees) indicates femoral anteversion
- To test for tibial torsion, measure the thigh-foot angle, the axis of the neutral foot relative to the axis of the thigh with the knee flexed to 90 degrees
  - An angle <10 degrees indicates tibial torsion
  - To test for metatarsus adductus, grading is based on the heel bisector line, which normally bisects the heel and crosses the forefoot between the second and third toes
  - Mild deformity: Heel bisector line crosses the third toe
  - Moderate deformity: Heel bisector crosses between the third and forth toes
  - Severe deformity: Heel bisector crosses between the fourth and fifth toes

TREATMENT & MANAGEMENT

- Education and reassurance are the mainstays of treatment
- Rotational variations will gradually normalize
  - Nonsurgical methods (eg, orthotics, shoe modifications, or exercises) are ineffective
  - Femoral anteversion may spontaneously correct by age 10
  - Tibial torsion usually spontaneously resolves by age 4–6
  - Surgical correction is reserved for children with severe gait deformity into adolescence who find their gait appearance unacceptable
- Metatarsus adductus, when present, is treated by physical therapy and stretching exercises, orthotics, serial casting, or surgery in severe cases

PROGNOSIS & COMPLICATIONS

- Most cases of rotational variations will gradually improve; parents/families should be clearly educated on the natural progression
- Internal rotation variations have not been associated with premature degenerative joint disease
- Risks and complications of rotational deformities are related to the surgical treatment, not the rotational disturbance

Clubfoot

INTRODUCTION

- Clubfoot is the most common congenital orthopedic condition that requires treatment
- The diagnosis is usually made early, often prenatally by ultrasound
- Untreated children with clubfoot develop severe disabilities with poor ambulation, poorly fitting shoes, and impaired self-image
- Successful treatment allows the child to perform normal daily activities without pain; however, some residual abnormality may remain
- Initial treatment is nonoperative
- The support and participation of family and orthopedic surgeon are crucial in achieving an acceptable outcome

ETIOLOGY, EPIDEMIOLOGY, & RISK FACTORS

- Idiopathic clubfoot, or talipes equinovarus, is a congenital foot deformity that results in a downward and inward pointed foot
- Many theories exist to pinpoint the etiology of congenital clubfoot; however, no single theory is able to fully explain the foot deformity
- The insult is thought to occur early in limb bud development
- Most cases are probably multifactorial
- Various syndromes and neuromuscular conditions (eg, Down syndrome, Larsen syndrome, arthrogryposis, diastrophic dysplasia, constriction band syndrome, Freemen-Sheldon syndrome, chromosomal deletions, Mobius syndrome) increase the prevalence of having clubfoot
  - Clubfoot associated with these syndromes generally has a worse prognosis than idiopathic clubfoot
- Half of cases are bilateral
- Twice as common in males than females
- Family history is important; subsequent siblings have an increased risk (3–4% chance if only one child has clubfoot; 25% chance if a parent and child are affected)

PATIENT PRESENTATION

- Clinical appearance is highly suggestive
- The classic appearance is downward and inward pointed foot or feet
  - Varus of heel (displacement of the navicular and calcaneus bones produce an inverted, or varus, hindfoot)
  - Ankle plantar flexion
  - Forefoot adduction
  - Midfoot inversion

DIFFERENTIAL DX

- Congenital constriction band syndrome
- Deformed (spontaneously correctable) foot due to intrauterine positioning
- Spinal cord disorders

DIAGNOSTIC EVALUATION

- Clinical examination is usually diagnostic
  - Motor strength and sensory exam should be performed to determine the presence of spinal cord disorders
  - Clubfoot is associated with many other anomalies and syndromes; thus, a thorough physical exam allows for accurate diagnosis of syndromic versus idiopathic clubfoot
- X-rays are not necessary but may be helpful if the diagnosis is unclear

TREATMENT & MANAGEMENT

- Nonoperative treatment is usually preferred, although the treatment protocols and casting techniques vary
- Passive manipulation and serial casting should be initiated immediately
  - Early treatment may improve outcome due to the viscoelastic nature of newborns' tissue
  - The casts are changed at 1- to 2-week intervals for up to 2 years
- Therapy is continued with casts and orthoses until the patient is walking well
- Surgical therapy to lengthen contracted tendons and ligaments and allow normal alignment of bones is required if conservative treatment fails
  - Surgery is a last resort that must be carefully weighed
  - After the first surgery, the foot develops thickened scar and hardened soft tissues that make subsequent surgery much more difficult

PROGNOSIS & COMPLICATIONS

- The success of nonoperative treatment protocols depends largely on compliance and is assisted by intense and focused programs with social, economic, and logistical support for patients and their families
- Even with appropriate treatment, many patients will have some residual lower extremity abnormality and impairment
- Surgical correction may lead to severe flatfoot with lateral heel translation
- Incomplete or loss of surgical correction may require further intervention later in life
- Other complications include valgus overcorrection, dorsal bunion, and dorsal subluxation of the navicular
- Deformity may recur whether treatment is operative or nonoperative

Idiopathic Scoliosis

INTRODUCTION

- Scoliosis is defined as a measured lateral deviation of the normal vertical orientation of the spine greater than 10 degrees
- Idiopathic scoliosis accounts for 80% of patients with structural scoliosis
- Idiopathic scoliosis is divided into three groups: infantile, juvenile, and adolescent (most common)
- School-based screening programs facilitate early diagnosis

ETIOLOGY, EPIDEMIOLOGY, & RISK FACTORS

- Scoliosis is defined as a lateral deviation or curvature of the thoracic or lumbar spine greater than 10 degrees
  - Right thoracic curve is most common
- Females are more likely to have increased curve magnitude
- The etiology is unknown; may be related to neurologic, hormonal, proprioceptive, or connective tissue disorders
- There is a strong family history; possible autosomal dominant inheritance
- The Scoliosis Research Society recommends screening children between 10 and 14 years of age; the American Academy of Pediatrics recommends screening at ages 10, 12, 14, and 16 years old
- A measurement of 7 degrees of trunk rotation or more should prompt an orthopedic referral

PATIENT PRESENTATION

- Most patients do not present with pain; more commonly they are asymptomatic or have a physical deformity complaint (eg, drooping or high shoulder, protuberant hip)
- Although back pain is uncommon, it is a presenting complaint in 20% of patients
  - When a patient does complain of back pain, a thorough history and physical should be performed to rule out a more menacing problem, such as tumor or infection
- Rotational deformities become exaggerated when the patient flexes forward at the waist
- Associated signs may include rib rotation deformity, limb length discrepancy, shoulder slumping, or waistline asymmetry

DIFFERENTIAL DX

- Neuromuscular disorders (eg, cerebral palsy, muscular dystrophy, spinal muscular atrophy)
- Failure of spine formation or segmentation
- Tumor
- Infection
- Neurofibromatosis
- Metabolic bone disorders
- Marfan syndrome
- Limb length discrepancy (during exam, limb lengths should be equalized with blocks because limb length inequality may present like scoliosis)

DIAGNOSTIC EVALUATION

- Clinical examination
  - Back and shoulders should be fully exposed down to the iliac crests
  - Skin exam to evaluate for midline hair tufts, dimpling, or hemangiomas
  - Palpation of posterior spinous processes (absence may indicate spina bifida)
  - Adams forward bending test will help determine the degree and direction of spine rotation
  - Spinal balance is determined by assessing the relation of the head to the pelvis: A plumb line is dropped from the base of the skull or spinous process of C7; the plumb line should not deviate more than 1–2 cm from the gluteal crease
  - Perform a thorough neurologic evaluation by assessing limb reflexes, abdominal reflexes, and motor/sensory examination to rule out neural axis pathology
- Standing AP and lateral X-rays: Measure the curve size by Cobb angle (the angle made by a line drawn along the superior endplate of the uppermost tilted vertebra and a line drawn along the inferior endplate of the lowest vertebra in the curve)
- MRI is indicated in patients with neurologic compromise, excessive kyphosis, onset of scoliosis before age 11, rapid curve progression, structural abnormalities noted on plain X-ray, severe pain, or leftward curves

TREATMENT & MANAGEMENT

- Observation alone may be sufficient; many curves do not progress enough to require treatment
- No treatment is necessary for curves less than 25 degrees
- Treatment options include bracing or surgery
  - Bracing may slow curve progression but will not permanently reduce the magnitude of the curve
  - Bracing is indicated for 30- to 45-degree curves or 20- to 30-degree curves with 5 degrees of documented progression
  - Bracing is reserved for patients with apex of curve below T7
  - Full-time brace treatments (23 hours) are more effective than part-time bracing (<16 hours)
- Surgery (fusion of the involved vertebrae) is reserved for curves >50 degrees and progressive curves >40 degrees in skeletally immature patients
- Exercise and electrical stimulation have not been shown to alter the natural progression

PROGNOSIS & COMPLICATIONS

- Younger age (<12 years), larger curve (>20 degrees), skeletal immaturity, and female sex are risk factors for curve progression
- Curve progression may occur despite bracing
- Severe curves (>90 degrees) predispose the patient to pain, cardiopulmonary dysfunction, and early death
- Less severe curves may still result in restricted pulmonary function, neurologic compromise, back pain, and poor self-esteem
- Surgical complications include postoperative neurologic deficit

Fractures

INTRODUCTION

- Because children are generally active and adventurous, yet lack judgment to accurately predict potential injury, fractures are a relatively common pediatric injury
- Fractures are more common in children than sprains or dislocations because ligaments are typically stronger than bones, particularly at the growth plate
- When taking a history from a patient or parent of a child with a fracture, always consider the developmental stage of the child; an injury mechanism that is beyond the developmental level of the child is suspicious for nonaccidental trauma

ETIOLOGY, EPIDEMIOLOGY, & RISK FACTORS

- Pediatric fractures result in different fracture patterns than adult fractures:
  - Complete fracture: Bone failure along both cortices in oblique, spiral, transverse, or comminuted fashions
  - Greenstick fracture: Bone failure occurs on the tension side but remains partially intact on the compression side
  - Plastic deformity: Due to the relative elasticity of the bone
  - Buckle fracture: Compression of bone, usually in the metaphyseal area
  - Growth-plate disruption or epiphyseal fracture: Generally described by the Salter-Harris classification; refer to the Diagnostic Evaluation section
- 10–15% of all pediatric injuries involve fractures
- Fractures, or suspected fractures, are the cause of 40–50% of emergency and urgent care visits in children

PATIENT PRESENTATION

- History of a trauma is usually present
- Pain at rest
- Pain with range of motion
- Bruising and swelling
- Deformity
- Inability to use limb or bear weight
- Point tenderness to palpation
- Compartment syndrome: Hemorrhage and edema impair blood flow into an area enclosed by surrounding fascia, resulting in reduced circulation and oxygenation, which leads to nerve damage
  - Most common in tibial fractures; can also occur in forearm and displaced supracondylar fractures
  - Red flags that may signify compartment syndrome include severe pain at rest and with range of motion with a tense extremity or decreased pulses

DIFFERENTIAL DX

- Tendon injury
- Sprain
- Dislocation
- Avulsion injury
- Muscle or soft tissue injury
- Nonaccidental versus accidental trauma may be the most important aspect of the differential diagnosis

DIAGNOSTIC EVALUATION

- Clinical examination includes complete neurovascular exam, assessment of pulses and perfusion, assessment of motor and sensory function distal to the fracture, and evaluation for suspected compartment syndrome (intracompartmental pressure can be measured)
- Anterior-posterior and lateral X-rays of the limb, including a joint above and below
- CT scan or MRI may be required in some cases
- Salter-Harris classification is used to describe fractures of the growth plate and epiphysis
  - I: Fracture through the physis only
  - II: Fracture through part of the physis, into the metaphysis
  - III: Fracture through part of the physis, into the epiphysis
  - IV: Fracture through the metaphysis, physis, and epiphysis
  - V: Crush of the physis

TREATMENT & MANAGEMENT

- As with any trauma, assess airway, breathing, and circulation
- First aid for suspected fractures includes immobilization and cold packs
- Reduction and immobilization with splint or cast is possible in most routine childhood fractures
- Surgical indications include open fractures, displaced epiphyseal fractures, displaced intra-articular fractures, and unstable fracture patterns
- Compartment syndrome may require surgical fasciotomy
  - Outcome is satisfactory if fasciotomy is done within 6 hours of time of onset
  - Adjunctive therapy may include increased fluid administration and urine alkalinization to prevent rhabdomyolysis

PROGNOSIS & COMPLICATIONS

- Fracture healing in children is much better than in adults due to anatomic and biochemical differences of the skeletal system
- Younger children have greater remodeling potential; thus, perfect anatomic alignment is not always necessary
- Complications of fractures include altered growth (especially with epiphyseal fractures—Salter-Harris types III and IV), nerve damage, and vascular damage

Osteogenesis Imperfecta

INTRODUCTION

- Osteogenesis imperfecta is a genetic connective tissue disorder affecting collagen production that results in brittle, fragile bones
- There is a wide spectrum of clinical manifestations: Affected infants may have broken or crushed bones at birth, whereas other patients may have only a few fractures that occur later in life
- The severity of disease dictates the degree of orthopedic intervention and prognosis; many patients require treatment for long bone fracture or deformity

ETIOLOGY, EPIDEMIOLOGY, & RISK FACTORS

- Osteogenesis imperfecta represents a group of disorders caused by mutations in the genes responsible for type I collagen production, resulting in abnormal collagen cross-linking
  - Type I collagen is present in bones, sclerae, ears, skin, and teeth
  - Qualitative and/or quantitative problems of type I collagen formation may represent the underlying basis for the wide clinical manifestations
- Sillence described four types of disease: Types I and IV are autosomal dominant disorders, and types II and III are autosomal recessive
- Affects all racial and ethnic groups
- Incidence varies among ethnic groups but may be as high as 4 per 100,000 people for the most common type (Sillence type I)
- Although the disease is usually genetically transmitted, it may also occur as a spontaneous mutation

PATIENT PRESENTATION

- Type I (mild) presents at preschool age with hearing loss, blue sclerae, and long bone deformities
  - Teeth may also be affected due to dentin deficiency (dentinogenesis imperfecta)
- Type II is lethal within a few days to a year; presents with blue sclerae and crumbled bones
- Type III (severe) presents with severe bone fragility, fractures in utero or at birth, short stature, and wheelchair dependence
  - Associated with decreased lifespan
- Type IV presents with normal hearing, normal sclerae, and moderate bone fragility

DIFFERENTIAL DX

- At birth:
  - Achondroplasia
  - Achondrogenesis
  - Hypophosphatasia
- During infancy:
  - Nonaccidental trauma
  - Scurvy
  - Congenital syphilis
- During childhood:
  - Nonaccidental trauma
  - Adrenal cortical tumor
  - Glucocorticoid therapy
  - Celiac disease

DIAGNOSTIC EVALUATION

- History and physical examination suggest the diagnosis
  - Bone fragility, especially of the long bones
  - Fractures early in childhood may lead to suspicion of nonaccidental trauma; a good history may help differentiate osteogenesis imperfecta from child abuse
  - Clinical examination may reveal multiple fractures, limb deformities, dental deformities, blue sclerae, and positive family history
- X-rays findings vary based on the severity of disease
  - Milder forms may only result in thin cortices and generalized osteopenia
  - Fractures are common; the initial healing phase is normal, followed by abnormal bone remodeling
  - Fractures may be in varying stages of healing
  - Skull may appear with thin cortices with a mushroom appearance
  - Fractures occur less frequently with advancing age
- Histologic evaluation: Disorganized, thin bony trabeculae with an increased Haversian canal diameter and osteocyte lacunae; wide osteoid seams with replicated cement lines and increased cell number due to large number of osteoblasts and osteoclasts

TREATMENT & MANAGEMENT

- Patient education to prevent fractures
- Treatment is aimed at fracture management, long-term rehabilitation, and counseling
- Hormone treatments, fluoride, calcium, growth hormones, and vitamin supplementation do not appear to significantly affect the underlying collagen disorder; however, recent studies suggest that bisphosphonates may have a beneficial effect
- Early bracing of extremities to prevent deformities, maximize function, and minimize fractures
- Long bone fractures are treated according to the nature of the fracture and age of the patient
- Scoliosis is common; corrective surgery is indicated for deformities exceeding 50 degrees
  - Bracing is ineffective at inhibiting progression

PROGNOSIS & COMPLICATIONS

- Survival depends on the severity and location of fractures at birth
  - Ribcage and skull fractures are often incompatible with life
- Types I and IV are milder forms
  - Patients usually live full lives with limitations based on deformities of the long bones, vertebrae, and other fractures
  - Multiple fractures beginning in childhood may lead to severe bowing deformities of the femur or tibia
- Type II disease results in death within days to a year
- Type III disease results in decreased lifespan and dependence on wheelchair

Achondroplasia

INTRODUCTION

- Achondroplasia is the most common form of dwarfism
- Common features include frontal bossing with apparent enlargement of the head and short stature due to shortened proximal limbs
- More than 90% of cases occur due to spontaneous genetic mutations
- Expected height on average for males is 4 feet 3 inches
- Patients with achondroplasia usually have normal intelligence

ETIOLOGY, EPIDEMIOLOGY, & RISK FACTORS

- Caused by abnormal cartilage calcification, which leads to short-limbed, rhizomelic (normal trunk with short limbs) dwarfism
- The most common form of disproportionate dwarfism; incidence is 1.3–1.5 per 100,000 births
- 80% of cases are due to spontaneous mutations
- Mutations in the fibroblast growth factor receptor (FGFR) gene on chromosome 4p cause overactivity of the receptor and failure of endochondral ossification
- Failure of endochondral ossification leads to shortened bones; however, bones are of normal diameter because the width of bones is controlled by intramembranous periosteal calcification, which is normal
- May be related to older paternal age (>40 years)

PATIENT PRESENTATION

- Rhizomelic appearance (normal trunk with short limbs)
  - The proximal limbs (eg, femur, humerus) are shortened (in contrast, mesomelic describes shortening of the midportion of the limb, and acromelic describes shortening of the distal limb)
- Shortened stature
  - Normally, the midpoint of stature is the umbilicus; in achondroplasia, the midpoint may be at the inferior sternum
- Persistent hypotonia at birth, which may last up to 1 year
- Delayed motor milestones
- Frontal bossing
- Nasal bridge depression
- Button nose
- Trident hands

DIFFERENTIAL DX

- Other forms of dwarfism
- Lethal forms of dwarfism (eg, achondrogenesis, thanatophoric dwarfism)
- Hypochondroplasia

DIAGNOSTIC EVALUATION

- Physical appearance is diagnostic
  - At birth, the diagnosis is usually apparent
  - The most striking feature is short stature and limb anomalies
  - Normal trunk height but shortened proximal limbs (either the humerus or femur)
  - Usually, fingertips reach down to the midthigh level; in affected patients, the fingertips usually do not extend further than the hip or greater trochanter
  - Prominent facial features include apparent head enlargement, frontal bossing, prominent mandible, and flattened nasal bridge
  - Due to the shortened upper limbs, the elbows may be contracted, and the radial head may be dislocated
  - Lower limbs may demonstrate genu varum and a waddling gait
- Radiographic findings include widened metaphysis and shortening of the long bones, sometimes with bowing; short and thickened phalanges of the fingers; and small foramen magnum
  - The pelvis may appear as a "champagne glass"
  - The spinal canal is narrowed, with decreased interpedicular distance from L1 to L5 in more than 60% of affected patients

TREATMENT & MANAGEMENT

- Most problems related to achondroplasia involve the spine:
  - In infancy, the size of the foramen magnum is small and may predispose to cervical cord compression and sudden death
  - Sleep apnea and hypotonia may be the presenting symptoms; treat central sleep apnea with neurosurgical decompression
  - Patients may also present with cervical spine instability
- Surgical correction of thoracolumbar kyphosis may be necessary
  - Kyphosis is noticed when the patient is in an upright sitting position
  - Indications for surgery include progressive kyphosis and kyphosis >30 degrees at the thoracolumbar junction
- Patients with achondroplasia are predisposed to lumbar stenosis due to the shortened pedicles and narrowed interpedicular distance
  - Patients may present with lower extremity weakness and clonus
  - Spinal decompression and fusion may be indicated for cervical myelopathy or spinal stenosis
- Lower extremity angular deformities (eg, genu varum) may occur early in life
  - Symptomatic treatment and reassurance are usually sufficient
  - Proximal tibial and fibular osteotomy may provide cosmetic relief

PROGNOSIS & COMPLICATIONS

- Life expectancy and intelligence are generally normal
- Although it is common for infants with achondroplasia to have hypotonia and developmental delay for the initial 3–6 months of life, it is uncommon for infants to present with limb hyperreflexia and clonus; therefore, evidence of cord compression should necessitate a neurologic workup to assess for a small foramen magnum
- Surgical decompression of lumbar spine stenosis usually reverses the neurologic deficit
  - Lumbar fusion may accelerate stenosis of the adjacent lumbar level
  - Recurrence of compression requires revision of surgical decompression

Rheumatology

Juvenile Idiopathic Arthritis

INTRODUCTION

- Previously known as juvenile rheumatoid arthritis, the disease has undergone multiple changes in classification schemes
- One of the common chronic illnesses in children
- An important cause of short- and long-term disability
- Follows complex genetic traits, like most of the autoimmune diseases

ETIOLOGY, EPIDEMIOLOGY, & RISK FACTORS

- An autoimmune disease of unknown etiology
- At least three different distinct presentations: Oligoarticular, polyarticular, and systemic (Still disease)
- Oligoarticular disease is more common than polyarticular disease; systemic disease is least common
- There are no significant risk factors, but strong associations with certain HLA types exist, particularly with oligoarticular disease
- Pathogenesis involves elements of both B- and T-cell pathways
- Suspicion for a viral trigger exists (eg, rubella)
- The most common rheumatic disease in childhood, with incidence of up to 20 cases per 100,000 children
- Bimodal peaks at 2 and 9 years old
- Girls more often affected than boys (2:1)
- More common in whites
- Functional classification: (I) normal function; (II) minor limitations in function; (III) significant limitations in function; (IV) wheelchair-bound

PATIENT PRESENTATION

- Oligoarticular disease occurs in 55% of cases
  - 1–4 inflamed joints (50% have monoarthritis)
  - Knees > ankles > elbows > hips
  - No systemic symptoms
  - Uveitis (may be asymptomatic)
- Polyarticular disease occurs in 30% of cases
  - Symmetric involvement of more than 4–5 joints
  - May have systemic involvement
- Systemic disease in 15% of cases
  - Systemic illness with high fever
  - Salmon-colored, 2- to 5-mm macules
  - Visceral involvement includes hepatosplenomegaly, lymphadenopathy, and pericarditis

DIFFERENTIAL DX

- **Oligoarticular Disease**
  - Infection (Lyme disease, tuberculosis, parvovirus B19, septic arthritis, reactive arthritis, synovitis)
  - Psoriatic arthritis
  - Traumatic effusion
  - Malignancy
- **Polyarticular Disease**
  - Gonorrhea
  - Systemic lupus erythematosus
  - Spondyloarthropathy
- **Systemic Disease**
  - Malignancy
  - Inflammatory bowel disease
  - Dermatomyositis
  - Systemic lupus erythematosus
  - Vasculitis

DIAGNOSTIC EVALUATION

- Defined as a clinical constellation of signs and symptoms for greater than 6 weeks in children less than 16 years old at onset
- No lab test is diagnostic, although there may be evidence of inflammation, particularly in the systemic and polyarticular forms
- Anemia of chronic disease and leukocytosis (up to 40,000–50,000 WBC/mm^3) occur
- Acute-phase reactants (ESR, C-reactive protein, hypergammaglobulinemia) may reflect disease activity in children with active arthritis
- ANA is commonly positive in oligoarthritis; sometimes positive in polyarthritis; rarely positive in systemic arthritis
- Rheumatoid factor (RF) is generally negative except in the RF-positive polyarticular subtype
- X-ray may be helpful in untreated patients with long duration of disease
- MRI with gadolinium is more sensitive to show synovial inflammation
- Mainly a clinical diagnosis that relies on good history taking and physical exam
- Timing of pain during the day (worse in the mornings), relation to activity (worse with inactivity), and morning stiffness (gelling phenomenon) are cardinal features of inflammatory arthritis
- Patients should be carefully examined for overgrowth around joints, asymmetric growth, leg length discrepancy, and micrognathia

TREATMENT & MANAGEMENT

- Early aggressive therapy to fully control the underlying inflammation is becoming more and more favorable since better outcomes have been shown in recent years
- Anti-inflammatory medications are the mainstay of treatment, including NSAIDs, steroids, disease-modifying antirheumatic drugs (eg, methotrexate, sulfasalazine, hydroxychloroquine), and biologics, such as anti-TNF agents (etanercept, infliximab), anakinra, and rituximab
- Physical and occupational therapy are aimed at preserving joint mobility and general function
- Ophthalmologic evaluation and surveillance for uveitis
- Surgery (functional, cosmetic, and/or joint replacement)
- Psychosocial support

PROGNOSIS & COMPLICATIONS

- Recently, prognosis has improved significantly due to newer, more effective medications
- Oligoarticular disease has very good prognoses unless uveitis is present
- Vision loss due to uveitis (20%) is the most important long-term cause of morbidity
- Systemic disease follows a chronic course with some disability
  - There is an association with macrophage activation syndrome (MAS) in patients with the systemic form; MAS is almost 50% lethal if not recognized and treated early in the course
  - Infections and certain medications (eg, sulfasalazine, NSAIDs) are known to trigger MAS
- Functional disability limiting lifestyle or work options occurs in less than 10–15% of cases
- Death from disease or treatment complications occurs in less than 1% of cases in North America

Kawasaki Disease

INTRODUCTION

- Also known as mucocutaneous lymph node syndrome
- Generally a self-limited, systemic inflammation primarily affecting the blood vessels
- Fever is the cardinal feature of the disease, which usually lasts about 12 days
- Morbidity and mortality are mainly related to the degree of coronary artery involvement
- Since the start of intravenous immunoglobulin (IVIG) treatment, the incidence of coronary artery aneurysms has been significantly decreased
- Incomplete Kawasaki disease has been described in which patients do not meet the diagnostic criteria, yet are at risk for coronary artery disease

ETIOLOGY, EPIDEMIOLOGY, & RISK FACTORS

- A systemic vasculitis primarily involving the mucous membranes, skin, lymph nodes, and coronary artery vessels
- Etiology is unknown; possibly infectious or toxic agents causing an aberrant immune response, which leads to endothelial injury in genetically predisposed individuals
  - Superantigen toxins from *Staphylococcus aureus* or *Streptococcus pyogenes*
  - There is a possible association with a novel *Coronavirus*
  - Various HLA genes have been associated with disease
- One of the most common vasculitides of childhood; incidence in children less than 5 years is 100 cases per 100,000 children per year
- Higher risk in Asians and males
- Occurs year-round, with clusters in late winter and summer
- Peaks between ages 2–3; much less frequent in children older than 5 years
- Increased risk of aneurysms in children less than 1 year old and especially less than 6 months old, who often present with incomplete disease
- Rare in children younger than 3 months, suggesting maternal transfer of passive immunity

PATIENT PRESENTATION

- The acute phase of disease is characterized by high fevers, irritability, cervical adenitis, conjunctivitis, rash, mucous membrane changes, edema or erythema of the of the hands and feet, desquamation in the diaper area, and occasionally abdominal pain and diarrhea
- The subacute phase is characterized by resolving fever, desquamation of digits starting under the nails, and occasionally arthritis; coronary artery aneurysms may occur in 20% of untreated patients
- The convalescent phase is usually asymptomatic; however, patients with coronary artery aneurysms may develop coronary artery stenosis and myocardial infarction
- Uveitis, hearing loss, and hydrops gallbladder occur in a minority of patients

DIFFERENTIAL DX

- Infectious agents (eg, adenovirus, measles, Epstein-Barr virus, rocky mountain spotted fever, leptospirosis, enterovirus)
- *Staphylococcus* or *Streptococcus* toxin-mediated disease
- Toxic reaction to medication (eg, Stevens-Johnson syndrome, serum sickness)
- Other rheumatic diseases (eg, polyarteritis nodosa, systemic juvenile idiopathic arthritis)
- Mercury hypersensitivity reaction

DIAGNOSTIC EVALUATION

- Diagnosis requires the presence of fever for at least 5 days, plus four out of five of the following criteria (not all criteria must be met before initiating therapy):
  - Bilateral conjunctivitis, usually bulbar and with limbal sparing
  - Unilateral cervical lymphadenopathy >1.5 cm (less common in patients in North America)
  - Nonvesicular rash, usually on the trunk
  - Mucous membrane changes, such as erythema, cracked lips, strawberry tongue, or palatal petechiae
  - Extremity changes, such as erythema of palms and soles, dorsal edema, or finger desquamation
- Laboratory evaluation during the acute phase may reveal increased ESR or C-reactive protein, elevated WBC count with slight left shift, elevated liver function tests, mild normochromic anemia, sterile pyuria, and cerebrospinal fluid pleocytosis with mononuclear predominance
  - During the subacute phase, increased platelet count and declining ESR may occur
- Cardiac evaluation requires baseline echocardiography, chest X-ray, and EKG
  - Up to 50% of patients have cardiac manifestations, including myocarditis, pericarditis, conduction disturbances, mitral/aortic regurgitation, and coronary artery aneurysm (may occur as early as day 7)

TREATMENT & MANAGEMENT

- Intravenous immunoglobin (IVIG) at high dose (2 g/kg) is the mainstay of therapy
  - 10% of patients require a second dose
  - About 1% of patients do not respond to IVIG
- Aspirin is initially used at high anti-inflammatory doses (80–100 mg/kg/d) during the acute phase until 48 hours after being afebrile
  - Then used at lower dose (3–5 mg/kg/d) as antiplatelet therapy until inflammatory markers and platelet counts are normalized (or longer depending on the degree of coronary artery involvement)
- Steroids are sometimes used; they have been associated with increased frequency of aneurysms, although this is somewhat controversial and needs further study
- Active management of coronary thrombosis (eg, heparin, angioplasty)
- Other immunosuppressive therapies (infliximab, cyclophosphamide) may be used in cases resistant to IVIG
- Newer anti-platelet agents (abciximab, clopidogrel) have also been used in severe cases

PROGNOSIS & COMPLICATIONS

- 4% of patients develop coronary artery aneurysms despite adequate therapy
- Some children may have recurrence of the disease, usually within 12 years of first episode
- Most children survive without any sequelae
- Poor prognostic indicators include age less than 1 year, male gender, fever lasting longer than 2 weeks, and recurrence of fever
- Some children die of cardiac complications during the acute or subacute stages
- In children with aneurysms, sudden death (often associated with exertion) may occur many years later, usually due to myocardial infarctions or arrhythmias
- Children with cardiac involvement may be at higher risk of coronary artery disease during adulthood

Henoch-Schönlein Purpura

INTRODUCTION

- Henoch-Schönlein purpura (HSP), also known as anaphylactoid purpura, is primarily a childhood disease (90% of all cases occur in childhood)
- The disease primarily affects small blood vessels
- One of the most common vasculitides in children
- The classic tetrad includes palpable, nonthrombocytopenic purpura; arthritis and arthralgias; abdominal pain and gastrointestinal disease; and renal disease

ETIOLOGY, EPIDEMIOLOGY, & RISK FACTORS

- The etiology is unknown, but infectious causes have been implicated
  - Beta-hemolytic *Streptococcus* may be a triggering agent
  - 50% of cases are preceded by a reparatory illness
- The disease is autoimmune-mediated: IgA deposition in vessel walls initiates an inflammatory cascade leading to vessel necrosis
  - Elevated levels of IgA anticardiolipin antibodies and TGF-beta occur
- Multiple organ involvement occurs, including disease of the skin, kidneys, gastrointestinal tract, and joints
- There may be a genetic component; there have been reports of familial occurrences
- Occurs primarily in the fall, winter, and spring
- Affects children 3–15 years of age (peak age, 4–7)
- Annual incidence of 20 per 100,000 in children
- Males more commonly affected than females

PATIENT PRESENTATION

- Manifestations occur over days to weeks
- Skin: Distinctive rash with generalized urticarial wheals that become macules then petechiae and purpura; purpuric lesions are palpable, nonpruritic, and located on dependent areas (eg, legs, thighs, buttocks)
- GI tract: Colicky abdominal pain with tenderness but no rebound; vomiting or ileus may occur
  - GI bleeding and intussusception are common
- Renal: Microscopic or gross hematuria, nephritic syndrome, mild proteinuria, acute nephritis with hypertension
- Genitourinary: Painful, tender testicle or scrotum due to localized vasculitis
- Neurologic: Headache, behavioral change, seizures
- Arthritis: Painful periarticular swelling and transient arthritis usually of lower extremity joints

DIFFERENTIAL DX

- Septicemia or DIC
- Hemolytic-uremic syndrome
- Bacterial endocarditis
- Acute postinfectious glomerulonephritis
- Rheumatic fever
- Acute surgical abdomen
- ITP
- AHEI
- Thrombotic thrombocytopenic purpura
- Leukemia
- SLE
- Polyarteritis nodosa
- Wegener granulomatosis
- Juvenile arthritis
- Berger disease
- Meningococcemia

DIAGNOSTIC EVALUATION

- There is no confirmatory test or diagnostic laboratory abnormalities
- At least two of the following diagnostic criteria must be present for diagnosis: palpable purpura, age less than 20 at onset, bowel angina, or vessel wall granulocytes
- Abnormal lab findings (nondiagnostic) include leukocytosis with left shift, anemia, elevated IgA (50–70% of patients), elevated ESR, and prolonged PT or PTT
  - C3 and C4 are generally normal
  - Antinuclear antibody and rheumatoid factor are usually negative (normal)
  - Urinalysis may show RBC or WBC casts and protein
- Kidney biopsy is not indicated unless nephrotic syndrome, persistent nephritic syndrome with gross hematuria, hypertension, or renal insufficiency occurs
- If the gastrointestinal tract is involved, an upper GI series with small bowel follow-through is indicated and shows thickened folds, pseudotumors, hypomotility, and thumbprinting
  - If intussusception is suspected, more than 50% are ileo-ileo and are not visualized by contrast enema
- If the scrotal area is involved, a Doppler can differentiate HSP from testicular torsion

TREATMENT & MANAGEMENT

- Outpatient management is usually sufficient
- Hospitalization is indicated if the patient cannot maintain hydration and for severe abdominal pain, gastrointestinal bleeding, change in mental status, severe joint involvement limiting ambulation, renal insufficiency, hypertension, or nephritic syndrome
- Supportive care with hydration, pain control, and nutritional support
  - NSAIDs can be used but are contraindicated in the presence of glomerulonephritis due to the risk of renal insufficiency
- Monitor electrolytes, BUN/creatinine, and blood pressures for renal insufficiency
- Severe disease requires frequent assessment of vital signs, hematocrit, stool guaiac testing, and abdominal exams
  - Acute change in mental status requires consideration of head CT scan to evaluate for intracranial hemorrhage
  - Consider corticosteroids for relief in patients with severe abdominal pain

PROGNOSIS & COMPLICATIONS

- The disease is usually self-limited
- Symptoms generally persist for about a month; younger children have shorter courses and fewer recurrences
- Reoccurrences occur in about 40% of patients; each episode is usually shorter and milder
- Abdominal complications may be noted by acute changes in symptoms or exam findings (eg, bowel infarction or perforation, intussusception, gallbladder hydrops, and pancreatitis)
- Morbidity is primarily associated with renal complications
  - Patients with microhematuria and mild proteinuria tend to have a good outcome
  - Patients with nephrotic or nephritic syndrome may develop long-term renal insufficiency
  - End-stage renal failure develops in 2–5%; long-term mortality rate is less than 1%

Systemic Lupus Erythematosus

INTRODUCTION

- A multisystem, episodic autoimmune disease
- Can present with a multitude of signs and symptoms mimicking many other diseases; therefore, the diagnosis may be delayed, especially in children
- Usually a clinical diagnosis supported by laboratory abnormalities; the characteristic laboratory finding is positive antinuclear antibody (ANA)
- Apart from drug-induced lupus, the etiology is unknown
- Complex genetic traits and environmental factors play a role, causing the end result of immune dysregulation

ETIOLOGY, EPIDEMIOLOGY, & RISK FACTORS

- A chronic inflammatory disease of uncertain etiology characterized by B-cell hyperreactivity, activation of complement, and T-cell defects
- Probable genetic contribution; 10% of patients have a first-degree relative with SLE
- Some drugs that cause lupus are procainamide, isoniazid, hydralazine, and minocycline
- 15–20% of cases have onset in childhood
- Peak onset in teens and middle age; rare before 5 years of age
- More common in girls and during adolescence
  - Female-to-male ratio before puberty is 3:1; after puberty, it is 9:1
- Native-Americans are more sensitive, followed by African-Americans and Hispanics
- Disease tends to be more severe in African-Americans and Hispanics
- Renal involvement is the major cause of morbidity
- Increased susceptibility to infections due to both active disease and immunosuppression

PATIENT PRESENTATION

- Constitutional: Fever, weight loss, malaise
- Mucocutaneous symptoms: Malar (butterfly) rash, diffuse alopecia, photosensitivity, vasculitic lesions, ulcers
- Musculoskeletal: Episodic painful large or small joint arthritis (nonerosive)
- CNS: Depression, falling grades, psychosis, chorea, stroke
- Cardiac: Chest pain or murmur due to pericarditis, myocarditis, myocardial infarction, endocarditis, or valvular sterile vegetations (Libman-Sacks endocarditis)
- Pulmonary: Increased work of breathing or cough due to pleural effusions, pneumonitis, pulmonary hemorrhage, or pulmonary hypertension
- GI: Abdominal pain due to hepatosplenomegaly, mesenteric vasculitis, peritonitis, or pancreatitis
- Ocular: Cotton-wool spots

DIFFERENTIAL DX

- Juvenile arthritis
- Dermatomyositis
- Polyarteritis
- Mixed connective tissue diseases (eg, scleroderma, polymyositis)
- Malignancy
- Thrombocytopenic purpura
- Hemolytic anemia
- Evan syndrome

DIAGNOSTIC EVALUATION

- American College of Rheumatology suggests 4 of 11 classification criteria should be present for diagnosis (all at once or separately); these diagnostic criteria provide more than 95% sensitivity and specificity
  - Malar rash (butterfly rash)
  - Discoid rash
  - Photosensitivity
  - Painless mouth ulcers
  - Arthritis in more than two joints
  - Pleural or pericardial effusion/inflammation
  - Proteinuria at least 3+ or >0.5 g/day
  - Seizure activity not attributable to other causes or psychosis
  - Anemia, leukopenia, or thrombocytopenia
  - Anti-DNA, anti-Smith, or antiphospholipid antibodies or false-positive VDRL
  - Antinuclear antibodies (positive in 98%); positive ANA can be seen in normal healthy children (low titer, relative of person with SLE), infections (viral, bacterial, TB, parasitic), malignancy (lymphoma, leukemia), hematologic disease (ITP, autoimmune hemolytic anemia), hepatic disease (chronic active hepatitis, primary biliary cirrhosis, autoimmune hepatitis), idiopathic pulmonary fibrosis, diabetes, thyroiditis, drug induced, rheumatologic disease (juvenile rheumatoid arthritis, myositis, Sjögren syndrome, scleroderma vasculitis)
- Low levels of C3, C4, and CH_{50} often represent active disease

TREATMENT & MANAGEMENT

- Long-term daily and pulse glucocorticoids
- Hydroxychloroquine as an adjunct to steroids, especially for mucocutaneous features and arthritis
- Cytotoxic drugs (eg, cyclophosphamide, azathioprine, mycophenolate, methotrexate)
- Biologics (eg, rituximab)
- Intravenous immunoglobulin for acute thrombocytopenia and hemolytic anemia
- NSAIDs for musculoskeletal complaints
- Dialysis with transplantation for severe lupus nephritis
- All patients should use sunscreen to prevent photosensitivity rash
- Appropriate vaccinations (eg, Pneumovax) may help avoid infectious complications
- A multidisciplinary team approach is essential; a special focus should be on the psychosocial aspects of the disease on the teenage population because poor compliance adversely affects outcome

PROGNOSIS & COMPLICATIONS

- Follows a chronic course with exacerbations and remissions
- The main prognostic indicator is the extent of major organ involvement
- Major causes of death include CNS lupus, nephritis, infections, pulmonary lupus, and myocardial infarctions
- Recurrent infections contribute significantly to morbidity
- Predictions about prognosis are fairly unreliable until later in the course of disease
- Prognosis is the poorest in CNS or renal disease
- Premature atherosclerosis is a major cause of death in adults with SLE
- 5-year survival is greater than 90%, 10-year survival is 85%

Dermatomyositis

INTRODUCTION

- A rare, chronic multisystem inflammatory disease affecting primarily the skin and muscle
- The most common cause of acquired muscle weakness
- The clinical presentation and course can be variable
- Childhood forms of the disease are distinct from adult presentations; one major difference in the childhood form is the development of calcinosis in patients with recalcitrant disease (20–30%)
- It used to have poor prognosis in the presteroid era; however, in recent years, the outcomes have dramatically improved, most likely as a result of early aggressive therapy

ETIOLOGY, EPIDEMIOLOGY, & RISK FACTORS

- An immune complex vasculitis of the skin, striated muscle, and gastrointestinal tract
- An upper respiratory infection (coxsackievirus B, influenza, *Streptococcus*) usually precedes the onset of disease, triggering an autoimmune process that attacks muscle cells
  - A number of other organisms such as *Toxoplasma*, parvovirus, hepatitis B virus, and *Borrelia* have also been implicated as inciting agents
- Complement activation and immune complex deposition have been demonstrated in the blood vessel walls of the muscles
- The etiology is unknown; both genetic and environmental factors appear to play a role
- Bimodal distribution with a peak in childhood and a larger peak at age 50 (16–20% of patients with dermatomyositis have onset in childhood)
- Average age of childhood onset is 7 years
- Up to five times more common in girls
- May be associated with mixed connective tissue diseases and other autoimmune diseases (eg, scleroderma, rheumatoid arthritis, systemic lupus erythematosus)
- Associated malignancies occur in adult dermatomyositis

PATIENT PRESENTATION

- Patients initially present with proximal, bilateral muscle weakness (eg, difficulty combing hair, rising from prone or seated position)
- Fever, malaise, weight loss
- Purplish discoloration of the upper eyelids (heliotrope rash)
- Scaly plaques on knuckles (Gottron papules) and other extensor surfaces with scarring
- Periungual capillary changes
- Respiratory and oropharyngeal muscle weakness
- Arthralgia, arthritis
- Dysphagia, hepatosplenomegaly
- Visceral vasculitis (signifies poor prognosis)
- Cardiopulmonary disease
- Calcinosis (calcium deposits in the soft tissues and under the skin) usually occurs under pressure areas and can protrude through the skin; may disappear spontaneously in some patients

DIFFERENTIAL DX

- Infectious or postinfectious myositis
- Neuromuscular diseases and myopathies (eg, muscular dystrophy)
- Myositis with other connective tissue diseases (eg, scleroderma)
- Rhabdomyolysis
- Guillain-Barré syndrome (weakness starts distally)
- Hypothyroidism
- Steroid use
- Trauma
- Drugs (penicillamine, statins, cocaine, alcohol)
- Fibrodysplasia ossificans progressiva

DIAGNOSTIC EVALUATION

- Diagnosis requires the presence of the pathognomonic rash and two of the following criteria:
  - Proximal muscle weakness
  - Elevated muscle enzymes (CK, LDH, aldolase, AST) and elevated factor VIII–related antigen indicative of endothelial damage
  - Characteristically abnormal EMG pattern indicating increased membrane irritability (increased insertional activity, abnormal myopathic motor potentials, bizarre high-frequency discharges)
  - Muscle biopsy showing inflammation or necrosis of muscle and vasculitis
- Elevated ESR and/or C-reactive protein (may be normal and thus have questionable value)
- Some patients will be antinuclear antigen (ANA) positive
- MRI of the muscles has been increasingly used to demonstrate muscle inflammation
- P-31 magnetic resonance spectroscopy can be used to demonstrate abnormal muscle metabolism
- Myositis-specific antibodies (MSA) and myositis-associated antigens (MAA) are rarely positive in children

TREATMENT & MANAGEMENT

- Treatment goals are to control the underlying inflammation and prevent complications
- Early and adequate glucocorticoid therapy is the mainstay of therapy
- Methotrexate is useful as a steroid-sparing agent and is being used much earlier in the course of the disease
- Other immunosuppressives or immunomodulatory agents (eg, IVIG, cyclosporine A, cyclophosphamide, rituximab) are used in therapy-resistant cases
- Hydroxychloroquine is used to treat the skin disease; topical tacrolimus has also been used for skin disease with some success
- Physical therapy to prevent contractures and preserve strength
- Respiratory support for patients with oropharyngeal and respiratory muscle weakness
- Dysphagia can lead to aspiration; if present, patient needs dietary and positional changes
- There is no effective medical management for treating well-established calcinosis
  - Low-dose warfarin may help with early calcinosis or for prevention
  - Aluminum hydroxide has improved diffuse calcinosis by lowering serum phosphate
  - Local surgical excision may be needed for motion-limiting, painful, or draining lesions
- Intestinal perforation should be managed with judicious surgical intervention

PROGNOSIS & COMPLICATIONS

- After an initial period of progressive weakness, most children stabilize and eventually recover with excellent functional outcome within 8 months to 2 years
- There is better than 90% survival rate
- Some children will have one or more relapses
- Unremitting, severe disease occurs in a small group of children
- Death occurs in less than 10% of children and is usually secondary to acute gastrointestinal ulceration and bleeding, respiratory insufficiency, or pneumonitis
- 5% of survivors will be wheelchair dependent; 5–10% have moderate to severe disability
- 20–30% have calcinosis, usually in patients with severe and unremitting disease
- Lipodystrophy occurs in 25%; hypertriglyceridemia and insulin resistance occur in 50%

Environmental Hazards and Toxicology

Burns

INTRODUCTION

- Flame, chemical, and scald (most frequent) burns are common in children
- Burns cause damage to the skin barrier and induce systemic immunosuppression (decreased T_h cells and immunoglobulin levels with increased T_s cell levels), which predisposes to infection (eg, *Staphylococcus*, *Streptococcus*, *Pseudomonas*)
- Postburn fluid shifts occur in which increased fluid flow to burned and normal tissue occurs due to endothelial damage, vasoactive substances, and other mediators
- First-degree burn (superficial): Sunburn
- Second-degree burn (partial-thickness): Scalding or chemical burn
- Third-degree burn (full-thickness): Flame burns

ETIOLOGY, EPIDEMIOLOGY, & RISK FACTORS

- Burns are the third most frequent type of injury in children and the second leading cause of accidental death
- Burns and complications from burns are a leading cause of morbidity and mortality in the pediatric population, especially under age 4
- Over 2 million cases per year occur with 70,000 hospital admissions (20,000 to burn units)
- The average age of a pediatric burn victim is under 3 years because toddlers are mobile, impulsive, unpredictable, and curious at these ages
- Scald burns are the most frequent type of burn in children (85% of cases)
- Burns may be the result of accidents or nonaccidental trauma; about 15% of burns are thought to be due to child abuse
- Preventive efforts such as public health campaigns, widespread use of smoke detectors, reduction of indoor smoking, legislation to lower the preset temperature of hot water tanks (at 120°), and the Federal Flammable Fabric Act (flame-resistant sleepwear) have reduced the number and severity of burns

PATIENT PRESENTATION

- First-degree (superficial): painful erythema, dry skin without blistering, minimal to no edema
- Second-degree (partial-thickness): moistened blisters, mottled gray or erythematous, extremely painful
- Third-degree (full-thickness): eschar formation; leathery or waxy appearance; dry, painless, white, pearly, and darkened lesions; hair easily removed; visible thrombosed vessels are pathognomonic
- Signs of infected burn wound: conversion of partial-thickness burn to full-thickness; increased erythema or edema at margins; sudden separation of eschar from underlying tissue; fever; purulent drainage
- Extracutaneous manifestations may include inhalational injury with upper airway edema, gastric ileus, and hematologic sequelae

DIFFERENTIAL DX

- Scald burns
- Flame burns
- Contact burns
- Electrical burns
- Chemical burns
- Accidental burns must be distinguished from inflicted burns
- Conditions resembling burns (eg, scalded skin syndrome, bullous impetigo)

DIAGNOSTIC EVALUATION

- Immediate management of airway, breathing, circulation, disability, and exposure (the ABCDE of trauma management)
- History and physical are the basis of diagnosis
- Patterns of injury and plausibility of history differentiate accidental burns from inflicted burns; findings concerning for child abuse include a history given by a caregiver that would not result in the injury, a reported injury mechanism that is beyond the developmental capabilities of the child, and circumferential or stocking-glove burn distribution that is concerning for an immersion injury
- Infection is diagnosed by wound culture or biopsy demonstrating $>10^5$ organisms
- Calculate the burn size
  - One "rule of thumb" is that the area of a patient's palm is equal to 1% of body surface area
  - The size of burn (in adults and older children) may also be estimated by the "rule of 9s": dorsal trunk (18%), ventral trunk (18%), each arm (9%), each leg (18%), head/neck (9%), and perineum (1%)
  - The "rule of 9s" is less accurate in infants and young children; trauma and burn centers use a detailed chart stratified by age to estimate body burn surface area in children younger than 12

TREATMENT & MANAGEMENT

- Treatment is aimed at acute management, prevention of complications, and rehabilitation
- Local wound care includes:
  - Aggressive debridement of devitalized tissue
  - Topical agents to decrease infectious burden on tissue (eg, silver sulfadiazine)
  - Prompt excision and grafting of third-degree burns may prevent infection; burn coverage can be accomplished by autograft, allograft, and artificial substitutes
- Fluid maintenance and nutrition are important due to massive fluid shifts (burn edema) and increased metabolic demands of stressed state
  - Replete fluids using Parkland formula (for initial 24 hours): 4 mL crystalloid/kg/% body surface area burned, plus maintenance fluids; then monitor for urine output >0.5 cc/kg/hr
  - Children <2 require glucose in IV fluids because they have low glucose stores
  - Do not include potassium in IV fluids; monitor serum potassium closely
  - Nutrition: Increased metabolic demands and needs for protein, fat, vitamins, and minerals may be as high as twice normal
- Tetanus prophylaxis
- Pain control with analgesics, including narcotics, particularly during dressing changes
- Intensive care admission for patients with profound metabolic or fluid derangements, inhalational injuries, hemodynamic instability, or suspected sepsis

PROGNOSIS & COMPLICATIONS

- First-degree burns tend to be uncomplicated and heal within 5–7 days
- Second-degree burns heal in 3–4 weeks unless deep invasion or superimposed infection occurs
- All burned skin is at increased risk of sunburn for 1 year and may also show pigmentary changes
- Complications include local infection (most important), pneumonia, pulmonary emboli, urinary tract infections, endocarditis, suppurative thrombophlebitis, contractures, and scarring
- Patients should be admitted to specialized burn units for smoke inhalation, electrical burns, large burn areas (>20% of body surface involved), circumferential burns, and second-degree burns to the hands, feet, face, or perineum

Lead Poisoning

INTRODUCTION

- Environmental sources of lead include gasoline, paint, and food can soldering (before 1970s); household fixtures from homes built before 1960; demolition or rehabilitation of old housing; industrial emissions from metal and battery plants; ceramic glazes and lead crystal; folk remedies; and mineral supplements
- Ingestion is the usual route of lead toxicity, although it can occur by inhalation or absorption as well
- Lead displaces calcium and iron, leading to deficiency of these nutrients
- Lead deposits in the bone and interferes with hematopoiesis
- Lead may cause acute lead encephalopathy

ETIOLOGY, EPIDEMIOLOGY, & RISK FACTORS

- Lead is usually picked up on the hands and transmitted to the mouth by young children's oral habits; large particles (such as paint chips) are less hazardous than lead in soil or household dust
- Risk factors include:
  - Poverty and substandard housing
  - Urban dwelling
  - Poor nutrition (deficiency of iron, calcium, and protein and high-fat diet)
  - Minority ethnicity
  - Age younger than 6 years
  - Pica and hand-to-mouth behaviors
- A protective factor is a diet high in green leafy vegetables because the phytins in these plants bind lead and assist in excretion
- Prevalence has been decreasing since 1978 when lead paint was disallowed and a decline occurred in the use of leaded gasoline; the current prevalence is well below 1% due to universal screening in at-risk populations and targeted screening in other populations

PATIENT PRESENTATION

- Low levels are asymptomatic
- Anorexia, nausea, vomiting, abdominal pain, or constipation
- Growth failure
- Anemia
- Hearing deficit
- Behavior problems, attention difficulties
- Ataxia
- Change in mental status, seizures
- Signs and symptoms of increased intracranial pressure may be present
- Encephalopathy, coma
- Fanconi-like syndrome with renal tubular dysfunction

DIFFERENTIAL DX

- Consider lead poisoning in the differential diagnosis of:
  - Anemia
  - Acute encephalopathy
  - Recurrent abdominal pain
  - Seizures and coma
  - Nausea and vomiting
  - Mental retardation
  - Attentional difficulties
  - Growth failure

DIAGNOSTIC EVALUATION

- Because lead is ubiquitous, few patients have a lead level of zero; therefore, most people have some degree of lead exposure
- Generally subclinical or asymptomatic; diagnosis is usually made as a result of routine screening
- Laboratory testing:
  - Serum lead level <10 μg/dL is considered tolerable (venous level is considerably more accurate than capillary level)
  - Hair samples are collected and tested but are less accurate than serum samples
  - Complete blood count may reveal basophilic stippling and anemia
  - Electrolytes, calcium, magnesium, and phosphorous should be measured
- Abdominal X-ray to assess bone lead content
- Long-bone films may reveal "lead lines" at the distal metaphyses
- Head CT scan is indicated if altered mental status
- Siblings or other children exposed to the same conditions should be evaluated when one child has an elevated lead level

TREATMENT & MANAGEMENT

- Prevention is accomplished by maintenance of painted surfaces in homes, rigorous household cleaning, and frequent handwashing, especially before meals
- Blood lead level 10–19 μg/dL: Environmental evaluation and retesting
- Blood lead level 20–44 μg/dL: Environmental evaluation and retesting; consider chelation therapy if levels cannot be effectively reduced
- Blood lead level 45–69 μg/dL: Environmental evaluation and outpatient chelation therapy with succimer
- Blood lead level >70 μg/dL: Urgent inpatient chelation therapy with succimer and EDTA
- Adequate nutrition with supplementation for optimal intake of essential minerals, such as iron and calcium
- The chelated lead complex is excreted in the urine, requiring a high urine flow to prevent renal damage
- Acute lead encephalopathy may require intubation and ventilation and may be accompanied by seizures, requiring benzodiazepines, and measures such as hyperventilation and mannitol for increased intracranial pressure

PROGNOSIS & COMPLICATIONS

- The detrimental effect of lead toxicity on cognitive function in the preschool years is reflected in cognitive testing throughout school-aged years and beyond
- Behavioral problems such as ADHD are more frequent in patients with lead toxicity and may persist beyond the resolution of the lead burden
- Other long-term neurologic sequelae may include static encephalopathy, hearing deficit, and cerebral palsy
- Some researchers believe that even modest levels of lead (near 10 mg/dL) may have a cumulative detrimental developmental effect

Iron Poisoning

INTRODUCTION

- Iron poisoning is the most common cause of death from poisoning in young children (30% of fatal pediatric ingestions)
- Iron-containing substances are easily available and are found in many households (eg, prenatal iron supplements, iron-fortified multivitamin and mineral supplements)
- Because children's chewable vitamins are made to taste good, they may be eaten as candy by small children; liquid iron preparations have a much less appealing flavor

ETIOLOGY, EPIDEMIOLOGY, & RISK FACTORS

- The majority of iron in the body exists within red blood cells
- Non–heme-bound iron is absorbed mainly in the duodenum and proximal jejunum and is bound to ferritin
- Physiologic amounts of iron do not cause injury due to presence of transport (transferrin) and storage (ferritin) proteins; however, these become overwhelmed in an overdose
- Iron is a potent oxidizer and catalyst of free radical formation; the free radicals damage mitochondrial membranes, interfering with oxidative phosphorylation
- To estimate the size of the ingestion, use milligrams of elemental iron times the number of pills ingested
- Toxicity occurs more often in younger children because they can more easily supersede the safe range with just a few tablets
- Even 20 mg/kg of elemental iron will result in symptoms; 60 mg/kg of elemental iron will result in serious toxicity; >250 mg/kg is likely to be lethal

PATIENT PRESENTATION

- Stage I: Gastrointestinal symptoms (abdominal pain, vomiting, hematochezia, and hematemesis), usually within 2 hours of ingestion
- Stage II: Relative apparent stability; however, iron may be accumulating within cells, and hypotension and acidosis may be impending
- Stage III: Shock due to hypovolemia and decreased cardiac output, acidosis, and coagulopathy
- Stage IV: Hepatotoxicity, usually within 48 hours of ingestion
- Stage V: Bowel obstruction from inflammation and stricture formation, occurring 2–4 weeks after ingestion

DIFFERENTIAL DX

- Other causes of abdominal pain, nausea, and vomiting (eg, infections, obstructions)
- Other causes of metabolic acidosis (eg, aspirin overdose, organophosphate ingestion)
- Other heavy metal intoxication
- Theophylline overdose
- Mushroom ingestion
- Colchicine intoxication

DIAGNOSTIC EVALUATION

- History of accidental iron ingestion (eg, an open or empty bottle of iron tablets or iron-fortified vitamins) and intentional iron overdose (eg, suicide gesture or attempt)
- Iron studies, including free serum iron, total serum iron, and total serum iron-binding capacity
  - After occupation of all iron-binding sites, free iron will accumulate in the plasma
  - Serum iron concentration peaks 4 hours after ingestion
  - Risk for significant toxicity exists if free iron concentration exceeds 50 mg/dL or if total iron concentration is >350 mg/dL
- Abdominal X-ray shows radiopaque iron in the gastrointestinal tract, although liquid and chewable preparations may not be observable

TREATMENT & MANAGEMENT

- Gastric decontamination by gastric lavage is usually indicated, especially if iron tablets were swallowed (because they may be slow to absorb)
  - Induced vomiting by syrup of ipecac is no longer recommended due to risk of aspiration
  - Iron is poorly absorbed by charcoal
  - Whole-bowel irrigation (GoLYTELY) may be used when there are retained intestinal iron pills
- Chelation with IV deferoxamine if systemic toxicity or metabolic acidosis occurs
  - Less severe cases are treated with 90 mg/kg every 8 hours for three doses
  - Severe, life-threatening cases may be treated with a continuous infusion of 10–50 mg/kg/hr
- Supportive care and volume support for systemic signs and symptoms, such as hypotension and hyperglycemia
- Endoscopy may be used to remove iron tablets or an iron tablet agglutination/bezoar

PROGNOSIS & COMPLICATIONS

- Patients may develop renal failure, ARDS, shock, and/or coma
- Sequelae may include liver failure and cirrhosis
- Long-term complications may include bowel stricture formation and obstruction

Acetaminophen Overdose

INTRODUCTION

- Acetaminophen is present in a wide variety of prescription and over-the-counter preparations, including pain relievers, sleep aids, and respiratory infection preparations
- It has become the most commonly used pain reliever and fever reducer in children since recommendations began to warn against use of aspirin in children due to Reye syndrome
- Acetaminophen is metabolized almost entirely in the liver, where it is converted into non-toxic forms and excreted in the urine
- One of the pathways for metabolism uses the cytochrome P450/glutathione system; when glutathione reserve in the liver is partially depleted, this pathway for metabolism is impaired, and buildup of toxic metabolites results in liver damage

ETIOLOGY, EPIDEMIOLOGY, & RISK FACTORS

- Although acetaminophen has a large therapeutic index and is safe when given in recommended dosages, acute overdose or excessive chronic use can result in significant hepatic injury
- Young children are less likely to suffer toxicity than adolescents and adults; this is because they metabolize acetaminophen through several alternate pathways and because they are unlikely to make an intentional overdose
- Nevertheless, accidental overdose may occur in children younger than 6 years when administered frequently to control high fevers or when using mixed preparations that contain acetaminophen
- Adults and adolescents are more likely to develop toxic acetaminophen levels than children
  - Severe toxicity in adolescents can occur in overdoses of as low as 10–15 g
  - Acute or chronic alcohol use potentiates the hepatotoxicity
  - In adolescents, overdose is commonly related to suicide attempts

PATIENT PRESENTATION

- May be asymptomatic initially
- The natural history of acetaminophen ingestion follows a predictable course:
  - Initial 24 hours: malaise, nausea, vomiting
  - 24–48 hours: nausea and vomiting diminish, right upper quadrant pain ensues, and liver enzymes become elevated
  - 72–96 hours: "time bomb effect" with worsening of liver enzymes; the patient may become more symptomatic
  - 4–14 days: gradual resolution of symptoms

DIFFERENTIAL DX

- Ingestion of other hepatotoxic substances
- Should be considered in the differential diagnosis of abdominal pain, nausea, and vomiting

DIAGNOSTIC EVALUATION

- Careful patient history, including prescription and over-the-counter medications as well as specific doses and dosing intervals; evaluate if the patient is taking more than one medicine that contains acetaminophen
- Unless overdose occurs as a suicide gesture or attempt, overdose may occur in the context of another illness, and symptoms may be attributed to that illness rather than acetaminophen toxicity
- Postingestion acetaminophen level directs the care provided:
  - Level should be measured at 4 hours after ingestion and plotted on the Rumack-Matthew nomogram, which shows serum level plotted against time since ingestion; this helps to predict the probability of hepatic toxicity and identify candidates for antidosis
  - The utility of serum levels and the nomogram is reduced if the ingestion occurred in several doses or over a period of time
- Liver function tests become elevated after 24 hours
- Testing for other ingested toxins (eg, alcohol, aspirin) and drugs of abuse is generally warranted

TREATMENT & MANAGEMENT

- Gastrointestinal decontamination via activated charcoal administration within 2 hours after ingestion; however, the potential benefits of gastric lavage may not be worth the risk of aspiration or esophageal perforation, unless the ingestion was extremely recent
  - Induced vomiting with syrup of ipecac is no longer recommended
- Use Rumack-Matthew nomogram to depict the risk of hepatotoxicity from acetaminophen
  - Patients with acetaminophen level within the safety range require no therapy
  - Patients with acetaminophen level (>150 $\mu g/mL$ at 4 hours after ingestion require antidotal therapy with N-acetylcysteine [NAC])
  - NAC may be given IV or orally; for oral administration, consider pre-medication with ondansetron or another antiemetic
  - NAC must be initiated before 16 hours after ingestion
  - After a loading dose, NAC is administered every 4 hours for 17 doses
- Liver function studies should be followed daily
- Psychiatric intervention is indicated if the ingestion was a suicide gesture or attempt; a one-on-one sitter may be warranted

PROGNOSIS & COMPLICATIONS

- The number of fatalities from acetaminophen intoxication has declined due to use of NAC
- Otherwise healthy patients who are promptly treated generally have a full recovery
- If treatment is delayed, hepatic failure and death may occur
- A few patients, mostly those who have delayed treatment, suffer significant hepatic injury and become transplantation candidates

Aspirin Overdose

INTRODUCTION

- Aspirin (acetylsalicylic acid) is found in many prescription and over-the-counter preparations, including plain aspirin, headache medications combined with caffeine, pain tablets with narcotics, and bismuth GI preparations; it may also be present in combination with antihistamines, decongestants, antidiarrheals, herbal medications, oil of wintergreen, and some creams and lotions
- The use of aspirin has declined in the pediatric population due to concern regarding Reye syndrome, but acute and chronic poisonings still remain a problem
- Reye syndrome is a disease of unknown etiology; typically occurs after a viral syndrome, particularly varicella; it is more likely to occur when the viral syndrome is treated with aspirin

ETIOLOGY, EPIDEMIOLOGY, & RISK FACTORS

- Salicylates stimulate the respiratory center of the medulla causing hyperventilation, increased oxygen consumption and carbon dioxide production, and respiratory alkalosis; compensatory bicarbonate excretion and increased pyruvate and lactate production ultimately result in metabolic acidosis
- Aspirin overdose is potentially toxic with ingestion 150 mg/kg; this is the equivalent of about twenty 325-mg tablets
- Approximately 35 deaths per year are due to salicylate overdose, resulting in higher mortality than ibuprofen and acetaminophen overdoses
- Adolescents are more likely to ingest large amounts of aspirin, often as a suicide attempt
- Children and the elderly are more likely to develop toxicity
  - Young children are at risk because a smaller dose is more likely to reach the toxic range
  - Elderly are at risk because of reduced renal clearance
- Acute overdose occurs when a child takes more than the therapeutic dose of aspirin, either accidentally or on purpose
- Chronic aspirin overdose can occur as a result of a patient on aspirin having reduced renal clearance, but this is uncommon in pediatrics since aspirin is not typically used

PATIENT PRESENTATION

- Nausea, vomiting, and diaphoresis
- CNS disturbances
  - Tinnitus and temporary hearing impairment or deafness due to vasoconstriction of auditory microvasculature
  - Dizziness and drowsiness
  - Cerebral edema, delirium, seizures, and coma may occur in severe cases
- Tachypnea
- Hyperpyrexia
- Hypotension
- Oliguria
- Pulmonary edema
- Aspirin overdose should be considered in the evaluation of a patient with altered mental status
- Presentation of Reye syndrome includes nausea, vomiting, lethargy, delirium, and hepatic failure

DIFFERENTIAL DX

- Other analgesic overdose
- Other cause of anion gap metabolic acidosis (refer to the Metabolic Acidosis entry)
- Reye syndrome
- Sepsis
- Encephalopathy
- Diabetic ketoacidosis
- Renal failure

DIAGNOSTIC EVALUATION

- Aspirin overdose is usually elicited by history
  - The patient may admit to intentional ingestion
  - A caregiver may find evidence of ingestion (empty bottles, vomited pill fragments)
  - Careful review of the patient's medications, including over-the-counter medications, may reveal excessive use of bismuth, pain, or upper respiratory infection medications
- Serial serum salicylate levels immediately and every 2–4 hours
  - Less than 50 mg/dL is usually asymptomatic with minimal physiologic impact
  - 51–110 mg/dL results in mild-to-moderate toxicity with metabolic acidosis
  - Greater than 110 mg/dL results in severe toxicity with potential sequelae
  - Consider the possibility of ingestions of sustained-release preparations
- Acetaminophen level should be checked if the patient is unsure about what was ingested because patients sometimes confuse aspirin and acetaminophen and acetaminophen toxicity can cause severe liver damage
- Electrolytes and arterial blood gas to monitor the degree of acidosis; usually repeated at least twice daily until acidosis resolves
  - Potassium can remain low due to loss of potassium in urine
- Bedside testing is available for salicylates in the urine
- Chest X-ray or CT scan if pulmonary or cerebral edema is suspected

TREATMENT & MANAGEMENT

- Attention to airway, breathing, and circulation; some patients, particularly those with altered mental status, may have CNS disturbances that make them unable to protect the airway, requiring airway management
- Endotracheal intubation may also be necessary to control hyperventilation or protect the airway during gastric decontamination
- Gastric lavage if patient presents within 1 hour of ingestion
- GI decontamination with activated charcoal, which absorbs aspirin from the GI tract
- Laxatives/cathartics enhance excretion of aspirin and charcoal
- Proper fluid resuscitation, sometimes to include potassium and sodium bicarbonate, depending on electrolyte derangement and degree of acidosis
- Urinary alkalinization to enhance elimination of salicylates if level is >40 mg/dL
- Hemodialysis in severe overdoses, renal failure, or CNS disturbances
- Proper airway management for patients with altered mentation
- Psychiatric intervention if the ingestion was intentional
- Patient may be discharged if serial salicylate levels are <30 mg/dL and declining
- Patient should be admitted to hospital if levels are persistently above 40 mg/dL or if acidosis, CNS changes, or renal abnormalities are present

PROGNOSIS & COMPLICATIONS

- Usually no long-term effects from drug after proper management of mild acute or chronic toxicity in the 30–40 mg/dL range
- Acute intoxications have a 1% mortality rate, whereas chronic intoxications have up to a 25% mortality rate
- ICU admission for those with intractable seizures, those in need of airway management, and those with severe acid-base or electrolyte derangement or pulmonary edema

Carbon Monoxide Poisoning

INTRODUCTION

- Carbon monoxide is a colorless, odorless gas found in various fuels (eg, kerosene, natural gas, oil), automobile exhaust, and smoke
- It easily crosses cell membranes throughout the body to cause multisystem toxicity
- Carbon monoxide is the leading cause of death from poisoning
- More common in the winter season because of furnace use and automobile garage use; a classic case is when all or most of a family become ill after sleeping in a poorly ventilated space with a fuel-burning heater

ETIOLOGY, EPIDEMIOLOGY, & RISK FACTORS

- Carbon monoxide binds to heme proteins with 200 times greater affinity than oxygen, thereby making less oxygen available to cells; also it decreases the transfer of oxygen into cells (it shifts the oxygen dissociation curve to the left)
- Can also bind to myoglobin, causing cardiac disturbances
- Carbon monoxide interferes with the electron-transport chain in the mitochondria, limiting oxidative phosphorylation
- Exposure may be accidental, intentional, occupational, or recreational
  - Accidental exposures usually occur as a result of house fires, the use of kerosene heaters without adequate ventilation, and generators
  - Intentional exposure as a means of suicide is usually via exhaust pipe emissions in a closed space (eg, garage), although this may result in accidental exposure as well
  - Occupational exposures occur when using degreasers, solvents, and other occupational chemicals because absorbed vapors are metabolized in the liver into carbon monoxide
  - Recreational exposures may occur (eg, "huffing" of solvents)
- A significant risk factor is low socioeconomic status because patients living in poverty are more likely to have inadequate or unsafe heating systems and occupational exposures

PATIENT PRESENTATION

- Symptoms are nonspecific; headache, dizziness, nausea, and weakness are frequent symptoms
- Flu-like illness
- Confusion, dizziness, headache, ataxia
- Nausea
- Weakness
- Chest pain, arrhythmias
- Syncope, coma
- Cherry-red skin coloration is not typically a bed-side observation, except in severe cases; it is more likely to be seen on autopsy

DIFFERENTIAL DX

- Influenza or other viral illness
- Meningitis or encephalitis
- Gastroenteritis
- Asphyxia
- Cerebrovascular accident
- Hypothermia
- Other toxicities
- Drugs of abuse
- Alcohol poisoning
- Cyanide ingestion

DIAGNOSTIC EVALUATION

- History should include intentional exposures and potential for unintentional exposures (eg, occupation, living and sleeping arrangement, house heating methods)
- Physical exam should include vital signs (may be variable, including hyperpyrexia, tachypnea and hyperventilation, tachycardia, alterations in blood pressure) and retinal exam (may have bright red vessels or retinal hemorrhages)
  - Pulse oximetry is not a reliable measure of oxygenation because the meter may not be able to distinguish between oxyhemoglobin and carboxyhemoglobin
- Laboratory testing includes complete blood count, complete metabolic profile and chemistries, arterial or venous blood gas measurement, carboxyhemoglobin level, cardiac enzymes, urinalysis, and CPK level
  - Carboxyhemoglobin level is useful if elevated but may not correlate with clinical severity or have predictive value
  - Assess for metabolic acidosis via arterial or venous blood gas measurement
  - Anemic patients are at increased risk
  - Assess anion gap and renal function
  - Cardiac enzymes for patients of any age with cardiac-localizing symptoms
  - Urinalysis and CPK to assess for rhabdomyolysis
- Head CT scan or MRI may show white matter and globus pallidus changes in acute or chronic poisonings

TREATMENT & MANAGEMENT

- Attention to airway, breathing, and circulation
- Immediate high-flow oxygen therapy until the patient is asymptomatic
- Those with mild symptoms that resolve with oxygen therapy may be safely discharged
- Patients without full resolution of symptoms must be further monitored and treated
- Telemetry to monitor for cardiac depression, ischemia, or arrhythmia
- Intubation and ventilation if mental status changes are pronounced or respiratory compromise ensues
- Hyperbaric oxygen therapy may be indicated for severe poisonings (eg, loss of consciousness, seizures, coma); it is also indicated for pregnant women because the fetal hemoglobin has even greater affinity for carbon monoxide than regular adult hemoglobin
- Patients should be monitored and treated as necessary for ARDS, acute tubular necrosis, and disseminated intravascular coagulation

PROGNOSIS & COMPLICATIONS

- Encephalopathy with long-term sequelae occurs in more than a one-third of patients with severe poisoning
- Severe exposures can leave patients with persistent neurologic symptoms, including chronic headache and subtle learning difficulties
- Occasionally, there may be residual effects of white matter, basal ganglia, and cerebellum
- Acute myocardial injury can lead to long-term congestive heart failure

Organophosphate Poisoning

INTRODUCTION

- Organophosphate is the term for chemicals made by the chemical reaction of phosphoric acid and alcohol; they are used primarily as pesticides and insecticides, sometimes herbicides
- They have also been used as a method of chemical warfare, or "nerve gas"
- Organophosphates act as acetylcholinesterase inhibitors; they prevent the normal break-down and removal of acetylcholine from the postsynaptic junction
- As a result of organophosphate poisoning, acetylcholine accumulates in the nervous system, activating nicotinic and muscarinic receptors and resulting in autonomic and central nervous system outflow

ETIOLOGY, EPIDEMIOLOGY, & RISK FACTORS

- Absorbed rapidly through the skin, respiratory and gastrointestinal tracts, and conjunctiva
- Quickest onset of symptoms occurs when inhaled or injected
- In the U.S., the use of organophosphates is restricted; about 4% of poisonings are due to insecticides
- In other countries, these compounds are used more frequently; therefore, the incidence of morbidity and mortality is higher
- Occurs most often in children younger than 6 who are playing in areas treated with insecticides
- Occupational exposure (eg, exterminator, crop duster, farmer) can affect the exposed adult as well as household members due to exposure to contaminated clothing
- In adolescents and adults, poisoning may occur from suicidal ingestions as well as occupational exposure
- Used as nerve gas, with several notable episodes of chemical warfare related to terrorist acts

PATIENT PRESENTATION

- The most common and earliest symptoms are often gastrointestinal (eg, nausea, vomiting, diarrhea, abdominal pain)
- The most important symptoms are neurologic:
  - Clonus, tremor
  - Weakness, neuropathy
  - Delirium, confusion, coma, seizures, psychosis
  - Optic neuritis and ototoxicity
- Muscarinic effects:
  - DUMBBELLS (diarrhea; urinary incontinence; miosis and muscle fasciculations; bronchor-rhea, bronchospasm, and bradycardia; eme-sis; lacrimation; salivation)
  - SLUDGE (salivation, lacrimation, urinary incontinence, diarrhea, gastrointestinal dis-tress, emesis)
- Cardiac arrhythmias, hypertension

DIFFERENTIAL DX

- Opioid overdose
- Salicylate overdose
- Mushroom poisoning
- Botulism
- Myasthenia gravis
- Guillain-Barré
- Other causes of seizures (metabolic, infectious, structural)
- Sedative-hypnotic withdrawal

DIAGNOSTIC EVALUATION

- Organophosphate poisoning is a clinical diagnosis; there is no readily available test
- Cholinesterase levels in red blood cells or plasma may be useful if available but are of variable reliability and do not correlate with clinical findings
- History of known exposure provides the best clinical clue
- Initial examination may be normal, and patient may be asymptomatic
- Patients may present initially with either of two dichotomous pictures: hypotension, bradycardia, and decreased respiratory effort, or hypertension, tachycardia, and hyperventilation
- Clinical response to administration of atropine and pralidoxime is suggestive of the diagnosis
- EKG may show sinus tachycardia, sinus bradycardia, reentrant arrhythmias, ventricular fibrillation, and ventricular tachycardia
- EMG shows a characteristic pattern
- There are several types of paralytic syndromes resulting from organophosphate toxicity
  - Proximal palsy involving the cranial nerves and muscles of respiration, resulting in respiratory failure and requiring mechanical ventilation, but with expectation of recovery within a few weeks
  - Distal palsy of the extremities, sparing the respiratory muscles, but with a protracted course

TREATMENT & MANAGEMENT

- Health care workers must wear gloves to avoid contamination
- Immediate decontamination: Remove and discard clothing, wash the patient with soap and water
- After decontamination and evaluation, the patient may be discharged if asymptomatic for 6–12 hours; symptomatic patients should be admitted for monitoring
- Attention to airway, breathing, and circulation
  - Frequently recheck the patient's status because patients are at risk for respiratory failure and life-threatening arrhythmias
  - Mechanical ventilation should be instituted sooner rather than later if respiratory compromise is evolving
  - Effective ventilation can be impaired by profuse respiratory secretions
  - Continuous cardiac monitoring and pulse oximetry
- Medical management includes atropine, which is a competitive inhibitor at autonomic postganglionic cholinergic receptors and helps with bronchorrhea and oxygenation
- Antidotal treatment with pralidoxime, which is synergistic with atropine; it reactivates acetylcholinesterase and may reverse some degree of muscle paralysis
- If CNS manifestations occur, consider diazepam in addition to atropine and pralidoxime

PROGNOSIS & COMPLICATIONS

- Morbidity and mortality are most dependent on type and dose of organophosphate, as well as prompt, appropriate respiratory support
- In fatal cases, the cause of death is usually respiratory failure
- Memory impairment, confusion, peripheral neuropathy, and changes in personality have been reported as long-term effects

Miscellaneous

Eating Disorders

INTRODUCTION

- American culture prizes thinness; dieting, weight loss, and body shape are predominant themes in the media; perhaps as a result, eating disorders have been steadily on the rise since the 1980s
- Eating disorders include anorexia nervosa, bulimia nervosa, binge eating disorder, and eating disorders with mixed features or not otherwise specified

ETIOLOGY, EPIDEMIOLOGY, & RISK FACTORS

- Anorexia nervosa: Purposeful excessive weight loss, distorted body image, and fear of obesity with secondary physiologic derangements
- Bulimia nervosa: Cycles of binge eating alternating with unhealthy weight loss strategies, including fasting, vomiting, abuse of diuretics or laxatives, or intense exercise
- Binge eating disorder: Once considered an "eating disorder not otherwise specified," it is now defined as recurrent episodes of binge eating in the absence of the regular use of compensatory behaviors seen in bulimia nervosa (eg, self-induced vomiting)
- Risk factors include family history, low self-esteem, immaturity, and overly critical family dynamics
- Incidence is highest in adolescent females of developed nations
- Far more common in females (9:1 female-to-male ratio)
- Also more common in individuals participating in sports in which thinness is an advantage (eg, dancing, swimming, gymnastics, wrestling)
- The female athletic triad is a common manifestation of eating disorders and is characterized by disordered eating, amenorrhea, and osteoporosis

PATIENT PRESENTATION

Anorexia Nervosa
- Weight loss and cachexia
- Amenorrhea
- Hypothermia, cold intolerance
- Bradycardia
- Orthostatic hypotension
- Hair loss, lanugo
- Abdominal bloating, discomfort, and constipation

Bulimia Nervosa
- Fatigue, decreased energy level
- Headache
- Abdominal fullness, nausea
- Callus on knuckles, salivary gland hypertrophy, and dental erosions may occur secondary to self-induced vomiting

DIFFERENTIAL DX

- Body dysmorphic disorder
- Food faddism
- Fat phobia (culturally influenced dietary patterns of avoiding fat intake)
- Systemic disorder resulting in weight loss (eg, malignancy, tuberculosis, inflammatory bowel disease)

DIAGNOSTIC EVALUATION

Anorexia Nervosa

- History and physical examination can reveal disturbance in perception of body weight and refusal to maintain normal body weight (<85% of ideal body weight)
- Primary or secondary amenorrhea may occur
- Laboratory studies may reveal elevated BUN, AST, and ALT; decreased levels of serum sodium, potassium, magnesium, and calcium; and decreased zinc, vitamin A, and copper
- EKG may show T wave inversion or ST depression

Bulimia Nervosa

- Recurrent binge eating twice a week for 3 months
- Binges are characterized by rapid, secretive consumption of large volumes of food associated with feelings of guilt, anxiety, and loss of control
- Compensatory weight loss activities, including purging (eg, self-induced vomiting, laxatives, enemas, diuretics) and nonpurging (eg, fasting, excessive exercise, use of agents to increase metabolism) types
- Serum amylase may be elevated
- Dental referral is necessary because bulimic patients often have poor dentition due to frequent self-induced vomiting, which exposes the teeth to excessive acid, which erodes enamel

TREATMENT & MANAGEMENT

Anorexia Nervosa

- Nutritional repletion focuses on replenishing glycogen, fat, protein, calcium, and iron stores; this must take place in an incremental fashion for several reasons
  - Anorexics are very oppositional; it is often necessary to employ both positive and negative reinforcement and a stepwise method of gaining privileges for gaining weight
  - Refeeding syndrome may occur if repletion occurs too rapidly (see below)
- Correct hematologic and electrolyte abnormalities, as necessary: Chronic hypokalemia, hypochloremia, and hyponatremia are dangerous; the cause of death in anorexia may be hypokalemia resulting in fatal arrhythmias
- Inpatient admission and therapy may be necessary for acute crises or severe cases
- Behavioral therapy (eg, make contracts to negotiate increased privileges for weight gain)
- Family therapy to address contributing dynamics

Bulimia Nervosa

- Nutritional consultation for instruction and eating plans with three structured meals daily
- Behavior therapy: Practice slow eating and enjoyment of food, eating with other people, supervision after eating, reinforcement of education surrounding the caloric content of food chosen and the body's nutritional needs

PROGNOSIS & COMPLICATIONS

- Depression and other major affective disorders are common comorbidities
- Anorexia nervosa patients are frequently resistant to undergoing therapy
- Bulimia patients are more likely to accept therapy and maintain a normal weight but have a high relapse rate
- Care must be taken in anorexia nervosa patients when introducing calories to avoid the severe electrolyte disturbances that occur with refeeding syndrome (a shift from fat to carbohydrate metabolism raises the basal metabolic rate and causes intracellular shifts of electrolytes; low serum phosphate, magnesium, and glucose are common and dangerous)
- Best prognosis occurs in patients who are treated in specialized eating disorders clinics that offer multidisciplinary care involving medical, psychiatric, nutritional, and family services

Failure to Thrive

INTRODUCTION

- Failure to thrive is a common problem in pediatrics; 5% of pediatric hospital admissions are to evaluate failure to thrive
- The term is used to describe a failure to gain weight at an adequate rate in children younger than 2 years of age
- Defined as the downward crossing of any two lines in a growth curve
- Failure to thrive must be aggressively evaluated, managed, and followed to prevent developmental sequelae in the vulnerable first 2 years of life

ETIOLOGY, EPIDEMIOLOGY, & RISK FACTORS

- More common in children of families with low socioeconomic status, complex medical or social problems, or substance abuse
- Psychosocial etiologies are more common than organic disorders
- A wide variety of childhood illnesses may manifest as failure to thrive, including genetic syndromes (eg, Prader-Willi syndrome), metabolic disorders (eg, inborn errors of metabolism, renal tubular acidosis), endocrine abnormalities (eg, rickets, hypothyroidism), malabsorption disorders (eg, celiac disease, cystic fibrosis), conditions with increased energy needs (eg, congenital heart disease, chronic infection), and structural defects (eg, GERD, tracheoesophageal fistula)

PATIENT PRESENTATION

- Typical growth curve pattern shows flattening of the weight curve and a decline in linear growth, with a relative preservation of head growth
- Fatigue and irritability are common
- Subcutaneous fat loss, wasting of the limbs and buttocks, and an anxious expression are common
- Edema may be seen in severe cases of protein-energy malnutrition

DIFFERENTIAL DX

- Neglect or inadequate parenting (also called psychosocial failure to thrive)
- Genetic short stature
- Growth deceleration due to genetic potential
- Normal variant

DIAGNOSTIC EVALUATION

- History and physical examination should include detailed nutritional, developmental, and social histories and serial growth measurements and analysis of growth charting
- Complete blood count to evaluate for anemia, leukocytosis, or leukopenia, which may be indicative of malignancy, chronic infection, toxic exposure, or rheumatic disease
- BUN, creatinine, and urine studies to rule out glomerular disease (hematuria or proteinuria), diabetes mellitus (glucosuria), and chronic urinary tract infection (pyuria)
- Stool studies should include fecal fat and reducing substances (malabsorption disorders) and heme test (inflammatory reaction, milk-protein or food allergy)
- Electrolytes, carbon dioxide, pyruvate, lactate, and ammonia levels to screen for metabolic disorders; urine and serum organic acids and amino acids also may be indicated
- Total protein, albumin, and fat-soluble vitamin levels reflect nutritional status

TREATMENT & MANAGEMENT

- Complete nutritional consultation
  - Calorie count
  - Intake of a sufficient amount of calories, fat, vitamins, and minerals
  - Recommendations for dietary modification for children with organic disease
  - Parental education and dietary counseling
- Specific treatment for organic disorders with involvement of subspecialists, as appropriate
- Social work consultation to address family and economic factors

PROGNOSIS & COMPLICATIONS

- Early diagnosis of organic disorders may prevent a medical crisis and results in a better long-term prognosis
- Psychosocial failure to thrive may be difficult to treat due to parental resistance to outside intervention
- Reversal of failure to thrive is essential for adequate brain development during the first 2 years of life
- Lack of appropriate treatment may result in long-term cognitive, growth, and behavioral sequelae

Metabolic Acidosis

INTRODUCTION

- Metabolic acidosis is not an independent condition but rather a symptom of an underlying disorder in the body; it is one of the most commonly encountered laboratory abnormalities
- Compensation to buffer metabolic acidosis occurs by several means: Chemoreceptors that modulate respiration are stimulated, resulting in increased respirations and often respiratory alkalosis; intracellular uptake of excess hydrogen ions occurs; renal excretion of hydrogen ions is augmented by urinary acidification; and neutralization of hydrogen ions occurs by phosphate and carbonate in the bone

ETIOLOGY, EPIDEMIOLOGY, & RISK FACTORS

- Normal pH is maintained in a careful balance (7.35–7.45) by intracellular and extracellular buffers (common buffers include sodium [Na^+], potassium [K^+], bicarbonate [HCO^{3-}], calcium carbonate [$CaCO_3$], phosphate [PO^{4-}], and serum proteins)
- The lungs and kidneys compensate by altering respiration and urinary excretion, respectively, to modify arterial partial pressure of carbon dioxide ($PaCO_2$) and HCO^{3-}
- Hyperventilation results in decreased $PaCO_2$ (appropriate compensation will decrease $PaCO_2$ by 1.5 mmHg for every 1-mEq decrease in HCO^{3-})
- The kidneys increase the production and reabsorption of $HCO3-$ by the excretion of hydrogen (H^+) in the urine (bound to Na^+, K^+, ammonia [NH_3], and calcium [Ca^{++}])
- Acids produced include ketones (starvation, diabetes, or salicylates), lactate (tissue hypoxia or hypoperfusion), and sulfuric or phosphoric acid (renal failure)

PATIENT PRESENTATION

- May be relatively asymptomatic if acidosis develops slowly
- Hyperventilation results as the respiratory system tries to compensate for acidosis by blowing off carbon dioxide (CO_2)
- May present as respiratory distress
- Muscle weakness
- Altered mental status, ranging from mild intoxication to coma
- Dehydration, nausea, vomiting, or diarrhea
- Oliguria or anuria
- Hypoperfusion leading to shock
- Signs of underlying etiology (eg, tinnitus due to salicylate ingestion)

DIFFERENTIAL DX

Increased Anion Gap
- Methanol
- Uremia
- Diabetic ketoacidosis
- Paraldehyde
- Iron/isoniazid
- Lactic acidosis
- Ethanol-ethylene glycol
- Salicylates

Normal Anion Gap
- Gastrointestinal losses
- Renal tubular acidosis
- Hyperalimentation
- Hypoaldosteronism
- Potassium-sparing diuretics
- Carbonic anhydrase inhibitors

DIAGNOSTIC EVALUATION

- History and physical examination, including history of toxin ingestions
- Initial laboratory testing includes chemistries (hyperkalemia) and arterial blood gas (decreased pH, decreased HCO_3^-, normal or decreased $PaCO_2$)
- Toxicology screen for salicylates, ethylene glycol, ethanol, and methanol
- Osmolar gap (measured osmoles − calculated osmoles): If greater than 0, a toxin is likely present
- Calculate the serum anion gap: $(Na^+) - [(Cl^-) - (HCO_3^-)]$, which may help elucidate etiology (normal = 8 16)
- Urinalysis for pH and oxalate crystals
- Urine electrolytes: Calculation of urine anion gap may be useful if the serum anion gap is normal or decreased: $[(Na^+) - (K^+)] + (Cl^-)$
  - If greater than 0, suggests renal cause; if less than 0, suggests gastrointestinal cause

TREATMENT & MANAGEMENT

- Treat the underlying cause (eg, insulin for patients with diabetic ketoacidosis, dialysis for toxins and renal failure, gastric lavage and charcoal for toxin ingestions, specific drug antidotes)
- IV bicarbonate administration may be indicated if pH <7.20; if pH does not correct with bicarbonate administration, consider ongoing losses of base
- Volume resuscitation and cardiovascular support
- Respiratory support, including intubation and mechanical ventilation if necessary

PROGNOSIS & COMPLICATIONS

- The underlying disease state predicts the prognosis and overall clinical course
- Metabolic derangements may be well tolerated on a chronic basis (eg, chronic renal failure) or may contribute directly to morbidity and mortality (eg, septic shock)

Hyponatremia

INTRODUCTION

- Serum sodium concentration should range between 135–142 mmol/dL; serum osmolarity should range between 280–300 mOsm/kg
- Serum sodium concentration dependents on several factors, including:
  - Sodium (Na) intake
  - The renin-angiotensin-aldosterone system: Renal reabsorption of sodium at the distal renal tubule is stimulated by aldosterone
  - Water balance: Water conservation via antidiuretic hormone in response to hypovolemia or elevated serum osmolarity
- "Normal saline," when referring to IV fluid administration, is 0.9% sodium chloride

ETIOLOGY, EPIDEMIOLOGY, & RISK FACTORS

- Hyponatremia is defined as a sodium level less than 130 mEq/L
- It is a relatively common electrolyte derangement in infants and children
- Most commonly occurs due to dehydration with salt loss exceeding water loss (hypovolemic hyponatremia), overreplacement of water, or disease states that cause water retention (euvolemic or hypervolemic hyponatremia)
- May occur in patients who have been instructed to take clear liquids, many of which do not contain salt (eg, ice, water, apple juice, gelatin)
- More common in developing countries where diarrheal illnesses (eg, rotavirus, cholera) are common
- Hyponatremia is one of the most common electrolyte abnormalities in hospital settings, affecting approximately 2% of all patients

PATIENT PRESENTATION

- May be asymptomatic
- Nausea, irritability, malaise
- Lethargy, headaches
- Signs of dehydration may be present (dry mucous membranes, tachycardia, hypotension, decreased urine output, sunken eyes, sunken fontanelle)
- Signs of volume overload may be present (edema, ascites, pulmonary edema)
- Seizures, coma

DIFFERENTIAL DX

- Excess free water intake from excessive dilution of infant formula
- Congestive heart failure
- Nephrotic syndrome
- Syndrome of inappropriate antidiuretic hormone (SIADH)
- Hypothyroidism
- Gastrointestinal losses (eg, diarrhea)
- Psychogenic water intoxication (>10 L/day)
- Renal losses
- Diuretics
- Mineralocorticoid deficiency, Addison disease
- Cystic fibrosis

DIAGNOSTIC EVALUATION

- History and physical examination, including careful assessment of volume status (dehydrated, edematous, or normal)
- Routine serum chemistries and urinalysis
- Random urine sodium level
  - Na^+ <20 mEq/L suggests salt retention
  - Na^+ >20 mEq/L suggests salt wasting
- Serum and urine osmolality
- Calculate the sodium deficit: (140 + measured Na^+) × 0.6 × body weight (in kg)
- Pseudohyponatremia (a factitiously lowered lab value) may be caused by hyperglycemia, hypertriglyceridemia, or hyperproteinemia
  - Sodium level is falsely lowered by 1.6 mEq/L for each 100 mg/dL rise in glucose above 100 mg/dL

TREATMENT & MANAGEMENT

- Treatment depends on the etiology and volume status
- If the patient is asymptomatic and volume depleted, fluid restriction and/or normal saline administration may be used to correct the sodium level
- If symptomatic, volume depleted, and sodium is <120 mEq/L, administer 3% saline (usually 2 mL/kg) until sodium level rises above 120 mEq/L, then switch to normal saline
- If the patient is volume overloaded, diuretics and sodium replacement may be required
- Increase the sodium level by 0.5–1.0 mEq/L per hour until 120 mEq/L, then correct the remaining deficit over 48 hours
- If a seizure occurs as a result of hyponatremia, the immediate therapeutic goal is to rapidly stop the seizure (not to rapidly normalize the sodium) using IV or rectal barbiturates

PROGNOSIS & COMPLICATIONS

- Hyponatremia is usually well tolerated and rarely has any long-term sequelae
- Slow, chronic changes in sodium are usually asymptomatic and well tolerated
- Acute changes in sodium are generally symptomatic, but once the sodium is corrected, symptoms resolve
- Too rapid correction of hyponatremia may result in osmotically induced damage to the CNS, leading to central pontine myelinolysis (spastic quadriparesis, ataxia, abnormal extraocular movements, swallowing dysfunction, and mutism)

Physical Abuse

INTRODUCTION

- The approach to physical abuse in childhood entails a systematic methodology, including:
  - A high index of suspicion because physical abuse is unlikely to be the chief complaint
  - A careful history, with an interview performed by a trained advocate
  - A proper medical evaluation and documentation of findings
  - Treatment of injuries and planning for treatment follow-up
  - Addressing safety issues and appropriate disposition
  - Making a report to child protective services and law enforcement agencies

ETIOLOGY, EPIDEMIOLOGY, & RISK FACTORS

- Parental risk factors include social isolation, substance abuse, mental illness, poor parenting skills, and unrealistic expectations of a child's developmental level
- Risk factors related to the child include physical illness or disability, mental illness, and "difficult" temperament
- Situational factors include concurrent domestic violence, financial difficulties and other stressors, and concurrent domestic violence
- No gender predilection
- Physical abuse is the second most common form of child maltreatment (neglect is more common)
- Occurs at all socioeconomic levels, but increased rates occur in families with lower economic means

PATIENT PRESENTATION

- Bruising: Increased concern for abuse if bruising occurs in nonmobile infants and children, patterned marks, on unusual body areas (ears and face, abdomen, buttocks, genitals), covering many areas of the body, or in various stages of healing
- Burns: Increased concern for abuse or neglect if second- or third-degree burn, patterned burn, burn on child with limited developmental ability, or delay in seeking medical care
- Fracture: Consider abuse if the fracture is occult, if the fracture is old and in the healing stage at the time of discovery, if the child is not developmentally able to cause the injury, or if it is attributed to an accident too minor to cause a fracture
- Head injury: May present with lethargy, apnea, apparent sepsis, or history of minor or no trauma (especially infants)

DIFFERENTIAL DX

- Bruising: Coagulopathy, Mongolian spots, collagen vascular disorder, folk remedies (eg, "coining")
- Burns: Impetigo, streptococcal toxic shock syndrome, contact dermatitis, fixed drug eruption, folk remedies (eg, "cupping"), phytodermatitis
- Fractures: Birth trauma, skeletal dysplasias, infection, nutritional disorders, neoplasm, drug toxicity, neuromuscular disorder, accidental

DIAGNOSTIC EVALUATION

- Detailed historical information from caregiver(s)
- Private interview of the child, if possible
- Complete physical examination, including funduscopic examination for retinal hemorrhages consistent with shaken baby syndrome
- Assess the child's developmental level versus mechanism of injury (eg, a child who does not yet walk will not likely have a fall injury)
- Detailed written and photographic documentation of all injuries
- Complete laboratory evaluation for possible medical conditions that could account for physical finding/injury (eg, coagulopathy)
- Complete skeletal survey for all cases involving fracture(s), suspected head injury, or other significant physical injury in all children younger than 3
- Cranial imaging (CT scan or MRI) of all children with suspected head injury, fracture of unknown origin, or neurologic symptoms
- Consider abdominal imaging for occult trauma

TREATMENT & MANAGEMENT

- Medical treatment as necessary depending on the injury type and severity
- Consider consultation with medical personnel who specialize in cases of suspected child abuse
- Report all cases of suspected or confirmed physical abuse to local child protective service agency and local law enforcement agency to ensure the child's safety
- Provide support to children and caretakers throughout medical evaluation
- After the initial evaluation, provide referral for counseling and ongoing medical care as appropriate
- Maintain a professional, nonjudgmental attitude toward involved caretakers

PROGNOSIS & COMPLICATIONS

- Minor injuries, such as bruises and superficial burns, heal well with no physical sequelae
- Deep burns may leave permanent disfigurement and scarring, especially if medical care is delayed
- Fractures may result in asymmetric growth of bone, disfigurement, or permanent loss of function
- Head injury resulting in cerebral edema, intracranial hemorrhage, or "shear" injury may result in a wide spectrum of medical sequelae, including mild to severe developmental delays, coma, or death
- Child may experience anxiety, mistrust, aggressive or withdrawn behavior, and low self-esteem as a result of abuse

Sexual Abuse

INTRODUCTION

- The approach to sexual abuse in childhood entails a systematic methodology:
  - A high index of suspicion when sexual abuse is not the chief complaint
  - A careful history, with an interview performed by a trained advocate
  - A proper medical evaluation and documentation of findings that is best performed by a specifically trained physician
  - Treatment or prophylaxis of diseases or injuries and planning for treatment follow-up
  - Addressing safety issues and appropriate disposition
  - Making a report to child protective services and law enforcement agencies

ETIOLOGY, EPIDEMIOLOGY, & RISK FACTORS

- Children have inherent vulnerabilities that place them at risk (eg, children are taught to obey adults and conform to expectations; children are by nature vulnerable to bribes, coercion, and threats)
- Specific risk factors for sexual abuse include low self-esteem or unmet emotional needs, single-parent home and/or adult nonrelative male in the home, history of domestic violence in the home, and poor supervision or poor choice of caregivers
- Incidence is much higher in girls (4:1 female-to-male victim ratio)
- The majority of perpetrators are male
- Occurs at all ages and in all socioeconomic classes
- Perpetrator is known to the child in 60% of cases; 25–50% of perpetrators are relatives

PATIENT PRESENTATION

- Behavioral presentations vary widely and may include:
  - Anxiety, new phobias
  - Depression, regression, withdrawal
  - Appetite change, eating disorder
  - New-onset enuresis or encopresis
  - Nightmares, difficulty sleeping
  - Somatic complaints
  - Sexualized behaviors/acting out
  - Alcohol and drug use in adolescents
- Medical presentations may include:
  - Genital or anal itching, discharge, pain, bruising, bleeding, other injury
  - Sexually transmitted disease
  - Dysuria, recurrent urinary tract infections
  - Pregnancy

DIFFERENTIAL DX

Behavioral Symptoms
- New-onset mental health disorder
- Accidental exposure to sexual acts or materials

Physical Symptoms
- Vulvovaginitis
- Straddle injury
- Lichen sclerosus
- Urinary tract infection
- Urethral prolapse
- Rectal prolapse
- Pinworms
- Molluscum contagiosum
- Congenital sexually transmitted disease
- Crohn disease

DIAGNOSTIC EVALUATION

- Historical information provided by caregiver or witness
- Disclosure by child relating history of abuse
- Physical examination of external genitals and anus to document bruising, abrasions, bleeding, scars, or hymenal injuries; nonetheless, the majority of affected children will have normal genital and anal exams, even with a credible disclosure of abuse; thus, a normal exam does not rule out the possibility of abuse
- Diagnosis of suspected sexual abuse may be made based on the child's disclosure alone *or* an abnormal medical exam
- Testing for sexually transmitted diseases and pregnancy should be performed if medically indicated
- Sexual assault kit (rape kit) when medically indicated
- Refer to a center specializing in sexual abuse for second opinion on physical exam or colposcopic exam and interview by a specialist in child abuse

TREATMENT & MANAGEMENT

- Prophylaxis for sexually transmitted diseases and pregnancy if medically indicated, with consent of responsible caretaker and child
- Report all cases of suspected or confirmed sexual abuse to local child protective service agency and to local law enforcement
- Provide support to the child and caretakers throughout the medical evaluation
- Ensure that the child has adequate follow-up with age-appropriate counseling services
- Ensure the child's safety with assistance of local child protective service agency to stop ongoing contact with alleged perpetrator until complete evaluation and investigation is performed

PROGNOSIS & COMPLICATIONS

- Psychological adjustment following abuse may be related to many factors, including the child's perception of the abuse, the caregivers' response to abuse, child's and caregivers' preexisting psychosocial strengths and limits, and the outcome of the investigation
- Possible sequelae include low self-esteem, poor interpersonal relationships, repetition of sexual abuse, promiscuity/prostitution, depression, self-abuse, anxiety, and chronic infections and/or increased risk of genital cancer related to sexually transmitted infections

Appendices

Appendix A. Developmental Milestones

Age of Child	Fine Motor	Gross Motor	Personal/Social	Self-Help/Adaptive	Language
Newborn	Opens and closes hands	Moves limbs symmetrically	Regards caretaker	Quiets self	Cries
1 month	Visual tracking to midline	Lifts head	Smiles reflexively	May suck thumb	Vocalizes
2 months	Head stable	Lifts head and chest 45°	Smiles socially	Reacts to bottle or breast	Vowel sounds
3 months	Regards hand	Lifts head and chest 90°	Responds to caretakers	Reacts to toy	"Coos"
4 months	Hands to mouth	Attempts to roll	Frequent smile	Pursues toy visually	Squeals
5 months	Holds toy	Rolls over	Prefers familiar caregivers	Works for toy	Likes voices
6 months	Toy to mouth	Sits with support	Lifts arms to be held	Object permanence	Babbles
7 months	Transfers	Sits; supports self with hands	Cries if left alone	Holds bottle	Makes syllables
8 months	Holds 2 objects	Sits, scoots, "commando crawl"	Stranger anxiety	Feeds self teething biscuit	"Dada" or "mama" (nonspecific)
9 months	Pincer grasp	Pulls to stand, crawling	Waves bye-bye	Uses sippie cup	Combines syllables
10 months	Bangs toys together	Cruises	Plays peek-a-boo	Feeds self cereal	Early jargoning
11 months	Puts object in cup	Stands alone	Affectionate gestures	Uses cup well	Receptive language
12 months	Turns pages of book	Walks	Imitates caregiver	Holds spoon	"Dada" or "mama" (specific)
15 months	Marks on paper with crayon	Runs	Parallel play	Wants to feed self	Jargoning
18 months	Stacks 2–4 blocks	Walks up stairs	Engages caregiver to play	Undresses self	Gestures, uses few words
2 years	Scribbles repetitive circles	Climbs well	Representative play	Washes hands	Two-word phrases
3 years	Copies single circle	Rides tricycle	Plays with others	Brushes teeth	Learning colors, numbers
4 years	Copies "+" sign	Hops	Identifies with gender group	Dresses self	Speech understandable
5 years	Copies square	Skips	Plays simple games	Makes cereal	Writes name

Appendix B. Approach to Well-Child Care

General Guidelines for Working with Children and Families

- Family input is integral to the well-child encounter
- Allow parents to advocate for the child
- Observe parent-child interaction
- Allow child as much proximity to the parent as necessary for comfort during the examination
- To decrease threat of examination, proceed from less invasive to more invasive parts of the examination (eg, hands first, mouth and ears last) rather than from head to toe
- Children should be examined in an examining gown rather than street clothing; do not defer genital exam

Development

Infancy (0–12 months): Attachment to primary and secondary caregivers, early feeding skills, rapid acquisition of developmental milestones, self-regulation (eg, soothes self by thumb-sucking), rudimentary language skills, attending to and interacting with environment

Early childhood (1–5 years): Formation of distinct relationships, locomotion, toilet training, independent feeding, continuous expansion of language skills, establishing boundaries, establishing increasing autonomy, initial peer relationships

Later childhood (6–12 years): Family is more important than peer groups, solidification of self-awareness and self-esteem, dramatic increase in cognition, decision-making abilities increase and become more important, challenging established boundaries, physical skills and coordination increase, selective peer relationships, school success or failure affects child mightily

History

- Include birth history, past medical history, family history, interim history, and social history
- Interim history should include review of systems, feeding and diet history, sleep quality and habits, behavior and discipline, and developmental milestones for each age group (fine motor, gross motor, personal/social, language, self-help/adaptive)
- Social history should include home environment, family composition, primary caregivers, parental issues (eg, custodial relationships, spousal relationships, occupation, substance abuse, coping mechanisms), daycare or after-school arrangements, recreational activities, group associations (eg, scouts), potential for toxic exposures (eg, lead paint, type of home heating, water source, passive smoke)

Physical Examination

- Assess growth percentiles, head and neck (including dentition), cardiovascular (including femoral pulses), lungs, abdomen, breasts and genitalia with Tanner staging, lymphatic system, musculoskeletal (including spine), neurologic, skin, vision and hearing

Immunizations: Per current recommendations, including diphtheria, tetanus, and pertussis; inactivated polio; *Haemophilus influenza* type B; pneumococcus; hepatitis B; hepatitis A; varicella; measles, mumps and rubella; rotavirus

Screening: Consider screening for lead toxicity, anemia, and tuberculosis exposure

Anticipatory Guidance: Include discussion of nutrition (eg, when to start solids in infancy, minimum requirements for picky eaters), safety issues (eg, car seats, bicycle helmets), development (eg, normal development, anticipated milestones), family relationships (eg, sibling rivalry), psychosocial matters (eg, appropriate social exposures, discipline), and illness or symptom management (eg, acetaminophen dose) and health promotion (eg, brushing teeth)

Leading Causes of Morbidity: Unintentional injuries, acute mild infections (eg, otitis media, common cold), chronic illness (eg, asthma), child abuse or neglect, conditions related to poverty (eg, malnutrition, lack of health care)

Leading Causes of Mortality: Unintentional injuries, motor vehicle crashes, congenital or genetic conditions, malignancy

Appendix C. Approach to Adolescent Care

General Guidelines for Talking to Adolescents

- Meet with family first and then with the adolescent alone, if possible
- Explain confidentiality ("Everything stays private unless I feel like you might hurt yourself or others or someone has hurt you physically or sexually")
- Avoid surrogate parent role and adolescent role, and act as an advocate

History: Review of systems, past medical history, family history, allergies (may need parental input), menstrual history (menarche, number of days, intervals, cramps, missed school)

Social History: "HEADSSS" assessment (reassess at every visit)

- *Home:* Where he/she lives and with whom; nature of the relationships with people at home; history of running away; homelessness or incarceration; problems at home, including violence or exposure to violence
- *Education:* Grade level, mainstream versus special education, favorite and least favorite subjects, change in schools, number of schools, relationship with teachers/coaches, occupational and educational goals, reading level, history of skipping or repeating a grade, grades and grade trends, school misses and reasons, suspensions, ability to complete homework
- *Eating:* How he/she feels about his/her weight, what he/she does to try to change his/her weight, number of meals per day, nutrition and food choices
- *Activity:* What he/she does for fun with or without friends, involvement in community organizations/religious groups, exercise, school sports, amount of television watching
- *Drugs:* Tobacco, marijuana, alcohol, other drugs (how much and whether or not there is any interest in quitting), substance use with high-risk situations, how substances are obtained
- *Sleep:* Sleep amount and times, insomnia, night wakening, where patient sleeps
- *Sexual activity:* Sexual orientation, sexual partners, vaginal/oral/anal intercourse, condom use, history of sexually transmitted infections, prior testing for sexually transmitted diseases including HIV, consensual or forced intercourse, comfort with having sex, history of pregnancy
- *Suicidality:* History of psychiatric illness, concerns for depression, presence or history of thoughts of hurting and/or killing self
- *Safety:* Seatbelt, drinking and driving, night driving, bike helmet, guns

Physical Exam: Growth percentiles, head and neck (including dentition) cardiovascular (including femoral pulses), lungs, abdomen, breasts and genitalia with Tanner staging, lymphatic system, musculoskeletal (including spine to assess for scoliosis), neurologic, skin, vision and hearing, blood pressure

Immunizations: Tetanus booster (Td), measles-mumps-rubella booster, varicella booster, hepatitis B series; HPV (Gardasil) vaccine is now indicated for girls

Screenings: Consider screening for anemia in menstruating females; pregnancy and sexually transmitted infections in sexually active youth; and tuberculosis in patients with an exposure or a risk factor

Leading Causes of Morbidity: Sexually transmitted infections, pregnancy, substance use/abuse, school problems, illiteracy, depression

Leading Causes of Mortality: Unintentional injuries, motor vehicle accidents, homicide, suicide, malignancy, HIV infection

Psychosocial Development

Early adolescence (11–13): Less interest in parental activities, preoccupation with self and pubertal changes, uncertainty about appearance, intense relationships with same-sex friends, increased cognition, idealistic vocational goals, increased need for privacy, lack of impulse control

Middle adolescence (14–16): Peak of parental conflicts, general acceptance of body, concern over making body more attractive, peak of peer involvement, conformity of peer values, increased sexual activity and experimentation, feeling of omnipotence, risk-taking behavior

Late adolescence (17–19): Reacceptance of parental advice and values; acceptance of pubertal changes; more time spent in intimate relationships; practical, realistic, vocational goals; refinement of moral, religious, and sexual values; ability to compromise and set limits

Appendix D. Approach to Fluid and Electrolyte Management

Basic Concepts

Total Body Water

1. Total body water (TBW) can be estimated as a percentage of total body weight as follows:

   - Newborns: 75%
   - Infants/Children: 65%
   - Adolescents/Adults: 60%

2. TBW is separated into the intracellular space (ICF) and extracellular space (ECF): ICF makes up two-thirds of the TBW, and ECF makes up one-third of the TBW.
3. The ECF is further distributed between two subcompartments: plasma volume and interstitial space.
4. The distribution of fluids across the plasma and interstitium is controlled by both oncotic and osmotic mechanisms.

   - Oncotic control is the major factor for ECF distribution; it is determined by serum protein levels (ie, albumin).
   - Serum osmolarity also contributes to ECF distribution. Serum osmolarity can be estimated by the following equation (normal serum osmolarity is 285 mOsm/L):

   $$P_{osm} = 2[Na^+] + Gluc/18 + BUN/2.8$$

Electrolytes

1. Sodium (Na^+) is the primary cation in the ECF, with a concentration of about 140 mEq/L.
2. Sodium homeostasis is controlled by *thirst, antidiuretic hormone (ADH)*, and *aldosterone.*
3. Potassium (K^+) is the primary cation in the ICF, with a concentration of about 160 mEq/L.
4. Potassium homeostasis is controlled by *Na^+/K^+ pump* and *acid-base balance.*

Fluid Calculations

Fluid Requirements

$$\text{Fluid Requirement} = \text{Maintenance Fluid} + [\text{Fluid Deficit}] + [\text{Ongoing Fluid Losses}]$$

1. All patients have maintenance fluid needs, although not all patients will have a fluid deficit or ongoing fluid losses. These need only be calculated when applicable, which is why they are in brackets in the above equation.

2. Maintenance fluids are dictated by routine fluid loss, including mandatory urine losses (50%), insensible skin loss (30%), respiration loss (15%), and stool loss (5%).
3. Fluid deficit and ongoing losses may be due to GI losses (diarrhea, emesis, nasogastric suction), third spacing (burns, trauma, sepsis, abdominal surgery), and/or excessive urine losses (inappropriate water-saving mechanisms).

Maintenance Fluid Requirements

1. Newborns

Day 1	60 cc/kg/day
Day 2	80 cc/kg/day
Day 3	100 cc/kg/day
Day 4	120 cc/kg/day

2. Infants and children

First 10 kg body weight	100 cc/kg/day ($\sim$4 cc/kg/hr)
Second 10 kg body weight	50 cc/kg/day ($\sim$2 cc/kg/hr)
Everything over 20 kg	20 cc/kg/day ($\sim$1 cc/kg/hr)

3. Thus, a 25-kg child requires the following:
(100 cc/day $\times$ 10 kg) + (50 cc/day $\times$ 10 kg) + (20 cc/day $\times$ 5 kg) = 1600 cc/day

Fluid Deficit

1. The best and most accurate estimate of acute fluid losses is by acute changes in body weight; however, using weights is difficult because of differences in scales, lack of baseline weights, and continued growth during childhood. Thus, multiple clinical and laboratory findings are used to estimate fluid deficit.
2. We use these clinical and laboratory findings to classify the degree of dehydration (mild, moderate, or severe) and, ultimately, the amount of TBW loss; see Table A.1.
3. Once we correlate our physical findings into a degree of dehydration as in Table A.1, we must then quantify the dehydration, expressing it as a percentage of TBW.

- *Infants:* Mild dehydration correlates to a loss of 5% of TBW, moderate dehydration correlates to a loss of 10%, and severe dehydration correlates to a loss of 15%.
- *Children and adolescents:* Mild dehydration correlates to a loss of 3% of TBW, moderate dehydration correlates to a loss of 6%, and severe dehydration correlates to a loss of 9%.

Fluid Replacement

1. Maintenance fluids are given evenly over 24 hours.
2. Fluid losses are replaced at different rates depending on *type* of dehydration, which is determined by the Na^+ level.

Table A.1. Parameters for Estimating Fluid Deficit for Isotonic and Hypotonic Dehydration

	Mild Dehydration	Moderate Dehydration	Severe Dehydration
Renal			
Urine volume	Small (<1–2 cc/kg/hr)	Oliguria (<0.5 cc/kg/hr)	Anuria (no urine output)
Urine concentration	+ +	+ + + +	+ + + + + +
BUN	Normal	+ +	+ + + +
Cardiovascular			
Skin color/perfusion	Normal	Acrocyanosis	Mottled
Heart rate	Normal	Increased	Markedly increased
Blood pressure	Normal	Orthostatic	Hypotension
Other			
Tearing	Normal	Decreased	Absent
Mucosa	Normal	Dry	Parched
Eyes	Normal	Depressed	Sunken
Fontanelle	Normal	Depressed	Sunken
Mental status	Normal	Depressed	Obtunded

- *Isotonic and hypotonic dehydration* (eg, vomiting, diarrhea, and others) is usually corrected over 24 hours.
- *Hypertonic dehydration* (eg, seawater ingestion, improperly mixed formula, excess sodium in parenteral fluids, diabetes insipidus, and renal disorders) follows different rules for estimation of fluid losses, and fluid replacement is corrected over 48 hours (hypertonic dehydration is an advanced fluids topic and will not be discussed in this appendix).

3. Fluid deficit is replaced in three phases over 24 hours. In phase I, an immediate bolus of fluid is administered. In phases II and III, the remainder of the fluid deficit (total fluid deficit minus the amount administered as a bolus) and maintenance fluids are administered.

- *Phase I (immediate bolus administration)*: 10 cc/kg of normal saline is administered as a bolus. Repeat boluses may be administered until cardiovascular stability and urine output are established—regular reassessment of fluid status is imperative! Larger boluses may be given during a resuscitation.
- *Phase II (initial 8 hours)*: Following the fluid bolus administered in phase I, the remaining fluid deficit (RD) must be calculated:
    RD = Total Deficit − Amount of fluid given as a bolus in phase I
    Half of the remaining deficit is replaced over 8 hours in phase II. (*Note:* Maintenance fluids must also be replaced in phase II.)
- *Phase III (hours 8–24)*: The remainder of the RD is replaced over the next 16 hours. (*Note:* Maintenance fluids must also be replaced in phase III.)

4. Ongoing losses (if present) are replaced "cc per cc" with electrolytes in equal concentration to what is being lost.

Example 1: Fluid Rate Calculation

A 22-kg child is hospitalized with dehydration secondary to diarrhea. He presents with signs and symptoms of moderate dehydration (tachycardia, orthostatic hypotension, dry oral mucosa, and oliguria). He is thus estimated to have 10% dehydration. His serum [Na^+] is 140 mEq/L. Assume no ongoing losses once the child is made NPO. IV fluids are started as follows.

Maintenance: First 10 kg of body weight: 10 kg $\times$ 100 cc/kg = 1000 cc
Second 10 kg of body weight: 10 kg $\times$ 50 cc/kg = 500 cc
Remainder of body weight: 2 kg $\times$ 20 cc/kg = 40 cc
_____
Total Maintenance = 1540 cc

1540 cc/day $\div$ 24 hr = Maintenance rate of 64 cc/hr (round up to 65)

Total Deficit: 10% of 22 kg = 2.2 $\approx$ 2.2 L or 2200 cc

Phase I: The child does not adequately respond to a single bolus, so two 10-cc/kg boluses are administered.

10 cc/kg $\times$ 22 kg = 220 cc of NS
10 cc/kg $\times$ 22 kg = 220 cc of NS
_____
Total Bolus = 440 cc of NS

Remaining deficit is then 2200 cc − 440 cc = 1760 cc.

Phase II: Deficit replacement: ½ of RD over 8 hr = 880 $\div$ 8 hr = 110 cc/hr.

Maintenance replacement = 65 cc/hr.

Thus, total phase II replacement rate = 110 cc/hr + 65 cc/hr = 175 cc/hr.

Phase III   Deficit replacement: Second ½ of RD over 16 hr = 880 cc $\div$ 16 hr = 55 cc/hr.

Maintenance replacement = 65 cc/hr.

Thus, total phase III replacement rate = 55 cc/hr + 65 cc/hr = 120 cc/hr.

Electrolyte Requirements

Finally, we must determine what concentration of saline our replacement fluid should contain.

1. Sodium is the key electrolyte for determining which solution should be chosen.
2. There are four basic stock solutions available:

Normal saline (NS)   154 mEq/L of Na^+
½ Normal saline   77 mEq/L
⅓ Normal saline   51 mEq/L
¼ Normal saline   38 mEq/L

3. *Phase I bolus should always use normal saline* to allow for expansion of the intravascular volume and reperfusion of vital organs (surgeons prefer lactated Ringer's solution).

4. Again, we must calculate our maintenance and deficit needs, but now for sodium deficit rather than total water deficit.

- Maintenance Na^+ = 2 to 4 mEq/kg/day (we will use 3 mEq/kg/day).
- Deficit Na^+ is determined by the type of dehydration:

Hypertonic	Na^+ >150 mEq/L	2–4 mEq/kg
Isotonic	Na^+ = 135–150 mEq/L	8–10 mEq/kg
Hypotonic	Na^+ <135 mEq/L	10–12 mEq/kg

Example 2: Sodium Replacement and IV Fluid Selection

We will now determine the type of fluid to be used for the calculations performed in Example 1. Sodium requirement for a 24-hour period is assessed. Then, we determine the concentration of fluids that will deliver this amount of sodium.

Phase I: Initial bolus is always normal saline. 440 cc NS = 0.44 L × 154 mEq/kg = 68 mEq of Na^+.

Phase II: Na^+ maintenance: 22 kg × 3 mEq/kg = 66 mEq.

Na^+ deficit: 22 kg × 8 mEq/kg = 176 mEq (use 8 mEq because patient is isotonic).

Na^+ total = 242 mEq (over 24 hours).

Na^+ total minus phase I Na^+ = 242 mEq − 68 mEq = 174 mEq.

Remaining Na^+ to deliver to the patient = 174 mEq (over 24 hours).

Total fluids remaining:

Maintenance = 1540 cc

Remaining deficit = 1760 cc

Thus, we need to administer 174 mEq of sodium in 3300 cc (3.3 L) of fluid. $[Na^+]$ = 174 mEq/3.3 L = 52 mEq/L, which is closest to ⅓ normal saline.

Thus, following an initial bolus of normal saline, we will replace the patient's fluids and electrolytes over 24 hours (phases II and III) with ⅓ normal saline.

Other Fluid Facts

1. For every increase in the serum glucose of 100 above normal, there is a decrease in serum Na^+ of about 1.6 mEq.
2. Use of 3% saline solutions should be reserved for Na^+ <120 mEq/L and severe symptoms.

- Use only enough 3% saline to return the serum Na^+ to about 120 mEq/L, then correct the remainder slowly,
- 3% saline contains 0.5 mEq/cc.

3. Anion gaps can *never* be a negative number.

$$\text{Anion Gap} = \text{Sodium} - (\text{Chloride} + \text{Bicarbonate})$$

The differential diagnosis is shown in Table A.2.

Table A.2. Differential Diagnosis for Anion Gaps

Elevated Anion Gap	Normal Anion Gap	Decreased Anion Gap
A-Aspirin/alcohol	Renal tubular acidosis	Lab error
	Diarrhea	Hypoalbuminemia
M-Methanol	Hypoaldosteronism	Bromism
U-Uremia		Multiple myeloma
D-Diabetic ketoacidosis		Paraproteinemia
P-Paraldehyde		
I-Iron/INH		
L-Lactic acidosis		
E-Ethylene glycol		

4. Oral rehydration: The World Health Organization (WHO) recommends fluids that contain 2.0–2.5 g/dL glucose and 50–75 mEq/L sodium (see Table A.3).

Table A.3. Oral Rehydration Solutions

Solution	Glucose (g/dL)	Sodium (mEq/L)	Potassium (mEq/L)
Pedialyte®	2.5	45	20
Pedialyte RS®	2.5	75	20
Apple juice	12	0.4	25
Coke®	10	3.6	
Gatorade®	4	24	2.5
Ginger ale	7.5	4.5	0.1
Grape juice	18	0.8	30
Jello®	10	10	0.1
Kool Aid®	10	0.2	0.1
Milk	4.8	22	38
Orange juice	11	0.4	50
City water		3	0.5

References

Chesney RW, Zelikovic I. Pre- and postoperative fluid management in infancy. *Pediatr Rev* 1989;11:153–158.

Finberg L. Hypernatremic dehydration in infants. *N Engl J Med* 1973;289: 196–198.

Harrison HE. Dehydration in infancy: hospital treatment. *Pediatr Rev* 1989;11: 139–144.

Holliday MA, Segar WE. The maintenance need for water in parenteral fluid therapy. *Pediatrics* 1957;19:823–832.

Molteni KH. Initial management of hypernatremic dehydration in the breast-fed infant. *Clin Pediatr* 1994;33:731–740

Index